Carotid Interventions

Edited by

Peter A. Schneider

Hawaii Permanente Medical Group
Honolulu, Hawaii, U.S.A.

W. Todd Bohannon

Texas Tech University Health Sciences Center
Lubbock, Texas, U.S.A.

Michael B. Silva, Jr.

Texas Tech University Health Sciences Center
Lubbock, Texas, U.S.A.

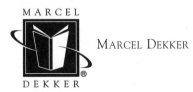

MARCEL DEKKER   NEW YORK

Library of Congress Cataloging-in-Publication Data
A catalog record for this book is available from the Library of Congress.

ISBN: 0-8247-5932-X

This book is printed on acid-free paper.

Headquarters
Marcel Dekker, 270 Madison Avenue, New York, NY 10016, U.S.A.
tel: 212-696-9000; fax: 212-685-4540

Distribution and Customer Service
Marcel Dekker, Cimarron Road, Monticello, New York 12701, U.S.A.
tel: 800-228-1160; fax: 845-796-1772

World Wide Web
http://www.dekker.com

The publisher offers discounts on this book when ordered in bulk quantities. For more information, write to Special Sales/Professional Marketing at the headquarters address above.

Current printing (last digit):

10 9 8 7 6 5 4 3 2

PRINTED IN THE UNITED STATES OF AMERICA

Foreword

This book on carotid interventions could not have been more appropriately timed with current clinical development and application of carotid stents plus protection as an alternative therapy to carotid endarterectomy. The book provides a contemporary, balanced, and expert approach to the understanding of carotid endovascular procedures and contains information that is essential for Interventionalists treating patients with carotid lesions. The text is an excellent companion book to Dr. Schneider's recently published *Endovascular Skills: Guidewire and Catheter Skills for Endovascular Surgery: Second Edition* and presents information related to carotid interventions that is not contained in the companion work. The breadth and value of Dr. Schneider's contributions exemplify his level of commitment to endovascular technologies. The editor's perspective on endovascular methods combined with his exceptional conventional vascular surgical technical expertise and skills provides a unique and invaluable perspective on this evolving field.

The initial chapters of *Carotid Interventions* contain a review of neurovascular and aortic arch anatomy, and equipment, inventory and facility requirements for carotid angioplasty and stenting. These chapters are written by experts on the topics and are concise and well illustrated. Subsequent chapters discuss more advanced topics such as advanced cerebrovascular arteriography, access challenges for carotid interventions, and the impact and appropriate consideration of comorbid factors in the successful treatment of complex patients. A chapter addresses technical components of the procedure, including a review of currently available and developing devices, catheters and imaging technologies. Techniques to optimize hemodynamics, recognize and treat neurological deficits, and react to clinical problems that present during procedures are reviewed in a clinically appropriate and comprehensive manner.

The final chapters of the text review data regarding the indications for and the success of carotid angioplasty and stenting compared to surgical and medical therapy. The discussion includes an overview of unresolved issues. A particularly valuable part of the text contains technical tips for angioplasty and stenting and management of complex issues and complications of carotid interventions. Ways to initiate a practice, obtain and develop skills, and confront unknown issues are summarized in a comprehensive and responsible manner. A very useful component of the text is the Appendix, which lists recommended inventory for carotid vascular procedures, contains a review of the National Institutes of Heath Neurologic Stroke Scale, and presents other useful technical information.

The book is not only expertly written and edited but addresses an important area of current interest in the evolution of vascular interventions. The challenges and responsibilities of adopting this new technology to treatment of carotid stenosis using surgical methods that have been developed to exceptional levels of success underline the importance of this work. Carotid angioplasty and stenting represents a particularly challenging area as it directly addresses highly feared clinical problems involving stroke, paralysis, and death. This book offers a comprehensive and responsible introduction and emphasizes the adoption and utilization of safe methods to gain maximal patient benefit.

This multi-authored text, with many of the pivotal chapters prepared by Dr. Schneider as sole author, represents a particularly significant contribution to the evolution and practice of endovascular interventions. The text is an invaluable source of critical information that is essential to the development, maintenance, and responsible practice of carotid interventions.

Rodney A. White, M.D.
Chief of Vascular Surgery
Harbor-UCLA Medical Center
Torrance, California

Preface

The purpose of this book is to assist the reader in the process of identifying, understanding, and improving the skills needed for incisionless treatment of carotid artery stenoses. Our emphasis is on technique and results but we have included practical advice on topics such as how to get started, what kind of training is needed, and how to safely and efficiently add carotid angioplasty and stenting to your therapeutic offerings.

The developing clinical utility of carotid angioplasty and stenting highlights the importance of a broader issue facing vascular surgery. Will vascular surgeons be able to adapt and retain our role as providers of full-service vascular care? We believe that vascular surgeons are ideally, if not uniquely, qualified to manage patients with extracranial cerebrovascular disease and to assess competing therapies.

Carotid stent placement represents the convergence of multiple factors at a time when we are rethinking our approach to vascular disease. Skills and technology developed in other, more forgiving, vascular beds have improved over the past few years. Carotid bifurcation atherosclerosis is more amenable to endovascular intervention than conventional wisdom would have predicted. Distal protection devices and other technical advances may be able to decrease stroke risk and make the neurological outcome of carotid stent placement competitive with carotid endarterectomy. Specialists in multiple disciplines represent an eager potential workforce ready to participate in the rapid dissemination of carotid stenting to an expanded pool of patients.

Among vascular surgeons, the traditional therapists of carotid occlusive disease, many offer only endarterectomy and have yet to perform carotid stent placement as an alternative therapy for their patients. Vascular surgeons who have honed their ability to offer effective therapy for carotid disease via carotid endarterectomy, but who do not have the experience that would allow them to participate in the performance of carotid angioplasty and stenting, are forced to choose between two unappealing alternatives:

abdicating their leadership role in the delivery of carotid therapeutics or emphasizing their skepticism and underscoring the flaws inherent to the process of carotid stenting trials conducted by other specialists.

Many cardiologists and radiologists have never managed carotid disease and face the challenges of learning and refining the clinical management paradigms for a complex medical problem. Since they do not have the skills necessary for performing carotid endarterectomy and no practical way of obtaining these skills, their options for treatment of carotid artery disease are limited to catheter interventions, medical management, or referring the patient to a surgeon. They have no reference for the importance of open surgical skills or even intimate clinical knowledge of carotid disease in adding to the effectiveness of a catheter-based interventionalist.

These factors make it difficult to obtain an objective assessment of the relative efficacy of the three competing therapeutic modalities: medical management, carotid angioplasty and stenting, and carotid endarterectomy. I assert that the ideal arbiter of the efficacy of competing treatments is a practitioner, capable of performing each with the highest possible level of skill and who has nothing to gain from the evident superiority of any one treatment. Endovascular surgeons possessing a combination of excellent endovascular skills and open surgical experience are the only specialists ideally positioned to evaluate the currently available carotid treatments.

Carotid stenting will assume a broad role in carotid disease management and is significantly different from other endovascular procedures. The cerebrovasculature is the last vascular bed to be significantly impacted by endovascular intervention. Vascular surgeons know too much; they are eyewitnesses to the friable carotid plaque contents that cause stroke. Carotid stenting is among the most sophisticated endovascular procedures and there is no open component, as there has been with endovascular grafts for aortic aneurysms. Carotid endarterectomy has been one of the most successful vascular procedures offered to patients over the years. For these reasons, vascular surgeons have been slow to adapt and other specialists have been eager to adapt this new technique. Despite the success and efficacy of carotid endarterectomy, further major improvements in the results of open repair are unlikely. In comparison, carotid stent placement is only in its first or second iteration, and is certain to improve with further enhancements in cerebral protection devices, access, miniaturization, and the accumulated knowledge garnered by continued endovascular work within the carotid bed.

We believe that if you are a clinician skilled in the management of carotid disease, you have experience with complex endovascular procedures, and you become an accomplished carotid angiographer, you are well prepared to master the skills of carotid stent placement. The incorporation of carotid stenting into vascular practice poses significant challenges and it is easy to get distracted by the logistics involved and the complexities of protectionism. However, the development of carotid stenting is likely to further the transition of vascular surgery from an open surgical specialty where many useful tools are ignored to a modern specialty where all available modalities are used to benefit the patients and provide a full spectrum of care. Old allegiances and nostalgia aside, carotid stenting is one of the most exciting developments ever in the management of vascular disease.

Peter A. Schneider, M.D.

W. Todd Bohannon, M.D.

Michael B. Silva, Jr., M.D.

April, 2004

Contents

Contributors

W. Todd Bohannon   Texas Tech University, Lubbock, Texas, U.S.A.

Marc Bosiers   AZ St. Blasius, Dendermonde, Belgium

Ruth L. Bush   Baylor College of Medicine, Houston, Texas, U.S.A.

Michael T. Caps   Hawaii Permanente Medical Group, Honolulu, Hawaii, U.S.A.

Daniel G. Clair   Cleveland Clinic Foundation, Cleveland, Ohio, U.S.A.

Mitchell W. Cox   Baylor College of Medicine, Houston, Texas, U.S.A.

Koen Deloose   AZ St. Blasius, Dendermonde, Belgium

Kim J. Hodgson   Southern Illinois University School of Medicine, Springfield, Illinois, U.S.A.

Karthikeshwar Kasirajan   The University of New Mexico, Albuquerque, New Mexico, U.S.A.

Peter H. Lin   Baylor College of Medicine, Houston, Texas, U.S.A.

Alan B. Lumsden   Baylor College of Medicine, Houston, Texas, U.S.A.

Robert B. McLafferty   Southern Illinois University School of Medicine, Springfield, Illinois, U.S.A.

Nicolas Nelken   Hawaii Permanente Medical Group, Honolulu, HI, U.S.A.

Patrick Peeters   Imelda Hospital, Bonheiden, Belgium

Peter A. Schneider   Hawaii Permanente Medical Group, Honolulu, Hawaii, U.S.A.

Michael B. Silva, Jr.   Texas Tech University, Lubbock, Texas, U.S.A.

Timothy M. Sullivan   Mayo Clinic, Rochester, Minnesota, U.S.A.

Jürgen Verbist   Imelda Hospital, Bonheiden, Belgium

1

Neurovascular Anatomy for Carotid Angiography and Interventions

MITCHELL W. COX, ALAN B. LUMSDEN, RUTH L. BUSH,
and PETER H. LIN

Baylor College of Medicine, Houston, Texas, U.S.A.

The purpose of this chapter is to review normal and variant vascular anatomy of the aortic arch and the extracranial and intracranial cerebrovasculature. There is specific emphasis placed on cerebrovascular anatomy as it pertains to carotid arteriography and carotid angioplasty. The ability to interpret cerebrovascular images is critical to providing high-quality patient care to patients with carotid occlusive disease. Variations in arch and intracerebral arch anatomy are usually irrelevant to open carotid surgery, but may be critical when performing carotid interventions. Understanding arch anatomy is integral to guiding sheath placement in the common carotid artery. Recognizing the presence of intracerebral variation or pathology may significantly influence periprocedural technique and patient management during carotid stent placement. There is a significant incidence of intracerebral pathology in patients having angiograms for extracranial occlusive disease, as high as 20% in some series (1). In the case of incidental findings, such as an aneurysm, it is critical to be able to localize the abnormality and communicate effectively with the consulting neurosurgeon or neurologist.

It has been debated whether arteriography should be routine for the evaluation of extracranial occlusive disease. Proponents of routine angiography cite a high incidence of unsuspected pathology on cerebral angiogram as justification for their position (1,2). Most vascular practices have moved away from routine angiography for extracranial occlusive disease, but the advent and popularization of carotid stenting may reverse this trend. Regardless of whether or not one believes in routine carotid arteriograms,

1

however, there is little justification for not getting cerebral views once the surgeon is in the angiography suite and the common carotid has been catheterized. A simple two-view cerebral angiogram obtained by injection of the common carotid is well within the scope of practice for an endovascular surgeon. The cerebral angiogram may diagnose incidental problems, demonstrate intracranial occlusive disease, and provide information that may be useful for operative planning (i.e., the degree of collateral filling) (3).

This review examines some common aortic arch variants that may complicate carotid angiography and interventions. The normal anatomy of the intracerebral vessels and commonly encountered pathology is also reviewed. The focus is on the anterior circulation since this is relevant to the management of extracranial carotid occlusive disease. The most common incidental findings are also discussed.

Aortic Arch Anatomy and Its Variants

Arch and carotid anatomy is familiar to vascular surgeons, but some normal anatomic variants may assume increased significance when planning carotid interventions. Figure 1 shows several classically described normal variants. Also important are

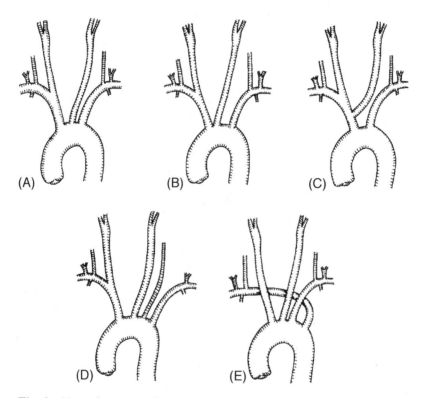

Fig. 1 Normal variants of the supra-aortic vessels are pictured including typical configuration (A), common origin of innominate and left CCA (bovine configuration) (B), origin of left CCA from innominate (C), aortic origin of vertebral (D), and aberrant right subclavian (E). (From Ref. 4.)

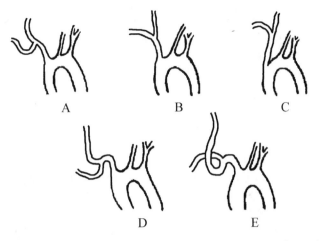

Fig. 2 Variations of innominate anatomy. C, D, and E will make angiography and intervention quite challenging. (From Ref. 5.)

subtle variations that can make cerebral angiography and carotid interventions extremely challenging. Figure 2 demonstrates minor variations in the angle and tortuosity of the innominate artery. In the case of Fig. 2A and B, it will likely be relatively straightforward to enter the innominate and right common carotid, but the configurations depicted in Fig. 2C–E are likely to make cannulation of the common carotid and any subsequent intervention much more challenging. Likewise, entering the left common carotid is often straightforward, but can be complicated by unusual angles or tortuosity. In Fig. 3, variants A and B will probably be possible to negotiate with a

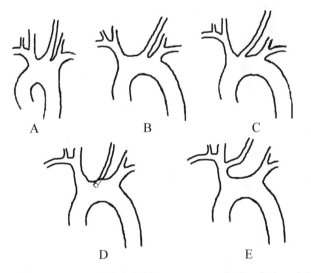

Fig. 3 Variants in left CCA anatomy are depicted. A and B will be easy to negotiate, while C, D, and E will be more difficult. (From Ref. 5.)

simple curve catheter, whereas C, D, and E will likely require additional maneuvering. There is more information about assessment and classification of the aortic arch in Chap. 2. This knowledge is applied to carotid stenting in Chap. 6, Access for Carotid Interventions.

Intracranial Angiography

After the common carotid artery has been selected and adequate views of the carotid bulb have been obtained, the next challenge is performing and interpreting the intracranial angiography. Standard anatomy texts are often not helpful as they usually focus on the Circle of Willis, which is not seen as a distinct structure angiographically. There are two systems of nomenclature, and vessels carry both a traditional name and an alphanumeric designation (A1, A2, M1, etc.). In order to sort out the anatomy, it is useful to look at the earlier portions of the subtraction study, where contrast has only filled the central arteries. It is easier to identify the major named vessels that have consistent locations before the innumerable terminal vessels have filled (Fig. 4). It is also important to look at both the AP and lateral views since some vessels will only be seen on one projection or the other.

Injection of the common carotid artery will mainly visualize the distribution of the ipsilateral anterior and middle cerebral arteries. The territories supplied by these arteries are clearly seen on the AP view with the anterior cerebral artery supplying the area between the two hemispheres along the falx and the middle cerebral artery supplying the outer cortex of the parietal and temporal lobes (Fig. 5).

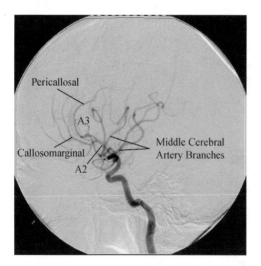

Fig. 4   On an early-phase lateral cerebral angiogram, major anterior cerebral (A2, A3, pericallosal, callosomarginal) and middle cerebral artery branches can be seen easily.

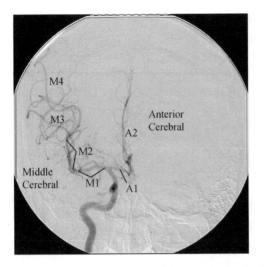

Fig. 5 Distribution supplied by anterior and middle cerebral arteries is clearly seen on this AP view. The first segment of the anterior and middle cerebral arteries (A1 and M1) is best seen with this projection.

Internal Carotid Artery

Evaluation of the intracerebral vessels begins with the internal carotid artery. The internal carotid artery is divided into cervical, petrosal, intracavernous, and cerebral segments. The short intracerebral segment gives off several smaller branches prior to the anterior and middle cerebral arteries, but only the ophthalmic and posterior-communicating arteries are likely to be visualized well. Both will be seen in the lateral projection, with the ophthalmic coming off first and running anteriorly and the posterior-communicating artery running posteriorly (Fig. 6).

One relatively rare variant that may be confusing is a persistent primitive trigeminal artery. This developmental abnormality, present in between 0.1% and 0.6% of patients, results in a large artery branching off the internal carotid and filling the basilar and posterior cerebral arteries. It is unlikely to be of clinical significance but may be associated with aneurysms of the posterior circulation. This variant is seen in Fig. 7.

Anterior Cerebral Artery

The first portion of the anterior cerebral artery (A1) is horizontal and best seen in the AP view (Fig. 5). As it curves upward, it gives off the anterior-communicating artery, which is usually short and may not be well visualized. What will be seen is filling of the contralateral anterior cerebral distribution if there is well-developed collateral circulation or occlusion of the contralateral internal carotid artery.

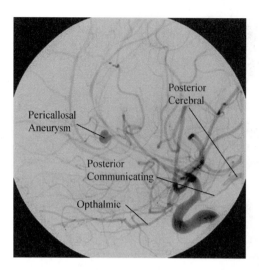

Fig. 6 Ophthalmic artery and posterior-communicating arteries are well seen in this angiogram, which also shows a pericallosal aneurysm. The posterior-communicating artery is seen to be filling the posterior cerebral artery.

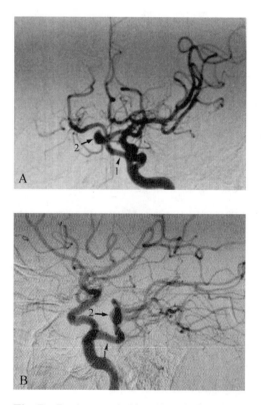

Fig. 7 Persistent primitive trigeminal artery is seen in AP (A) and lateral (B) projections. The artery (1) connects the ICA with the basilar artery. A basilar artery aneurysm is also seen (2). (From Ref. 6.)

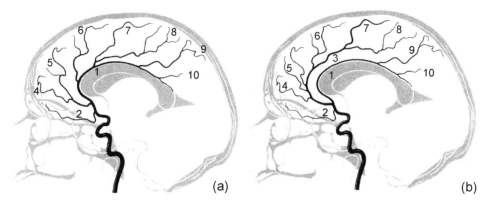

Fig. 8 Two typical anterior cerebral artery configurations are seen—absence of callosomarginal (a) and dominant callosomarginal (b). (1) Pericallosal; (2) frontoorbital; (3) callosomarginal; (4) frontopolar; (5) anterior internal frontal; (6) middle internal frontal; (7) posterior internal frontal; (8) paracentral; (9) parietal internal superior; (10) parietal internal inferior. (From Ref. 4.)

Once past the anterior-communicating artery, the anterior cerebral artery, now A2, starts to curve around the corpus callosum. Here it is visualized on a lateral projection as it makes a gentle curve in the central portion of the hemisphere (Fig. 4). It typically divides into two branches, the more central pericallosal and the outer callosomarginal, both designated A3. Either of these vessels may be diminutive or absent, with the other one becoming correspondingly enlarged (Fig. 8). Moving further toward the terminal branches, the course and origin of these vessels are highly variable and they are named for the portion of the brain that they supply. Typical locations of branches are noted in Fig. 8.

Middle Cerebral Artery

The middle cerebral artery originates at the internal carotid artery and courses laterally. This horizontal, or sphenoidal, segment is designated M1 and is only seen well in the AP projection (Fig. 5). At some point along the M1 segment, the middle cerebral artery divides into two or three trunks—all still M1 initially. The trunks then turn superiorly, becoming the M2 or insular portion of the middle cerebral artery (Fig. 9). The three separate trunks will be best seen on the lateral projection (Figs. 10 and 11). The branches then angle through the sylvian fissure that separates the temporal and parietal lobes, appearing more horizontal on the AP projection. This is referred to as the Opercular, or M3, segment. Finally, blood flow reaches the smaller branches along the outer cortex of the frontal and parietal lobes. These are the terminal (M4) branches and carry separate names reflecting the portion of the cortex that they supply. Main branches are seen diagrammatically in Fig. 10.

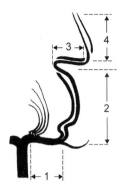

Fig. 9 Schematic of the middle cerebral artery in AP view. (1) Sphenoidal (M1) segment; (2) insular (M2) segment; (3) opercular (M3) segment; (4) terminal (M4) segment. (From Ref. 4.)

Posterior Cerebral Artery

The posterior cerebral artery is unlikely to fill from an injection of the common carotid artery, but may occasionally be opacified via a large posterior-communicating artery (Fig. 6). Since both posterior cerebral arteries arise from the basilar artery, contrast injection into one vertebral will opacify both sides. One or both sides may be visualized if the artery fills via the posterior communicating. The posterior cerebral artery is divided into P1, P2, P3, and P4 or precommunicating, ambient, quadrigeminal, and calcarine segments. Figures 12 and 13 show a diagrammatic representation and angiogram, respectively.

Pathologic Findings

Stenosis or occlusion of one or more intracerebral vessels is a common finding in patients with carotid stenosis and has been documented in up to 15% of patients undergoing carotid arteriography. If a patient develops a neurologic deficit during angiography or angioplasty and stenting, evaluation for evidence of new vessel occlusions is essential. Occlusions of A1, A2, M1, and M2 will likely be obvious, and occlusion of the anterior cerebral artery is seen in Fig. 11. There is complete absence of filling in the normal distribution of the vessel. More distal occlusions may not be obvious, but may also have less clinical relevance. Figure 14 shows a high-grade stenosis of the middle cerebral artery at M1.

As mentioned earlier, the anterior cerebral and anterior-communicating arteries are a major source of collateral flow in occlusive disease and are the major source of cross-filling visualized during carotid angiography. A large amount of cross-filling may be normal, but more commonly is the result of a stenotic or occluded internal carotid artery on the side receiving the collateral flow (Fig. 15). Look for a stenosis distally in the internal carotid that may result in symptoms even after endarterectomy or angioplasty

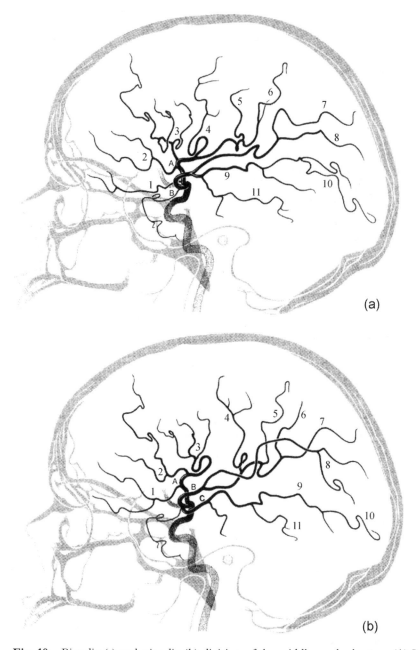

Fig. 10 Bipodic (a) and tripodic (b) division of the middle cerebral artery. (A) Upper trunk; (B) middle trunk; (C) lower trunk. (1) Fronto-orbital; (2) orbitofrontal; (3) prefrontal; (4) prerolandic; (5) rolandic; (6) anterior parietal; (7) posterior parietal; (8) angular; (9) posterior temporal; (10) temporooccipital; (11) middle temporal. (From Ref. 4.)

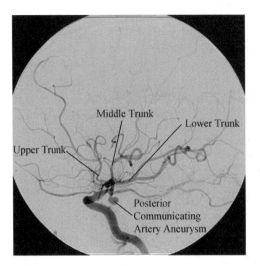

Fig. 11 Middle cerebral artery distribution is seen well because of anterior cerebral artery occlusion. A posterior-communicating artery aneurysm is also present.

and stenting. Collateral flow is best demonstrated on the AP projection and may be seen best later in the run.

Berry aneurysms are not uncommonly found during carotid angiography, and large series report an incidence of 1–3%, with a 3% incidence in the NASCET trial (7–9). These most commonly arise at bifurcations of the vessels comprising the Circle of Willis, but may be seen on any of the major-named vessels. Ninety percent of aneurysms are located in the anterior circulation, and those in the posterior circulation

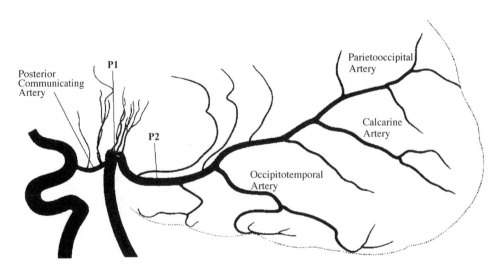

Fig. 12 Posterior cerebral artery is seen diagrammatically with major-named terminal branches and first two numbered segments. (From Ref. 4.)

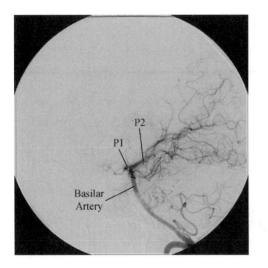

Fig. 13 Posterior cerebral artery is seen after injection of the vertebral artery. Identification of smaller branches is more difficult since both sides fill with contrast via the basilar artery.

are unlikely to be visualized without contrast injection in the vertebral arteries. One third of aneurysms are found on the anterior-communicating artery, one-third at the posterior-communicating–ICA (internal carotid artery) junction, and one fifth at the middle cerebral artery bifurcation. Aneurysms are multiple in 20–30% of patients and once one aneurysm is found, complete four-vessel angiography to look for a second aneurysm is mandatory. At a minimum, delineation of the aneurysm should include AP, lateral, and 30° oblique views. Figures 6, 11, and 16) demonstrate pericallosal, posterior-communicating, and anterior-communicating artery aneurysms, respectively.

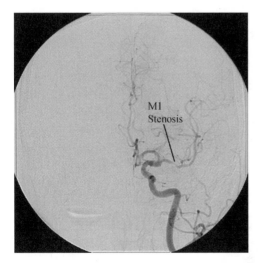

Fig. 14 High-grade stenosis of the M1 segment of the middle cerebral artery is seen well in this AP projection.

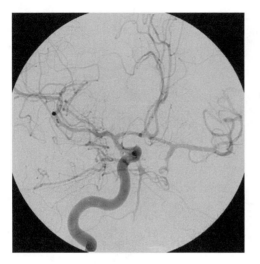

Fig. 15 Collateral filling of the contralateral anterior cerebral and middle cerebral arteries is seen after injection of the carotid.

Arteriovenous malformations (AVMs) may also be noted as incidental findings on angiography, but these are much more rare. Most series of angiograms for extracranial occlusive disease do not report this anomaly, but one series demonstrated two AVMs in 100 carotid angiograms (2). AVMs are visualized as an abnormal tangle of vessels and are classically associated with dilated feeding arteries and early venous filling. Findings suggestive of AVM should prompt further imaging with CT or MRI and neurosurgical referral. A dramatic example is seen in Fig. 17. Chap. 5 contains additional information about the management of pathologic findings on carotid arteriography.

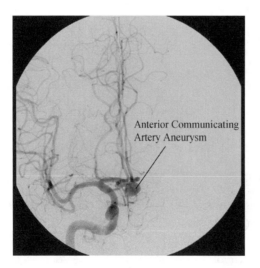

Anterior Communicating
Artery Aneurysm

Fig. 16 Large anterior-communicating artery aneurysm is seen well in this AP projection.

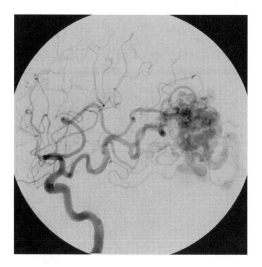

Fig. 17 Large posterior fossa AVM is clearly seen after injection of the carotid. Note the hypertrophied feeding vessels and early venous filling.

Summary

Recognition of normal and variant anatomy of the cerebral circulation is key to performing carotid angiography and endovascular intervention. Variant anatomy of the aortic arch and supra-aortic vessels is not infrequent and may dramatically increase the difficulty of angiography and interventions. Intracranial pathology is also relatively common in patients presenting for arteriogram prior to therapy of extracranial occlusive disease, and most patients should have cerebral views performed during a carotid angiogram. Incidental findings may include stenosis or occlusion of the intracerebral vessels, berry aneurysms, or, in rare cases, AVMs. Recognition of these lesions and further evaluation or appropriate referral are keys to providing the highest quality of patient care.

References

1. Long SM, Kern JA, Fiser SM, et al. Carotid arteriography impacts carotid stenosis management. Vasc Surg 2001; 35(4):251–256.
2. Griffiths PD, Worthy S, Gholkar A. Incidental intracranial vascular pathology in patients investigated for carotid stenosis. Neuroradiology 1996; 38(1):25–30.
3. Osborn AG. Diagnostic Cerebral Angiography. 2d ed. Philadelphia: Lippincott Williams & Wilkins, 1999.
4. Huber P. Cerebral Angiography. 2d ed. New York: Georg Thieme Verlag, 1982.
5. Vitek, J. Abnormal arch and intracranial pathology, from www.tctmd.com, 2002.
6. Ikushima I, Arikawa S, Korogi Y, et al. Basilar artery aneurysm treated with coil embolization via persistent primitive trigeminal artery. Cardiovasc Interv Radiol 2002; 25(1):70–71.

7. Yeung BK, Danielpour M, Matsumura JS, et al. Incidental asymptomatic cerebral aneurysms in patients with extracranial cerebrovascular disease: Is this a case against carotid endarterectomy without arteriography? Cadiovasc Surg 2000; 8(7):513–518.

8. Kappelle LJ, Eliasziw M, Fox AJ, et al. Small, unruptured intracranial aneurysms and management of symptomatic carotid artery stenosis. North American Symptomatic Carotid Endarterectomy Trial Group. Neurology 2000; 55(2):307–309.

9. Pappada G, Fiori L, Marina R, et al. Incidence of asymptomatic berry aneurysms among patients undergoing carotid endarterectomy. J Neurosurg Sci 1997; 41(3):257–262.

2

Aortic Arch Classification into Segments Facilitates Carotid Stenting

W. TODD BOHANNON and **MICHAEL B. SILVA, JR.**

Texas Tech University, Lubbock, Texas, U.S.A.

PETER A. SCHNEIDER

Hawaii Permanente Medical Group, Honolulu, Hawaii, U.S.A.

The purpose of this chapter is to present a simple method of describing aortic arch anatomy that correlates with the degree of complexity required to access a specific carotid artery for intervention. The anatomy of the aortic arch and its branches is an essential consideration when evaluating a patient for carotid angioplasty and stent placement (CAS). This chapter is intended to assist in planning the procedure and to help the physician in advising patients of the probability of success.

There are several categorization systems of the aortic arch that are well suited to describe conditions that affect the entire arch, such as dissection, aneurysm, and arch elongation and ectasia (1,2).

We propose a simple system not for describing the entire arch, but for describing the *segments* of the aortic arch as they pertain to carotid access to specific arteries (Fig. 1). The carotid stent operator needs to answer the following question: how complex will it be to place a sheath in a specific arch branch artery? This question can be answered by dividing the arch into segments, each one of which represents different degrees of challenge. This system is intended to offer additional information after the general shape of the arch has been assessed.

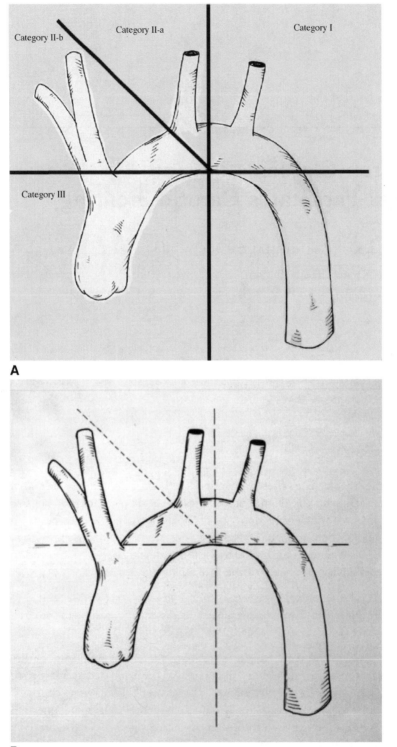

Category II-b

Category II-a

Category I

Category III

A

B

Arch Branch Access Is Determined by Segment of Origin ("Surf and Turf" Classification)

The arch aortogram is performed in the optimal left anterior oblique position. This is described in more detail in Chap. 4. A vertical line is drawn that bisects the arch into halves, one to the left and one to the right (Fig. 1). A horizontal line is drawn across the superior aspect of the inner curve of the aortic arch. This inner curve, or fulcrum, is a significant point that is not considered in any other classification system. This fulcrum is significant in negotiating turns toward arteries that have their origins to the right of the vertical line. Once the catheter or sheath reaches this fulcrum point (where the horizontal and vertical lines cross), it is the trajectory from there to the origin of the artery intended for catheterization that determines the conduct of the case. Segment I is located to the patient's left and above the horizontal line, segment II is to the patient's right and above the horizontal line, and segment III is to the patient's right and inferior to the horizontal line, extending into the ascending aorta. Although the configuration of the entire arch is important, on a case-by-case basis, it is the pathway to the carotid artery intended for treatment that influences the success of the procedure. Therefore the segment of the aortic arch in which the artery of interest arises is the key factor.

Access to an arch branch in segment I is simpler than in segments II or III since it is a straighter pathway from groin to carotid. A simple curve catheter may be used to cannulate the artery, and the sheath or guide catheter can usually be passed without a superstiff exchange guidewire. Segment II is further divided into a and b subdivisions. A diagonal line that extends through the middle of Segment II delineates these subdivisions. Segment IIa is located superiorly and segment IIb is located inferiorly. Sheath access into segment IIb is usually more challenging than segment IIa since it is further to the patient's right and closer to the horizontal line. From the fulcrum point, a segment IIb artery requires more angulation to reach the common carotid artery than a segment IIa vessel. A stiff exchange guidewire is usually required to pass the sheath. In progressing from segments IIa to IIb, the closer the origin of the common carotid artery is to the horizontal line, the more likelihood that a complex curve cerebral catheter will be required to cannulate the artery. Access to an artery in segment III (usually the innominate artery when this occurs) is even more

---

Fig. 1 Aortic arch segments: The "Surf and Turf" classification. (A) The aortic arch is divided into three segments. These represent categories of increasing levels of difficulty in obtaining sheath access into the target common carotid artery. Segment I access is the least technically demanding. Segment II access is more challenging, and this zone is bisected to delineate the increasing difficulty of access. As the target artery origin descends toward the ascending aorta, IIb is usually more challenging than IIa. Segment III access is the most difficult, as the origin of the target vessel is below the fulcrum point of the aortic arch. (B) Stylized version of the same arch showing that each of the branch arteries may originate from a different segment.

difficult and may be impossible. The catheter must clear the fulcrum, double back on itself in the caudal direction, and then reverse directions again to proceed in the cranial direction. A segment III artery may require multiple maneuvers to achieve sheath access. This system of describing the arch segments focuses on sheath access as the initial goal of the CAS procedure. Catheterization and sheath placement become progressively more challenging as one proceeds from segment I to segment III. There is more about access for carotid interventions in Chap. 6.

Rationale for Classification of Arch Anatomy into Segments

Myla (3) has developed a classification system for assessing the general shape of the entire arch. A line is drawn across the "top" of the arch. In a level 1 arch, the branches originate along this "arch line." If the arteries originate inferior to the arch line, it is a level 2 arch. When the arteries have their origins more than two common carotid artery diameters inferior to the arch line, it is considered a level 3 arch (Fig. 2). This system provides a useful assessment of the overall shape of the arch. The important concept is that the further inferiorly along the aorta the origin of the artery for cannulation is located, the greater the degree of difficulty in access placement. This system lumps all the arch branches together and also focuses on the apex of the aortic arch. However, the individual artery that requires access will determine the difficulty of the case. For example, the left common carotid artery may originate near the apex of a level 3 arch ("difficult") and not be very challenging to gain sheath access, while the innominate artery in the same patient may be very challenging to access. Although a general categorization of the entire arch is helpful, variability among the targeted branch arteries influences the approach.

The essential premise of estimating the increasing difficulty of arch access centers on the proximal origination of the target branch artery from the ascending aorta. When a horizontal line across the origin of the target artery becomes closer to the horizontal line of the lower apex of the aortic arch, the technical difficulty of sheath access into the carotid artery increases (Fig. 3). The window for catheter manipulation decreases as the two parallel lines become closer. This is a good conceptual exercise, but the location of the cranial-most point in the arch is not of direct value in the assessment process. This point does not influence guidewire, catheter, or sheath passage. It is the fulcrum over which these tools must work that determines the conduct of the case. The "surf and turf" classification provides a system for rapid but specific assessment without complicated measurements.

Optimal Arch Aortogram

After the pigtail catheter is in place in the arch, the image intensifier is rotated in the left anterior oblique (LAO) position until the pathway of the catheter forms as broad an arc as possible (Fig. 4). This is usually between 30° and 45° of LAO (Fig. 5). If the

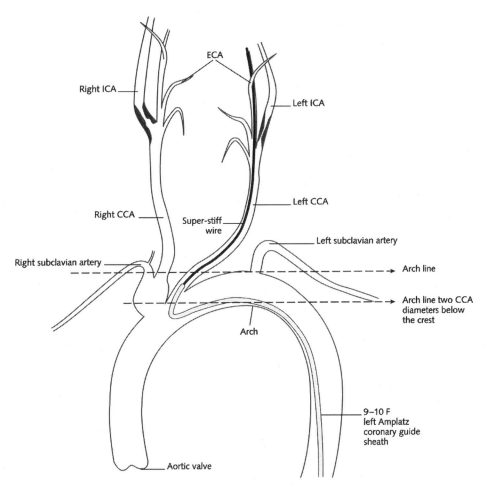

CCA: common carotid artery; ECA: external carotid artery; ICA: internal carotid artery.

Fig. 2 Classification of the entire arch using the Myla System. This is an example of the level 3 arch. A line is drawn across the top of the arch. If the origins of the arteries are more than 3 common carotid artery diameters inferior to the top of the arch, it is a level 3 arch. Examples of levels 1, 2, and 3 arches are presented in Fig. 1 of Chap. 7. (From Ref. 3.)

image intensifier is rotated too far, the arc of the catheter will begin to close again as the projection approaches the lateral position. The optimal LAO arch projection helps to identify the true length of the arch and also to separate the arch branch origins for arteriographic evaluation.

Other Access Options

Regardless of indication for carotid angioplasty and stent placement, if sheath access into the common carotid is not successful, the CAS procedure cannot be performed

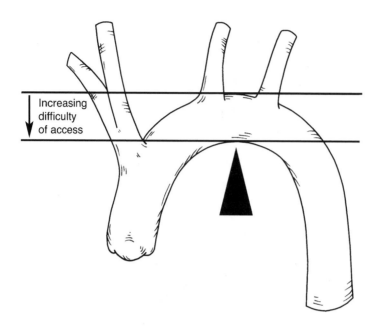

Fig. 3 The closer the parallel lines become, the more challenging the sheath access becomes. The arrow demonstrates the arch fulcrum point.

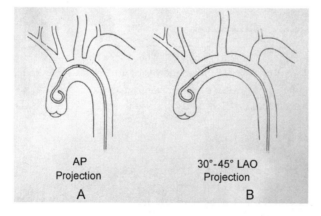

Fig. 4 Anterior oblique projection of the aortic arch. (A) An anteroposterior view does not adequately demonstrate the length and configuration of the arch. (B) As the image intensifier is rotated to the left anterior oblique position, the arch of the aorta unfolds and the catheter within the arch shows a broader arc. The image intensifier should be rotated until the course of the guidewire or catheter in the arch forms the broadest arc. (From Schneider PA, Endovascular Skills, Marcel Dekker, New York, 2003, pp. 91.)

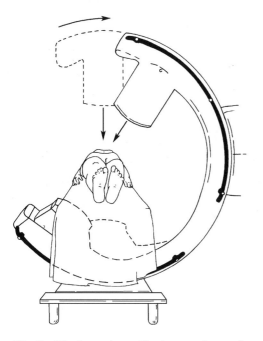

Fig. 5 The image intensifier is rotated away from the AP position and into the LAO to better visualize the widest arc of the aortic arch.

using a percutaneous femoral approach. Other access options must be explored, including brachial artery or direct common carotid access (4,5). Otherwise, the patient must be re-evaluated for carotid endarterectomy.

Technical Tips

1. The initial arch aortogram should be obtained in the optimum oblique projection to give the widest arch possible (Figs. 4 and 5, more about this in Chap. 4).
2. When planning the initial branch vessel catheterization, the relative complexity of the access can be estimated from the location of the vessel's origin as it relates to the fulcrum point of the arch (Fig. 1).
3. Segment I arteries are the most straightforward to catheterize and access with a high likelihood of success.
4. Segment II catheterizations are more challenging. This segment of the arch is bisected into IIa and IIb categories, with the degree of catheterization difficulty increasing from IIa to IIb subdivisions.
5. Segment III arteries are the most challenging to catheterize, with the origin of the target artery caudal to the horizontal line of the arch fulcrum.

Conclusion

The anatomy of the arch and its branches is an important predictor of the degree of difficulty of sheath access to the carotid artery. As described in this chapter, the segment of origin of aortic arch branch intended for catheterization helps to estimate the potential for technical success or the need for other access alternatives. Thus the preoperative counseling in the more difficult categories must stress the potential for the inability to achieve sheath access to the target common carotid artery. While there are many factors that contribute clinical significance in a given case, this simple system is useful for a quick assessment of arch anatomy and the development of strategy in planning a case.

References

1. Bosniak MA. An analysis of some anatomic-roentgenologic aspects of the brachiocephalic vessels. Am J Roentgenol, Radium Ther Nucl Med 1964; 91:1222–1231.
2. Mani RL, Eisenberg RL. Complications of catheter cerebral angiography: analysis of 5000 procedures. Am J Radiol 1978; 131:861–865.
3. Myla S. Carotid access techniques: an algorithmic approach. Carotid Interv 2001; 3:2–12.
4. Mubarak Al, Vitek JJ, Iyer SS, New G, Roubin GS. Carotid stenting with distal-balloon protection via the transbrachial approach. J Endovasc Ther 2001; 8(6):571–575.
5. Sievert H, Ensslen R, Fach A, et al. Brachial artery approach for transluminal angioplasty of the internal carotid artery. Catheter Cardiovasc Diagn 1996; 39:421–423.

3

Equipment, Inventory, and Facilities for Carotid Angioplasty and Stenting

DANIEL G. CLAIR

Cleveland Clinic Foundation, Cleveland, Ohio, U.S.A.

The purpose of this chapter is to provide an overview of the equipment, inventory, and facilities required for carotid stent placement. Preparation for a surgical procedure includes assuring the proper equipment is available to perform the operation. One would not attempt to perform a carotid endarterectomy without the availability of the proper clamps, shunts, endarterectomy spatulas, and other necessary items with which the surgeon is familiar. Likewise, it is necessary to assure the presence of the proper interventional equipment when performing percutaneous carotid interventions. The necessary catheters, guidewires, guiding catheters, and sheaths, balloons, and stents must be available to perform these procedures. One will need to assure that the room is equipped to adequately monitor the patient. Medications must be readily available, including anticoagulants, antiplatelet agents, hemodynamic medications as needed, and limited sedation as required. The assisting staff must be knowledgeable in the nomenclature of the catheters and equipment used during interventional procedures. This requires staff members who can work with both standard peripheral equipment and potentially either coronary or neurointerventional equipment, which tend to be based on smaller caliber guidewire systems.

The surgeon/interventionalist must be comfortable with the ability of the staff to assist in performing these procedures. Educating the assisting staff beforehand on the nature of the procedure to be performed, the important points of the case, and the specific assistance that will be necessary is critical to assuring smooth progression through the intervention. Assuring adequate monitoring for the patient permits rapid assessment of the patient's status, thereby allowing intervention for hemodynamic problems early and limiting their impact upon the outcome. Some surgeons find themselves more comfortable performing these procedures for this reason in an operating room setting with the assistance of an anesthesiologist or nurse anesthetist. It is important that the person performing the intervention be confident that the people assisting can quickly deal with hemodynamic or airway problems when they occur. The responsibility for the procedure and everything associated with it ultimately lie with the surgeon.

In outlining the required setup for performing carotid interventions, it is necessary to delineate distinctions between differing categories of equipment. Fixed imaging equipment in the endovascular room is not mandatory but is best and will facilitate performance of these procedures. In addition, a room stocked with adequate disposable inventory is highly desirable. Lastly, it is helpful to develop a method of arranging the room for these procedures. These issues are addressed below under the headings equipment, inventory, and room setup. More information is available from other sources about creating the right environment for performing carotid stenting and other endovascular procedures (1–4).

Equipment

One important aspect of performing these procedures safely is assuring that the patient is adequately monitored before, during, and after the procedure. For this reason, it is imperative to have monitoring equipment in both the procedure room and the recovery room. Monitoring will necessitate the presence of someone in the room whose primary responsibility is assessing the patient. This person has a significant role in assuring that the subject is stable and that the monitoring equipment is functioning appropriately. It is also mandatory that resuscitation equipment be available should it become necessary. This requirement is similar to what one should have available for procedural rooms for any peripheral intervention and includes a functioning suction device, oxygen, and intravenous solutions along with a cart equipped with standard emergency resuscitation material.

Monitoring equipment is similar to that available for the operating room or special procedures suite. One should have standard oxygen saturation monitoring equipment. This device should be attached to an extremity with adequate flow to assure continuous monitoring of the oxygenation status of the patient. It is often best to assure that this probe is placed away from the extremity in which arterial access is obtained to assure that distal vessel spasm or disease, if present, does not impair the readings of this monitor. In addition, it is necessary to have continuous monitoring of the electrocardiographic tracing. This is best performed with a 5-lead system, and in order to limit impingement upon the image being obtained, it is helpful to have radiolucent lead systems. The use of these leads allows imaging to be performed without having to adjust lead placement or wire position during the procedure, which can alter the appearance of the electrocardiographic waveform or, in some instances, cause loss of the tracing.

It is also mandatory to have the ability to continuously monitor the arterial pressure with both invasive and noninvasive means. In most cardiac catheterization laboratories, this arterial pressure system is part of the manifold system used to connect to the arterial sheath following insertion. It is helpful to have this additional port off the manifold that allows pressure monitoring. The pressure system can, however, be added to the sidearm of the sheath attaching the side port of the sheath to a separate pressure monitoring system. In addition to this invasive arterial pressure monitor, it is necessary to have a noninvasive method of monitoring the pressure in case the invasive system is not functioning or is impaired for a period of time during the procedure. It is extremely helpful to the interventionalist to have all this information available. Having a separate monitor facing the proceduralist with all of these things shown on a physiological monitor is immensely beneficial (Fig. 1).

Once the monitoring system for the patient is assured to be adequate, the next most important piece of equipment in the room is the imaging system. These systems may be either fixed or mobile systems and there are advantages and disadvantages to each. The most commonly used systems for these procedures are fixed imaging systems. These systems have the best images, the largest fields of view, and the ability to store imaging positions. They are, however, significantly more expensive than the

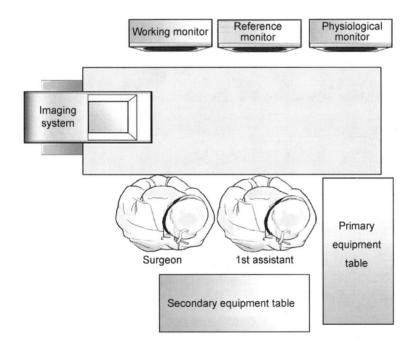

Fig. 1 This diagram shows an example of how the endovascular suite may be arranged to facilitate carotid stent placement.

mobile imaging systems and occupy more space than mobile units. Most interventionalists, if given the choice, would choose a fixed imaging system to use to perform these procedures. It is clear that the imaging is superior with fixed systems and the ability to position the image intensifier and the area in question in close proximity and to adjust the focal length of the radiation beam are options that are unavailable with a mobile system. It is imperative that the procedure be performed in a setting where both subtracted and unsubtracted digital runs can be obtained. This combination allows fine imaging and also imaging to still be obtained when the patient is not completely cooperative or when the surgeon wants the patient to be able to relax during the imaging. Especially early on in one's experience, the better the imaging, the easier the procedure will be to perform and the shorter the procedure will be. For these reasons, I favor a fixed imaging system when performing these procedures.

The table used for these procedures should be a floating-point table that is carbon fiber and allows imaging in all rotations. Attempting this procedure with a mobile system without a carbon fiber table adds to the complexity of the case and will limit the angles in which images can be obtained. This may limit the ability of the surgeon to use the best view to perform the intervention. Floating-point tables allow rapid surgeon positioning of the table and decreases the time necessary for performing the procedure. If one is using a mobile system, a floating-point, carbon fiber table will be helpful.

While not all interventionalists will use a power injector for carotid studies, it is necessary to have this piece of equipment to perform aortic arch injections and obtain anatomic detail of the aortic arch and its branches. Although hand injections of the carotid circulation are adequate and quick, the use of a power injector offers the ability to repeatedly inject the branch vessel with a small fixed amount of contrast without aspiration of the catheter or the risk associated with system disconnection while repositioning the image intensifier and the patient. Power injectors can be set to automatically reload for multiple injections where the same rates and amounts of contrast will be used. This reduces time to perform studies and can limit risk to the patient.

It is additionally helpful to have a sterile workspace upon which to work. In order to move expeditiously through the performance of these procedures, arranging two tables behind the team is helpful (Fig. 1). The space offered by an additional "back table" provides an area upon which the items to be used are prepared and placed, available in the order of use. The time saved not searching for an item on a crowded surface will easily offset the small space loss incurred by the additional table.

Inventory

Prior to performing a procedure, inventory items should be assembled. Thinking through the performance of the procedure allows the review of important points and assures that in preparing the equipment, one methodically assesses equipment needs. In attempting to review the inventory needed to perform these procedures, we will similarly progress through items as one would normally progress through the intervention.

ACCESS ITEMS

Access equipment is similar to what is needed to perform other peripheral interventions. The surgeon should be comfortable with access and the equipment needed for this. Needles (18 gauge), standard endovascular access guidewires, and short, working sheaths (4–8 Fr) should be the standard items with which one has become accustomed. A large number of the complications occurring perioperatively are related to arterial access, and for this reason, care should be taken to assure that the initial part of the procedure proceeds smoothly. This is not a good time to try a new access needle or guidewire or, for that matter, a closure device with which one is unfamiliar, as the aggressive use of antiplatelet agents mandate smooth access and easy, reliable sheath removal. The hypotension, which can accompany a difficult access or closure, may result in neurologic problems that are preventable.

CATHETERS

Normal progress of the procedure entails performance of an arch aortogram to assess directly the status of the great vessel origins. An adequate length, at least 90 cm, flush catheter should be available. Any of the standard flush catheters in the long length will serve. It is usually helpful to have a pressure monitor available from this point forward to check that both sheath and flush catheter are intraluminal by measuring pressure. While many diagnostic studies are performed with 4- or 5-Fr catheters, when planning to proceed to carotid stenting, it is often helpful to begin with a 6-Fr access sheath to allow monitoring of arterial pressure during the catheterization procedure. In addition, a 6-Fr access sheath may be easily exchanged for a 6-Fr guiding sheath.

Following the flush aortogram, selective catheterization of the vessel(s) in question is performed. This will require a variety of catheter shapes, varying from slightly angled (simple curve) to a completely reversed curvature (complex curve). A wide selection of catheters ranging from those with a slight angle such as the Berenstein or vertebral catheter to those with increased angulation such as the H1 Headhunter and JR4 catheters and those with reverse curvatures such as the VTK, Sos, and Simmons catheters should be available. Facility with an understanding of a basic variety of catheters is helpful in minimizing catheter switching. The fewer catheters advanced through an arterial system, the less likely damage or complication can occur. The size of catheter used to perform these selective views is usually 5 Fr. These catheters permit adequate contrast flow to view these vessels. Catheter selections and choices for varying anatomy are part of the ability to perform cerebral angiography. It is helpful to use the least-angled catheter possible to gain vessel access. Having minimal angle on the catheter will allow easy advancement of the catheter over the guidewire into the vessel selected. A large number of arch vessels can be catheterized utilizing an angled, Glide catheter (Boston Scientific) and a hydrophilic guidewire.

GUIDEWIRES

After engaging the orifice of the vessel with the catheter, it is often necessary to advance a guidewire into the vessel to advance the catheter over. If there is not a dramatic amount of tortuosity in the aortoiliac segment, a stiff, hydrophilic guidewire is helpful, as it allows the catheter to be advanced more easily into the vessel in question. When there is tortuosity in the system, either in the aortoiliac segment or the thoracic aorta, manipulating a rigid guidewire can be difficult and the guidewire and catheter can often be "popped out" of the vessel. In these situations, using a "floppy" hydrophilic guidewire can allow rotation of the tip of the guidewire without these kinds of difficulties. The less rigid guidewire does make it more difficult to advance the catheter with direct transmission of longitudinal movement to the tip of the catheter. This can tend to draw the guidewire back in the vessel in question. One way of overcoming this problem is to utilize a selective catheter in conjunction with either a long, braided, flexible sheath or a guide catheter. These items give "body" to the system without making it difficult to manipulate catheter or guidewire. These guide catheters or long sheaths are often advanced over a rigid guidewire.

In order to advance a sheath or guide catheter into the vessel to be treated, rigid guidewires may be necessary. When the angulation is more difficult to traverse, the use of a more rigid guidewire, such as the Amplatz superstiff (Boston Scientific), may be helpful. In some instances where long purchase of the guidewire into the vessel to be cannulated is unobtainable because of the proximity of the lesion, a 1-cm flexible-tipped Amplatz superstiff guidewire may be used. Careful advancement of these guidewires is mandatory to assure that the guidewire does not damage the vessel and to assure that the rigid portion of the guidewire advances beyond any area of tortuosity. The latter problem can result in migration of the catheter out of the vessel of interest.

GUIDING CATHETERS AND GUIDING SHEATHS

A wide variety of guide catheters and long sheaths are available for use in these procedures. The size of current stent systems remains the limiting factor in choosing the size of the guiding sheath or guiding catheter. Currently, the procedure is performed most commonly with either a 6-Fr sheath or an 8-Fr guide catheter. Sheaths that have commonly been used for this purpose include the Brite Tip sheath (Cordis), the Shuttle sheath (Cook), and the Raabe sheath (Cook). The first of these is a nonbraided sheath, which is fairly kink-resistant and has a smooth outer surface and an easily visible distal marker on the sheath. The next two sheaths are very flexible and kink-resistant and vary in the use of either a Tuohy–Borst type adaptor or a diaphragm at the working end of the sheath. The use of a standard diaphragm can decrease blood loss and minimize manipulations required of the sheath; however, the Tuohy–Borst adaptor allows the ability to back-bleed the sheath and to assure that the diaphragm does not damage any of the items being advanced into the sheath. The Raabe sheath, in particular, has a very short dilator tip, which limits the potential problems which may arise from the portion of the dilator tip extending beyond the sheath.

Guide catheters come in a variety of shapes and allow selective catheterization of vessels that would otherwise be difficult if not impossible to treat with a sheath alone. Similar to the recommendations for limiting angulation of the selective catheters, limited angulation of guide catheters allows smoother advancement into the vessel. When this can be performed over a selective catheter or with a dilator, the potential for injury to the proximal vessel or distal embolization is minimized. There is a vast array of guide catheters available for these purposes and providing an exhaustive list here would likely not be helpful. Many of the commercial producers of guide catheters provide a diagram and list of the guiding catheters available and their respective shapes. Some commonly used guides for this purpose include the H1 guide catheter and the JR4 guide catheter. It is important to remember that all guide catheters have their nomenclature related to the outer diameter, and inner lumen diameter of these can vary depending upon the thickness of the wall and the manufacturer. For most purposes, an 8-Fr guide catheter provides nearly the equivalent inner lumen as a 6-Fr sheath. One should be sure to check the specifications on the package beforehand to assure that all equipment utilized will fit through the intended guide catheter. These guides will all require the use of a Tuohy–Borst adaptor proximally.

PROTECTION DEVICES AND SMALLER DIAMETER GUIDEWIRES

After accessing the vessel to be treated with either the appropriate guide sheath or guide catheter, the placement of a protection device should be considered. We currently use protection for all cases of carotid stenting. The current designs vary from the use of either proximal or distal balloon occlusion to filter devices. In some patients, one form of device may be unusable either because of the lack of collateral circulation or the inability to advance the device into the area beyond the stenosis. Extremely tortuous vessels beyond the stenosis should prompt consideration of converting to standard surgical therapy or avoidance of filter protection devices unless there is adequate vessel length proximal to the tortuosity to utilize the protection device in this segment.

Additional small caliber guidewires should be available in the event they are needed to assist with the crossing of a high-grade stenosis of the vessel to be treated. Utilizing 0.014-in. guidewires will allow the use of either 0.014- or 0.018-in. balloon catheter systems.

BALLOON CATHETERS

Balloon systems and inflation devices will be necessary to treat stenoses. One should have both large (0.035 in.) and small (0.018/0.014 in.) balloon systems available so that any arterial process encountered can be treated. It is helpful to have monorail balloon systems for use as these can minimize the time necessary to advance and remove these devices. Balloons are available from a number of providers. Lower profile balloon systems can make crossing the lesion initially easier, while it is also helpful to have high-pressure balloons for dilatation of calcified difficult lesions. An inflation device with a pressure gauge is used to dilate the balloons and to assure monitoring of inflation for documentation and reporting.

STENTS

Flexible, self-expanding stent systems with low-profile, trackable delivery catheters and reliable deployment mechanisms are a necessary part of the armamentarium to perform carotid interventions. Many of these devices have been described elsewhere. The delivery systems should be low profile, 6 Fr or less, and trackable. Ideally, this would be a monorail system with a simple and reliable deployment mechanism that avoids movement of the stent during placement. It is also helpful to have a slight taper to the delivery catheter to allow imaging through the sheath or guide catheter around the delivery system to assure proper placement of the stent. There are a number of these systems currently available, and a variety of lengths should be available to treat different length lesions. Backup systems should also be available so that should mal-deployment or even contamination of the system occurs, a replacement is available.

MEDICATIONS

The cardiac and hemodynamic issues, which can arise in this setting, mandate the rapid availability of a variety of cardioactive medications and good intravenous access for the patient. Immediate availability of agents to manage hypotension, bradycardia, hypertension, and coronary symptoms along with glycoprotein IIb/IIIa inhibitors should be easily accessible by staff in the unit.

Atropine should be available in an easily injectable system to rapidly deal with the hypotension that can accompany inflation of the angioplasty balloon in the carotid bulb. In some instances, additional atropine beyond the initial dose may be needed and should be available. Pacing leads should be accessible in case the patient proves unresponsive to medical therapy for bradycardia. Hypertension is frequent in this patient population and should be treated promptly to limit the potential for intra-cranial hemorrhage. Continuous infusion of nitroglycerin is helpful for this issue as it can be rapidly titrated up or down to control blood pressure, and this agent will help with anginal symptoms in patients as well. Other agents, such as hydralazine and labetolol, should also be available; however, caution should be used when giving agents that may decrease heart rate as these can be detrimental to the patient who develops bradycardia later. It is also dangerous to give these patients a long-acting antihypertensive agent. Many of these patients will develop hypotension following the revascularization procedure, and reversal of these longer-acting agents can be difficult to achieve.

It is also mandatory to have medications available to treat hypotension rapidly. Many patients have a decrease in blood pressure soon after completion of the revascularization procedure and will require medications to maintain adequate blood pressure. Initial maneuvers to deal with this hypotension will often involve rapid volume infusion; however, with significant decreases in blood pressure, medical therapy with either dopamine or ephedrine may be necessary, and these should be readily available.

Facilities and Room Setup

It is important to have the facility and room arranged so that the surgeon is comfortable performing the procedure and has all equipment necessary for the procedure close at hand. Fig. 1 schematically represents the position of personnel and equipment in the room. The room should be large enough to allow movement around the patient and sterile field. The area around the head of the patient should be unobstructed so that assessment can be performed easily from both sides. The patient should be comfortably positioned. A cradle for head positioning is often helpful. Safety straps and side restraints help maintain patient position and safety especially in the event of periprocedural neurologic events. The interventionalist should be positioned tableside with easy access to the equipment tables. It is essential to have adequate assistance during these procedures and to assure that the assistant is well versed in the technique and equipment. The assistant should be positioned to the side of the interventionalist and should also have easy access to both of the tables. Monitoring cables should be positioned away from the head and shoulders to allow free visualization of the arteries in this region. The image system is best positioned at the head of the table with the monitor bank for images positioned at eye level opposite the surgeon. The monitor bank should include three monitors. The first should contain the working images. The second monitor is a reference monitor to allow posting of reference images that can be used to assist with positioning catheters and guidewires. The final monitor should be a physiological monitor which contains the output of the continuous hemodynamic measurements, oxygen saturation, electrocardiographic tracing, and noninvasive pressure measurements. While performing these procedures, it is necessary to constantly reassess these measurements and tracings.

References

1. Dietrich EB. Endovascular suite design. In: White RA, Fogarty TJ, eds. Peripheral Endovascular Interventions. St. Louis: Mosby, 1996:129–139.
2. Mansour MA. The new operating room environment. Surg Clin North Am 1999; 79:477–487.
3. Armonda RA, Thomas JE, Rosenwasser RH. The interventional neuroradiology suite as an operating room. Neurosurg Clin N Am 2000; 11:1–20.
4. Schneider PA. Where do we work? In: Schneider PA, ed. Endovascular Skills. New York: Marcel Dekker, 2003:175–181.

4

Carotid Arteriography

PETER A. SCHNEIDER

Hawaii Permanente Medical Group, Honolulu, Hawaii, U.S.A.

The purpose of this chapter is to provide a step-by-step guide to carotid arteriography. The components of a step-by-step approach to carotid arteriography are listed in Table 1. Carotid arteriography is the key prerequisite to gaining the experience required for carotid stent placement.

Role of Carotid Arteriography in Clinical Vascular Practice

Carotid arteriography in the evaluation of extracranial occlusive disease was performed for decades as the "gold standard" to determine the degree of stenosis. At a time when the role of arteriography is assuming less overall importance due to improved noninvasive methods of vascular imaging, the arteriography that is required is absolutely essential because it is used as a guide to determine methods and options for endovascular repair. Carotid arteriography in the era of stent placement is not about quantifying the degree of stenosis; we have better means of performing that task. Carotid arteriography is a pathway to treatment; it is a means for assessing whether carotid stent placement is possible and if so, how to get there. Arteriography is no longer diagnostic, it has become the basis for treatment. From the standpoint of endovascular skill development, if you can't "gram" it, you can't treat it. Vascular specialists need to be accomplished in carotid arteriography if they are going to participate in the future treatment of carotid disease.

Table 1 Step-by-Step Approach to Carotid Arteriography

Supplies
Arch aortogram
Arch assessment (more in Chapter 2)
Choose selective cerebral catheter
Selective catheterization of carotid artery
Selective arteriography in multiple projections
Filming and contrast administration sequences
Technical tips
Protocol
Qualifications

Clinical Evaluation of the Patient Before Carotid Arteriography

As with any instrumentation of the vasculature, carotid arteriography should be performed as a part of a patient's care only after a complete assessment of the risks and benefits of the procedure. Carotid arteriography has its own set of risks, some of which are probably unavoidable. The potential complication of concern to physicians and patients is stroke, and the procedure is planned and performed with emphasis on minimizing the likelihood of this complication. Prior to the development of carotid stent placement, most patients with carotid bifurcation stenosis were treated with carotid endarterectomy on the basis of duplex evaluation without carotid arteriography. In institutions where carotid duplex met quality assurance and accuracy criteria, arteriography was usually performed selectively for patients with carotid disease in whom history, physical examination, or noninvasive vascular studies suggested that carotid bifurcation endarterectomy would not be straightforward or would not solve the patient's problem. Examples of indications for carotid arteriography in this setting are included in Table 2. The development of carotid stent placement has promoted a move back toward arteriography. Whereas the usual obstacles to safe performance of carotid endarterectomy included medical comorbidities and some anatomical situations (such

Table 2 Indications for Proceeding to Carotid Arteriography in Patients with Carotid Occlusive Disease

History	Physical exam	Carotid duplex
Symptoms and disease don't match	Brachial blood pressure gradient	High bifurcation
	Noncardiac bruit at base of neck	Excessive tortuosity
Symptoms in different cerebrovascular beds	Diminished carotid pulse	CCA disease
	Subclavian or vertebral bruit	Reversed vertebral
Nonlocalizing symptoms	Diminished brachial pulse	Distal ICA disease

as high bifurcation), the primary obstacles to safe carotid stent placement are usually anatomical and lesion factors. At present, carotid arteriography is the best way to assess these factors related to anatomy and plan strategy for treatment. The operator must be cognizant of the introduction of the additional risk of carotid arteriography into the treatment regimen. At present, it is not an uncommon practice to perform carotid arteriography as a separate initial procedure to help decide whether carotid stent placement would be appropriate. As techniques improve, it is likely that arteriography and intervention will be performed more as a continuum during the same procedure and that decisions about anatomical and lesion-related obstacles, sizing, and planning will be made during the procedure.

Clinical evaluation of a patient's medical condition prior to carotid arteriography is similar to patient assessment prior to other types of arteriography. Carotid arteriography patients are more likely than others to be receiving antiplatelet agents at the time of the procedure. It is usually safe to perform arteriography in patients on antiplatelet therapy, as long as there are no other factors that are likely to promote hemorrhage, such as end-stage renal disease. If the antiplatelet agent must be stopped, it should be 10 days before the procedure. Arteriography is usually safe in patients on coumadin, but the size of the arteriotomy should be minimized and extra care and monitoring is required of the access site after the procedure. The usual sheath size for carotid arteriography is 4 or 5 Fr. Patients with renal insufficiency are managed with preoperative normal saline hydration and mucormyst. Thought should be given to which views and sequences are required in order to minimize the amount of contrast required in cases of renal insufficiency. Alternatives to standard iodinated contrast in carotid arteriography are limited. Carbon dioxide arteriography is contraindicated. Gadolinium is not known to be safe, but case reports of its use in the cerebral arteries are beginning to appear (1). Patients with contrast allergy are treated with prednisone and benedryl prior to the arteriogram.

Severe cardiac or pulmonary comorbidities add some risk to the procedure and may make the procedure more difficult. These patients may be unable to breath-hold for a few seconds. The pulmonary hyperinflation of chronic obstructive pulmonary disease may make arch and vessel origin visualization more difficult using fluoroscopy. Patients with congestive heart failure may be sensitive to the osmotic load of the contrast. Patients with long-standing hypertension tend to have an elongated arch that pushes the origins of the branch vessels down into the chest and causes more acute curvature of the distal arch (Fig. 1). Treatment of hypertension during the procedure is discussed in Chapter 8. Severe hypertension adds risk to the arteriogram. Blood pressure tends to be more labile during the procedure, patients are often somewhat dehydrated due to antihypertensive regimens, and the risk of stroke with any procedure is probably elevated.

Examination of the patient should include a neurological exam and an assessment of the vascular system. Specifically, a complete examination of the vasculature should include bilateral brachial blood pressures, palpation of pulses at the carotid, subclavian, axillary, brachial, and superficial temporal positions. Any difference in brachial blood

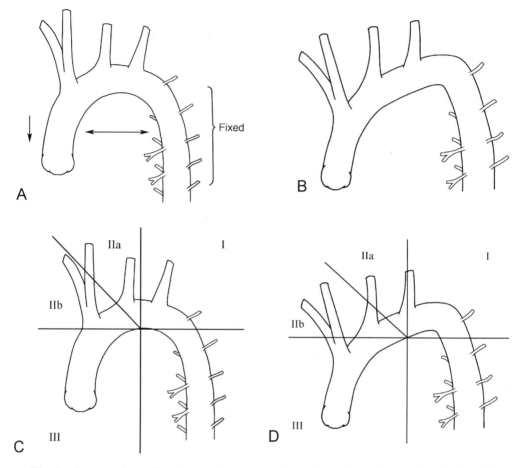

Fig. 1   Aortic arch configurations influence carotid arteriography: using the "surf and turf" classification. (A) This is a normal arch. (B) Some patients have an elongated arch that pushes the origins of the branch vessels down into the chest and causes more acute curvature of the distal arch. (C, D) By using the "surf and turf" classification, as described in Chapter 2, the differences between these two types of arches can be evaluated. In C, the innominate artery originates in segment IIb, and in D, it originates in segment III.

pressure of 10 mm Hg or more is likely to be significant. Avoid palpating the carotid bifurcation because of the potential for embolization or vagal stimulation. The index pulse for the extracranial cerebrovasculature is the right common carotid artery. The left common carotid artery has its origin more posteriorly than the right and, as a result, the left side is often slightly deeper. Subclavian artery pulses are often palpable just superior to the clavicle and lateral to the clavicular head. Axillary artery pulses are usually palpable inferior to the clavicle at the deltopectoral groove. If one side can be palpated and the other side cannot, it is usually a significant finding. Auscultation for bruits over the carotid, subclavian, and vertebral arteries should be performed. The quality of a carotid bruit often reveals something about the carotid lesion. In general, the higher the pitch the more narrow the residual lumen. Auscultation should be performed along the length of the sternocleidomastoid groove in the anterior neck to identify the location of greatest intensity. This helps to differentiate carotid and cardiac sounds and also helps to locate proximal common carotid artery lesions and high bifurcations. Subclavian and vertebral artery bruits may be heard at the base of the neck, especially in the supra-clavicular area.

A plan for arterial access should be made on the basis of the physical exam. The first choice is usually femoral artery access. The femoral pulses and the femoral arteries are palpated. It does not seem to matter for carotid arteriography which side is used. If there is no femoral access or it is contraindicated, the left brachial artery is the second choice for access. The right brachial artery is a third choice. Although direct, common carotid artery access, either percutaneous or open, is sometimes used for interventions, it is almost never required for carotid arteriography.

A brief neurological examination does not take much time but is essential. Included in the evaluation should be visual fields, cranial nerves III through XII, extremity motor and sensory function, and cerebellar function (balance and coordination). A deficit in any of these areas must be compared with the postangiography condition of the patient.

Informed consent is best obtained in the office, when patients are afforded time to consider the issues and to discuss with their families. Patients are often concerned about the possibility of stroke as a result of arteriography and this should be discussed directly. The potential for access site and other complications are also discussed.

Supplies for Carotid Arteriography

The basic supplies required for carotid arteriography are similar to those for other types of arteriography and are listed in Table 3. In addition to these supplies, a leaded apron, thyroid shield, and leaded glasses are used by the operator. Other accessories include arterial dilators, a sheath, guidewires, a flush catheter, and diagnostic catheters. These are discussed in the next few sections.

Arterial Access for Carotid Arteriography

Access is usually through the common femoral artery. Both femoral areas are prepared and draped. A towel is placed on the patient's lap holding the supplies required for puncture: a syringe for local anesthetic, a scalpel, a clamp, an arterial puncture needle, and a guidewire. Intravenous antibiotics are administered if the patient has a prosthetic graft or heart valve in place. The femoral artery is palpated and the inguinal ligament is traced from the anterior superior iliac spine to the pubic tubercle. After local anesthetic infiltration of the skin and subcutaneous tissue, the common femoral artery is punctured along its proximal few centimeters with the needle at an angle of approach of 45°. When

Table 3 Supplies for Carotid Arteriography

Entry needle	10- and 20-ml syringes
#11 Scalpel blade	Local anesthetic
Gauze pads	22-gauge needle
Clamp	Mechanism for discards
Drapes	Sterile connector tubing
Sterile cover for image intensifier	Heparinized saline
Gown	Guidewire
Gloves	Torque device

pulsatile backbleeding is achieved, the nondominant hand holds the needle and the dominant hand advances a general-purpose, floppy tip starting guidewire through the needle. Fluoroscopy is used to advance the guidewire into the abdominal aorta.

When access through the common femoral artery is not feasible, the brachial artery may be punctured using micropuncture technique. A micropuncture set (Cook, Inc., Bloomington, Ind.) includes a 22-gauge needle, a short 0.018-in. guidewire with a floppy tip, a 4 Fr short catheter with an inner dilator that passes over the 0.018-in. guidewire. The 21-gauge needle is placed in the artery. When backbleeding occurs, the 0.018-in guidewire is advanced through the needle. The needle is removed and the 4 Fr catheter with the inner dilator is passed over the guidewire. After the catheter is in place, the dilator and short guidewire are removed and the 4 Fr catheter provides access for the desired guidewire.

The most common complications following carotid arteriography occur at the access site. In the case of femoral access, the location of the inguinal ligament is essential in determining where the puncture should be. Fluoroscopy may be used prior to puncture to locate the head of the femur. The artery usually passes over the medial side of the femoral head and can sometimes be visualized under fluoroscopy. Most puncture site complications are related to arteriotomies that are too high, too low, or forced into an area too hostile for simple puncture. Puncture of the artery proximal to the femoral head is too far proximal. Puncture of the external iliac artery cannot be adequately compressed after the procedure. The proximal deep femoral artery is also difficult to compress because of its deep course and may bleed afterward. The proximal superficial femoral artery is often a site of plaque formation, and puncture at this location may cause thrombosis. The major concern about brachial artery access is the possibility that even a small sheath hematoma will cause an upper extremity neurological deficit.

Access Sheath for Carotid Arteriography

A short, hemostatic access sheath is not mandatory for carotid arteriography but is advisable. During catheter exchanges, the sheath provides protection of the arteriotomy from the catheters and also protection of the catheters from the skin and soft tissue. Catheter exchanges are simpler and safer with a sheath securing the arteriotomy. Since selective carotid artery catheterization requires simultaneous rotation and push/pull of the catheter, friction encountered at the access site can make these maneuvers more difficult. The access sheath reduces the friction at the access site. The sheath has a hemostatic valve, a dilator to stiffen it during placement, and a sidearm port for flushing. The sheath is advanced with the dilator in place to avoid uncontrolled end-arterectomy by the hollow sheath tip. A sheath is sized by its inside diameter, which is the same as the largest diameter catheter the sheath will accept (since catheters are sized by outside diameter).

Either a 4 or 5 Fr sheath is used depending upon the anticipated usage of 4 or 5 Fr catheters. The dilator and the sheath are irrigated and wiped with heparinized saline. Lock the dilator hub in place so that it does not back out while the sheath is being advanced. A small-caliber sheath can almost always be placed by using a starting guidewire. The guidewire in place should be advanced far enough so that the floppy tip is well inside the patient and that the entry site is crossed by the sheath while it is on the stiff portion of the guidewire shaft. The sheath is loaded onto the guidewire and advanced all the way to the entry site as the guidewire is pinned by the assistant. The sheath is held along its shaft near the tip so that it does not buckle while going through the skin and soft tissue. Sometimes it is helpful to rotate the sheath back and forth to get through the subcutaneous tissue. Place the sidearm port toward the operator. Pressure is maintained at the arteriotomy with the nondominant hand until the sheath goes into the artery. Advance the sheath to its hub. After the sheath is placed, take out the dilator, aspirate through the sidearm port and flush with heparinized saline. The sheath is flushed intermittently during the case.

Guidewires and Catheters for Carotid Arteriography

Some of the many possible choices for these guidewires and catheters that we commonly use are listed in Table 4. The minimum guidewire length is 180 cm and 0.035-in. platform guidewires are used. A starting guidewire is advanced initially into the aorta and the access sheath is placed. The starting guidewire has a floppy, atraumatic tip. A 180-cm long, 0.035-in. Newton or Bentson or another general-purpose guidewire is satisfactory. The starting guidewire is advanced into the arch of the aorta. The flush catheter is placed over the starting guidewire and the arch aortogram is performed. Fig. 2 shows some of the flush catheter head configurations available. The pigtail catheter is most often used for the flush aortogram. It has a curl-shaped head with an end hole and multiple side holes to minimize any jet or whip effect. The 4 and 5 Fr pigtail catheters, 100 cm in length, are capable of infusing at contrast 15 and 27 mL/sec, respectively. The arch is assessed and a selective catheter is chosen. This process is discussed in detail in the sections below. The flush catheter is exchanged for a selective catheter. Selective catheters have a single end hole, some type of shape at the tip, and are 90 to 125 cm in

Table 4 Guidewires and Catheters for Carotid Arteriography

Starting guidewire
   Newton 180 cm, floppy tip, 0.035 in.
   Bentson 180 cm, floppy tip, 0.035 in.
Selective guidewire
   Glidewire 260 cm, angled tip, 0.035 in.
Access sheath
   5 Fr, 15-cm length, hemostatic sheath
Flush catheter
   Pigtail 100 cm, 4 Fr (flow rate 15 mL/sec)
   Pigtail 100 cm, 5 Fr (flow rate 27 mL/sec)
Selective cerebral catheters (see Figure 2)
   Simple Curve
      Angled Glidecath 100 cm, 4 Fr, 5Fr
      Angled Glidecath 120 cm, 4 Fr
      Vert 120 cm, 5 Fr
      H1 Headhunter 100 cm, 5 Fr
   Complex curve
      Simmons 1 100 cm, 4 Fr, 5 Fr
      Simmons 2 100 cm, 4 Fr, 5 Fr
      Simmons 3 100 cm, 5 Fr
      JB 2 100 cm, 5 Fr
      Vitek 100 cm, 125 cm, 5 Fr

length (but most catheters are 100 cm in length). In comparison to flush catheters, a 5 Fr selective cerebral catheter with a single end hole is able to safely administer approximately 8 to 10 mL of contrast per second. The selective catheter is advanced into the branch vessel over the selective or steerable guidewire. The selective catheter may be a simple curve or a complex curve (Fig. 3) (2). There is more information about selective catheters in the section below on "Selective Cerebral Catheters."

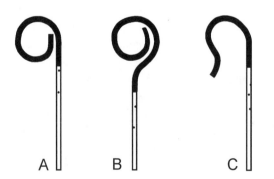

Fig. 2 Flush catheters for arch aortography. Flush catheters have an end hole and multiple side holes to permit rapid administration of contrast in the high-flow aortic arch. (A) Pigtail. (B) Tennis racket. (C) Omni flush (Angiodymanics).

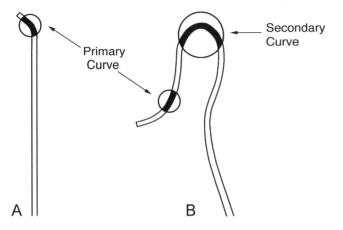

Fig. 3 Simple curve and complex curve cerebral catheters. (A) This is a simple curve catheter. There is a primary curve located near the tip of the catheter. (B) A complex curve catheter, in this case a Simmons catheter, has a primary curve near the tip and a secondary curve proximally along the shaft. The complex curve catheter must be reformed in the vasculature after the guidewire is removed.

Handling of Guidewires and Catheters During Carotid Arteriography

Guidewires are wiped with heparin–saline-soaked gauze or Telfa prior to and after each placement. Catheters are flushed and wiped in the usual manner prior to insertion and after each exchange. After placement, a catheter should be carefully aspirated, the syringe should be maintained in the vertical position to trap air bubbles, and the catheter should be flushed. Catheters should be flushed only sparingly and very gently after insertion. Extra caution must be exercised to be certain that no unintended solutions are infused. When connecting the catheter to the extension tubing for the power injector, care is taken to avoid generating or leaving air bubbles in the line. When removing a guidewire from the catheter, especially when the catheter is in a low-flow position, remove the guidewire steadily and without whipping it to avoid creating suction when the catheter fills slowly with backbleeding. If the selective catheter tip is against the arterial wall and it backfills slowly, pulling the guidewire too fast will create microbubbles that must be removed.

Selective catheters are handled using a series of maneuvers that includes pushing, pulling, and rotating the catheter shaft. The guidewire may be advanced for variable distances along the catheter shaft or protrude a distance beyond the selective catheter tip and each guidewire position changes the handling properties of the catheter. All catheters, but especially selective catheters, should be maneuvered carefully since any catheter tip, no matter how simple, could cause embolization. Areas of diffuse disease should be evaluated with caution. Occasionally it is prudent to avoid selective catheterization because of disease in the arch. The arch is one of the few places in the vasculature where a selective catheter may be maneuvered fairly regularly without the leading guidewire. This is because the selected catheter head will only take its shape if the guidewire is withdrawn into the catheter proximal to the catheter head. After the catheter tip is used to cannulate the artery, the guidewire is advanced. If the arch is free of disease, the selective catheter may be advanced from the distal arch to the proximal arch to cannulate one of the arch branches without the guidewire protruding from the end of the catheter. The tip of the catheter is turned away from the wall of the aorta as the catheter is advanced. Use a three-way stopcock to assist in clearing the line when cerebral catheters are connected to the injector tubing. After hook up, the third port of the stopcock is aspirated with a 10-mL syringe; first from the catheter side to remove a small amount of blood, then to the injector side to remove a small amount of contrast.

Anticoagulation During Carotid Arteriography

There is a wide range of acceptable practice with respect to heparin administration during carotid arteriography. Some operators do not administer heparin during carotid arteriography and some always do. The longer the catheter indwelling time, the more selective the catheterization, the more diseased the vasculature, and the lower the flow in the carotid artery, the more likely the patient is to benefit from anticoagulation. The authors use the following general guidelines. If an arch aortogram alone is planned, heparin is not used. Patients undergoing selective carotid arteriography are treated with 50 units of heparin per kilogram. Patients in whom the procedure will proceed to intervention are administered 75 to 100 units per kilogram. If a complete arteriogram is planned, including multiple obliques of the bilateral extracranial and intracranial circulation, it is likely that the catheter placement in the carotid artery will exceed the clotting time. In addition, a preocclusive lesion may cause a standing column in the proximal carotid artery and the introduction of contrast material may prompt thrombus formation.

Arch Aortography

After the femoral sheath is placed, the guidewire is advanced to a location where the floppy tip is at or beyond the intended location of the catheter head in the ascending aorta. The guidewire is pinned and the pigtail catheter is advanced into the ascending aorta. Avoid placing the guidewire in the left ventricle or into the coronary arteries. The image intensifier is rotated into the left anterior oblique (LAO) projection to a position in which the arc of the catheter-guidewire is as broad as possible, usually 30° to 45°. The guidewire is left in place in the flush catheter to help visualize the arc of the catheter until the optimal LAO position is obtained. A marker pigtail catheter with centimeter markers may also be used, and as the image intensifier rotates into the optimal position, the markers appear to become equidistant under fluoroscopy. There is further discussion about this maneuver in Chapter 2 (also see Figs. 4 and 5 of Chapter 2). Catheter placement for arch aortography is based upon fluoroscopically visible landmarks. Arch aortography is performed with the catheter head in the ascending aorta, well distal to the coronary ostia but proximal to the innominate artery. The arc shape of the catheter and the cardiac and mediastinal silhouette are used to position the head of the pigtail catheter. Following removal of the guidewire, the catheter head takes its preformed shape and the catheter shaft conforms somewhat to the general shape of the arch. If the arch is elongated, as in the example in Fig. 1B, the origin of the innominate may be fairly proximally located along the upslope of the arch in segment III. The course of the catheter shaft after guidewire removal usually reveals this less favorable arch shape prior to performing arch aortography. In this case, the pigtail may be advanced slightly before performing the arch aortogram to be sure to include the innominate artery in the contrast flow. If the pigtail catheter shaft takes a more evenly curved upside "u" shape, the catheter head does not need to be so close to the aortic valve since the innominate artery usually originates in segment II. The pigtail catheter is flushed with heparin–saline solution. The catheter is permitted to backbleed momentarily while the sterile tubing of the automated power injector is purged. After the air bubbles are removed from the system, the catheter is connected to the sterile tubing. The catheter is again aspirated through the power injector to check the system for microbubbles.

The catheter crossing the arch provides a marker for the inferior aspect of the field of view. A 12- or 14-in. field of view is usually adequate to evaluate from the proximal ascending aorta to beyond the carotid artery bifurcations. This field of view assists in selective catheterization. The arch aortogram demonstrates the location of the branch origins. The approximate location of the bifurcation on the upper part of the field of view will provide a guide for guidewire placement ahead of the advancing selective catheter during selective catheterization. The patient is asked to breath hold during image acquisition. Contrast injection is usually 15 for 30 (15 mL/sec for 2 consecutive seconds) or 20 for 40 (20 mL/sec for 2 sec). Table 5 provides a list of arteriographic

Table 5 Arteriographic Sequences for Arch Aortography and Carotid Arteriography: Contrast Administration and Image Acquisition

Arteriogram	Catheter head placement	Contrast administration			Image acquisition per second	Pressure (PSI)	Rate of rise
		Rate	Volume (ml)	Time (sec)			
Arch aortogram	Ascending aorta	15 for 30	30	2	4 to 8	1200	0
		20 for 40	40	2	4 to 8	1200	0
Innominate arteriogram	Innominate artery	6 for 18	18	3	4 to 8	600	0.2
		8 for 24	24	3	4 to 8	600	0.2
Carotid arteriogram	Proximal common carotid artery	4 for 8	8	2	4	300–500	0.2–0.5
		3 for 9	9	3	4	300–500	0.2–0.5
		4 for 12	12	3	4	300–500	0.2–0.5
Cerebral arteriogram	Proximal common carotid artery	3 for 12	12	3	8	300–500	0.2–0.5
		4 for 12	12	4	8	300–500	0.2–0.5
	Proximal internal carotid artery	3 for 6	6	2	8	250	0.5

sequences for arch aortography and carotid arteriography. Image acquisition is variable, but a common sequence would be 4 to 8 images per second for 4 to 6 sec or until contrast washes out. The LAO projection of the arch is used to establish the landmarks required for selective catheterization of the aortic arch branches.

Assessing the Aortic Arch

The aortic arch is assessed using the "surf and turf" classification as described in Chapter 2. The arch is bisected with a vertical line. A horizontal line is drawn across the upper inner aspect of the peak of the arch (Fig. 1 of Chapter 2). Segments I, II, and III represent increasing levels of challenge to catheterization and therefore dictate catheter choices. This approach assists in choosing a selective cerebral catheter that is well suited for catheterization of the aortic arch branches. Table 6 offers suggestions for cerebral catheter choices based upon arch segment classification. More detail about this is presented in the next two sections.

Selective Cerebral Catheters

Selective catheters have no side holes, only an end hole for passing the guidewire and administering contrast. There are dozens of catheter shapes used for cerebral arteriography, but they can generally be divided into simple curve and complex curve catheters (Fig. 3). Examples of simple curve and complex curve catheters we use commonly are listed in Table 4 and are shown in Fig. 4. Most surgeons have a couple of favorite choices in each of these two catheter-type categories and use these few catheters for most of the cases.

Table 6 Choosing a Cerebral Catheter Based Upon the Arch Configuration

	Selective Catheter Choices for Carotid Arteriography			
	Segment I	Segment IIa	Segment IIb	Segment III
First Choice	Angled taper glide-cath	Angled taper glide-cath	H1 Headhunter	JB2
Second Choice	H1 Headhunter	H1 Headhunter	JB2	Simmons 1or 2
Third Choice	JB2	JB2	Simmons 1 or 2	Vitek

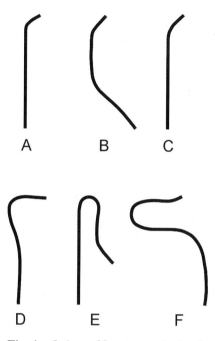

Fig. 4 Quiver of favorite cerebral catheters. Some of our favorite simple curve and complex curve catheters are included here. Simple curve (A) Angled taper Glidecath (MediTech). (B) H1 Headhunter. (C) Vertebral. Complex curve (D) JB2. (E) Simmons 2. (F) Vitek (Cook).

The simple curve catheter has a bend, or primary curve, near its tip that permits the guidewire to be directed into the side branch. A simple curve catheter is used to catheterize the carotid artery by passing the tip of the catheter proximal to the branch of interest, and then withdrawing the catheter as its tip is rotated superiorly into the origin of the artery (Fig. 5). The advantage of simple curve catheters is that they do not require reshaping of the head and their use is fairly straightforward. The disadvantage of simple curve catheters is that they are not shaped for working on segment III arteries.

Complex curve catheters have a minimum of two curves, a primary curve near its tip and a secondary curve more proximally along the catheter. In the case of the Simmons catheter, a commonly used complex curve catheter, the secondary curve, or elbow, forms a turn of approximately 180° (Fig. 3). This secondary turn of the catheter back on itself redirects the tip of the catheter in the opposite trajectory. This is the curve that must be reformed in the artery after the guidewire is removed in order for the catheter head to take its shape. A complex curve catheter may be reformed in the ascending aorta by bouncing the guidewire off the aortic valve or by using the subclavian artery to reform the elbow of the catheter before advancing it into the arch (Figs. 6 and 7). Because of this reverse curve, the catheter tip behaves differently than other catheter types. After the catheter is placed in the artery, if the catheter is advanced into the patient, the tip of a complex curve catheter comes out of the carotid artery and prolapses into the ascending aorta since the catheter tends to bend or reform at the secondary

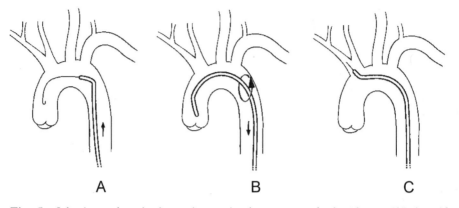

Fig. 5 Selective catheterization using a simple curve cerebral catheter. (A) A guidewire is introduced into the ascending aorta and a simple curve catheter is passed over it. (B) The guidewire is withdrawn into the catheter, allowing the catheter head to take its shape. The catheter is withdrawn and rotated. (C) The tip of the catheter enters the arch branch and the guidewire is advanced. (From Schneider PA. Endovascular Skills. New York: Marcel Dekker, 2003:93.)

curve (Fig. 8). If the catheter is withdrawn from the patient, the catheter tip distal to the secondary curve straightens and the catheter tip advances into the artery. This configuration is well suited to catheterization of branch arteries that originate in segment III, since the shaft of the catheter follows the arc of the aortic arch in one direction and the elbow or secondary curve allows the tip of the catheter to come back on itself and into the acutely angled origin of the segment III branch (Fig. 9). The primary curve at the catheter tip then points superiorly. The Simmons 1, 2, and 3 catheters are distinguished by the varying lengths of catheter extending beyond the secondary curve.

The tremendous utility of the complex curve catheter is that it can be used to catheterize vessels that are anatomically configured to be impossible for catheters with a simple curve. The disadvantages of complex curve catheters are twofold: (1) The catheter head must be reformed or reshaped. This is an extra maneuver; it requires a segment of aorta large enough to do it, and opportunities for embolization from a diseased arch are increased by both guidewire and catheter manipulation. (2) Since the secondary curve attempts to maintain its shape, the catheter does not easily track over the guidewire further into the branch artery. For routine carotid arteriography, this is not usually a problem since the arteriogram can be performed adequately with the tip of the complex curve catheter in the origin of the common carotid artery and the elbow of the complex curve catheter making the turn into the arch. However, when carotid stent placement is the goal, the selective cerebral catheter must be advanced into the external carotid artery to place the anchoring exchange guidewire. Advancing a complex curve catheter into the carotid artery requires that a significant length of guidewire be advanced, usually past the carotid bifurcation. For the complex curve catheter to follow the guidewire into the external carotid artery, the elbow or secondary curve must become almost straight. Since the complex curve is used in situations where the angle of

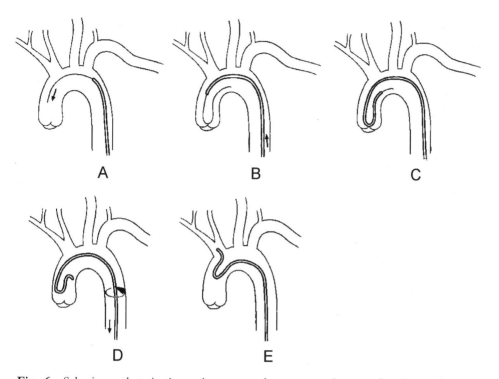

Fig. 6 Selective catheterization using a complex curve catheter: reforming a Simmons catheter in the ascending aorta. (A) A guidewire is introduced into the ascending aorta and a complex curve catheter is passed over it. (B) The guidewire is bounced off the aortic valve and back on itself into the arch. The catheter is advanced into the ascending aorta. (C) The catheter follows the guidewire antegrade into the aortic arch. (D) The guidewire is removed and the catheter head has reformed in the ascending aorta. The catheter is withdrawn and rotated. (E) The tip of the catheter engages the origin of the arch as the tip spins superiorly. (From: Schneider PA. Endovascular Skills. New York: Marcel Dekker, 2003:94.)

origin of the artery is fairly acute, such as segment III arteries, it may not be possible to straighten the elbow enough to permit the catheter to follow the guidewire. Therefore, during carotid stent placement, if a complex curve catheter is required to cannulate the common carotid artery, many operators will exchange the complex curve catheter for a simple curve, rather than attempt to advance the complex curve catheter.

When a vessel origin is cannulated with the tip of a selective catheter, the guidewire is advanced for at least a short distance so that the catheter may be advanced a few centimeters into the branch. This maneuver helps to secure the catheter so that it does not pop out during the recoil associated with high-pressure contrast administration. In this position, contrast may be administered into the branch vessel without losing contrast into the aortic arch through side holes. The tip of the selective catheter must be free of the artery wall and distant from unstable lesions prior to any pressure injection, since the only outlet for the contrast is the end hole and any jet effect may cause damage.

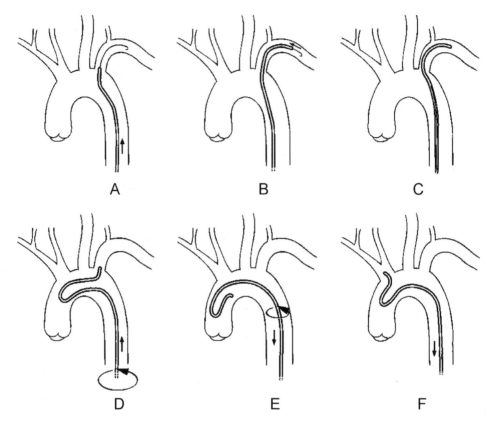

Fig. 7 Selective catheterization using a complex curve catheter: reforming a Simmons catheter in the subclavian artery. (A) A simple curve catheter is placed in the subclavian artery and exchanged for a complex curve catheter. (B) As the guidewire is withdrawn, the catheter head begins to take its curved shape. (C) The guidewire tip is withdrawn until it is just proximal to the secondary curve or elbow of the catheter. (D) Forward pressure on the catheter permits the head of the catheter to reform in the aortic arch. After reforming, the catheter is rotated and advanced into the ascending aorta. (E) The catheter is withdrawn and rotated to engage the arch branches. (F) After the tip of the catheter is in the artery, slight traction on the catheter helps to straighten the tip. (From Schneider PA. Endovascular Skills. New York: Marcel Dekker, 2003:95.)

It is usually best to puff contrast by hand into the catheter to check its position before connecting to the pressure injector.

Selective Catheterization of Aortic Arch Branches with Simple Curve Catheters

After the LAO arch aortogram is performed, the image intensifier and the table are kept stationary. The anatomy, configuration, and lumenal contour of the arch are evaluated. A selective cerebral catheter is chosen and exchanged for the pigtail over a long Glidewire

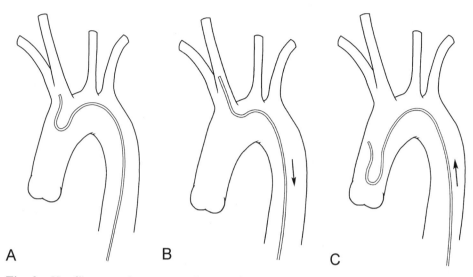

Fig. 8 Handling complex curve catheters. (A) The Simmons catheter is placed in the innominate artery. (B) Traction on the catheter tends to straighten the secondary curve or elbow of the catheter. This prompts the catheter tip to extend further into the artery. (C) Pushing on the catheter causes it to prolapse into the ascending aorta.

(Terumo, Medi-Tech). The selective catheter choice is based upon the shape of the arch and the segment of the arch from which the artery intended for catheterization originates. Although some operators choose to use complex curve catheters for most selective carotid arteriography, this approach is labor-intensive and is rarely required. Arch branches originating in segments I and II can almost always be cannulated with a simple curve catheter. Segment III arteries are more challenging since the catheter work is performed over the fulcrum of the peak of the inside wall of the aortic arch. A simple

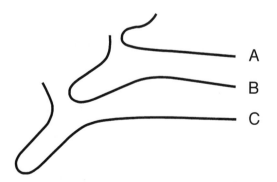

Fig. 9 Comparison of Simmons catheters. These catheters vary by the length of catheter from the secondary curve to the tip. (A) Simmons 1. (B) Simmons 2. (C) Simmons 3. The longer distance from secondary curve to catheter tip, as in Simmons 3, has a larger catheter head that must be reshaped. After catheter placement in the artery origin, the longer catheter tip extends farther into the artery.

curve catheter may be used to attempt to cannulate a segment III vessel, but if it does not go easily, switch soon to a complex curve catheter. There is more information about choosing a selective cerebral catheter in the sections that follow and in Table 6. When diffuse or shaggy disease is present in the roof of the aortic arch or there is occlusive or aneurysmal disease in the origins of the branches, selective catheterization of the arch branches may be contraindicated.

The approximate location of the vessel origin for cannulation is identified using bony landmarks (Fig. 10). For example, the position of the origin of the innominate artery may be juxtaposed in the LAO projection to the location of the head of the right clavicle. After the selective catheter is advanced into the ascending aorta, the guidewire is withdrawn into the shaft of the catheter and the catheter tip takes its shape. The simple curve catheter is rotated and withdrawn slightly so that its tip approaches the origin of the arch branch vessel (Fig. 5). The tip of the catheter is visualized using fluoroscopy and magnified views. The tip of the selective catheter tends to demonstrate a perceptible jump into the origin of the artery. A clockwise rotation of the catheter seems to work best to enter the innominate artery. When moving from the innominate artery to the left common carotid artery, a counterclockwise turn is usually best since the left common carotid artery origin is slightly posterior to the innominate origin.

After the catheter engages the artery origin, it is usually best to adjust the catheter tip slightly to secure it in the artery. This usually involves slight continued rotation and advancing the catheter a few millimeters. An angled tip, steerable Glidewire, 0.035 in and 180 cm or 260 cm long, usually sits somewhere in the shaft of the catheter during catheterization and is then advanced beyond the catheter tip. As the guidewire approaches the catheter tip, the catheter head will change shape, sometimes enough to push the catheter head out of the artery. Guidewire advancement through this segment should be performed steadily but slowly. If the guidewire tip hits the wall of the artery without making the full turn superiorly, continued forward pressure on the guidewire will cause the catheter to buckle and pop inferiorly into the arch. The guidewire should not be advanced far enough so that it encounters the carotid bifurcation or the carotid stenosis. Refer back to the LAO arch aortogram to estimate the approximate location of the carotid bifurcation. After the guidewire has been advanced into the artery, advance the catheter with steady but gentle forward pressure.

There are several factors that affect catheter trackability over the guidewire in this location. (1) The distance between the operator's hand and the head of the catheter is relatively long. (2) The length of guidewire permitted to extend beyond the catheter tip into the branch artery is relatively short. (3) The angle of origin of the arch branch may be fairly acute, that is, a tight turn for the catheter to pass further into the common carotid artery. (4) The pathway from groin to arch may be somewhat tortuous, creating some redundancy in the catheter length along this area. These factors set up a situation where the catheter may not track the guidewire immediately, but with increasing forward pressure will suddenly jump forward into the artery (Fig. 11). Vigilant guidewire control must be maintained since redundancy in the guidewire tends to gather and lurch forward

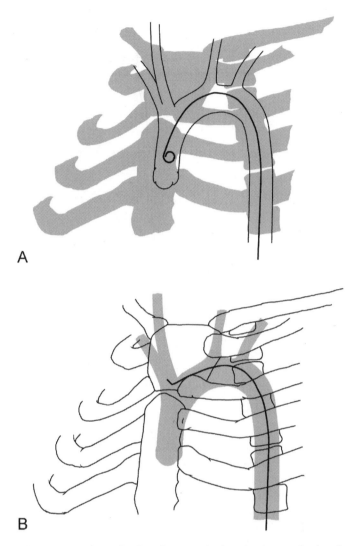

Fig. 10 Use bony landmarks to assist in selective cerebral catheterization. (A) The arch of the aorta and its branches are viewed through the framework of the bones of the thorax. These relationships change based upon the obliquity of the view. (B) The innominate artery is catheterized using these landmarks as a guide. Sternal wires and other foreign bodies may also be used when present.

as well. The operator must be ready, not just to pin the guidewire, but to also quickly pull the guidewire back if necessary. The catheter may also prolapse forward into the proximal aortic arch instead of following the guidewire around a sharp turn into the branch. The catheter may pull the guidewire out of the branch if it is pushed forward while it is not tracking the guidewire. When applying forward pressure on the catheter shaft to get the catheter to follow the guidewire, observe the catheter head carefully for

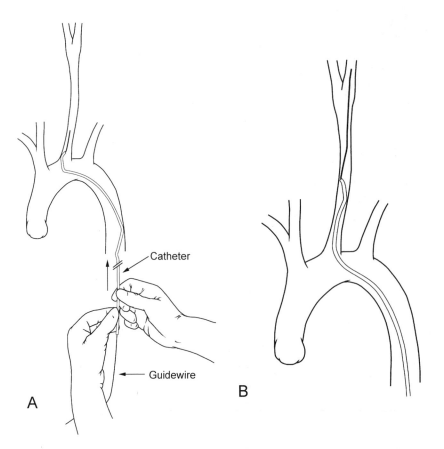

Fig. 11 The advancing selective cerebral tends to jump forward when advancing into the branch artery. (A) After catheterizing the origin of the common carotid artery and passing a guidewire, forward pressure is applied to the catheter. There is usually some redundancy along the course of the catheter, and forward pressure when the catheter head is not advancing tends to create more redundancy. (B) Continued pressure on the catheter to advance sometimes makes the catheter jump forward by suddenly straightening itself. The guidewire may also advance suddenly with the catheter.

signs that it is tracking the guidewire. If not, release pressure and consider the following maneuvers. If the guidewire can be advanced a few more centimeters, this will help to make the superior turn on a more solid segment of guidewire. If the carotid artery is tortuous or if it is a bovine configuration, it may be helpful to turn the patient's head to one side or the other to make the angle of entry into the artery less acute (Fig. 12). Having the patient take a deep breath and hold it for a few seconds may also improve the angle of curvature that the catheter must pass (Fig. 12).

When cannulation of the innominate artery is performed, it is usually clear by observing the catheter tip. It is a large artery and the catheter tip usually enters it with a noticeable jump. Often the guidewire advances directly into the common carotid artery. However, the innominate artery may be short or tortuous and the guidewire may prefer

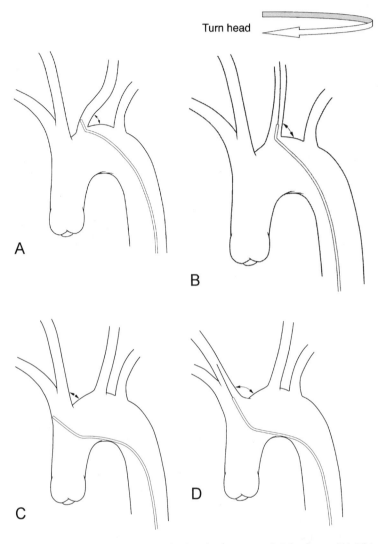

Fig. 12 Passing selective cerebral catheters around tight turns. (A) This shows a patient with a bovine arch configuration. In order to catheterize the left common carotid artery, the catheter must pass a sharp turn from the patient's right to the patient's left. (B) This turn to the patient's left can be made less acute if the patient's head is turned to the right. (C) The catheter must pass over the fulcrum of the aortic arch, then turn sharply into the origin of the innominate artery. (D) Having the patient take a deep breath and hold it momentarily will depress the arch and alter the angle of takeoff of the artery. This new angle often makes the turn into the artery less acute.

to go into the subclavian artery instead of the right common carotid artery. One option in this situation is to steer the guidewire into the proximal right subclavian artery. The catheter is advanced over the guidewire and into the right subclavian artery. Cannulation of the right common carotid artery is performed by withdrawing the guidewire into the catheter head and slowly pulling the catheter into the innominate artery. There is usually a small but perceptible jump inferiorly by the catheter tip as it is withdrawn from the origin of the right subclavian artery. The catheter head is rotated medially and anteriorly and the steerable guidewire is advanced into the right common carotid artery. The catheter is passed over the guidewire and into the right common carotid artery. Another option is to remove the guidewire and slowly withdraw the catheter. This must be done slowly since the catheter has very little internal support without the guidewire. Contrast is puffed by hand, and as the catheter tip approaches the innominate artery bifurcation, contrast will reflux into the right common carotid artery. The innominate artery bifurcation can then be road-mapped. A right anterior oblique projection of the image intensifier is often best.

The left common carotid artery usually originates in segments I or II of the arch and is generally simpler than the innominate artery. Bony landmarks and the LAO arch aortogram are used as a guide. The tip of the catheter is rotated superiorly. When the catheter tip extends superior to the arch profile, it is adjusted slightly and the guidewire is advanced. The distance along the aortic arch from the origin of one branch to the next may be short and it is occasionally a challenge to recognize which vessel has been entered. If there is any doubt, it is best to advance the guidewire a few centimeters, advance the catheter into the branch, remove the guidewire and puff contrast to identify the artery. When moving from one artery to the next, if they are very close together, the catheter sometimes tries to skip by the artery origin. The catheter is placed so that its tip is just proximal to the artery intended for catheterization. The catheter is withdrawn slightly and rotated. When the catheter tip pops into the artery, the guidewire is advanced using the same principles as outlined above.

Whenever a catheter is placed into the common carotid artery, be aware of anatomic landmarks that indicate that the catheter location so it is not permitted to advance too close to the bifurcation. After placement of the selective catheter in the common carotid artery, a few milliliters of contrast are puffed to check the position of the catheter tip before pressure injection is performed. The innominate artery, left common carotid artery, and left subclavian artery are cannulated in this manner when a simple curve catheter is used.

The simple curve catheters we use most commonly are shown in Fig. 4. They are the angled taper Glidecath, the H1 Headhunter, and the vertebral catheters. Each of these can be obtained in calibers of 4 or 5 Fr and lengths of 100 or 120 to 125 cm. These catheters are more similar to each other than they are different and most of their usage is based upon personal preference. There are multiple simple curve catheters from which to choose. The angled Glidecath has a hydrophilic coating and is very flexible. The shaft is straight and there is a short bend at the tip of approximately 45°. The angled portion of the tip is a centimeter in length. The advantage of this catheter is that it is atraumatic.

After cannulating the artery, it can usually be safely adjusted and even advanced for a very short distance without the guidewire. The disadvantage is that it is so flexible that passing the guidewire toward the catheter tip will often straighten the catheter tip enough so that its angle is gone and it comes out of the artery into which it has just been placed. Its surface is slick and its shaft lacks firmness; after the catheter is well inside the artery, passing a stiff guidewire may drag the catheter out of the artery. The shafts of the H1 and vertebral catheters are stiffer. The H1 catheter shaft has a long gentle curve followed by two bends. The working end of the catheter resembles a Satinsky clamp shape. The bend at the tip is similar to that of a Glidecath. Passing a guidewire through the tip of the H1 is less likely to completely straighten the catheter tip. The vertebral catheter has a straight shaft and a slightly stiffer tip.

Selective Catheterization of Aortic Arch Branches with Complex Curve Catheters

The complex-curve-shaped catheters may be used to cannulate any of the branch vessels but are most useful when the angle of origin of the arch branch is acute and the peak of the arch forms a fulcrum, as is the case in segment III. This occurs with some frequency in catheterization of the innominate artery. The double curvature of the catheter head gives these catheters a width that must be achieved prior to approaching the vessel by reforming or reshaping the catheter head. The catheter may reformed in the ascending aorta (Fig. 6) or the proximal descending aorta (Fig. 7).

In the ascending aorta, the guidewire is advanced and it bounces off the aortic valve and passes back down the arch. The catheter is advanced over the guidewire so that the elbow of the catheter, in this case a Simmons, is located in the ascending aorta just distal to the aortic valve (Fig. 6). The guidewire is withdrawn and the catheter is advanced slightly, permitting the catheter head to take its shape by assuming its full curvature at the secondary curve or elbow. The catheter is simultaneously withdrawn and rotated so that its tip lands inside the branch vessel origin. Aortic arch disease is a contraindication to this maneuver. The catheter tip is visualized using fluoroscopy as it engages the roof of the arch. The catheter tip usually pops into the vessel origin. If it does not, it can be dragged, tip up, along the arch until the branch artery is cannulated. Sometimes a slight clockwise angle is required to catheterize the innominate artery. After the tip enters the artery, it is usually best to adjust the catheter slightly. The catheter is observed using a smaller field of fluoroscopy. A slight pull on the catheter usually helps to secure it in the origin of the artery. The guidewire is advanced into the artery. Gently withdrawing the catheter removes some of its redundancy within the aortic arch and the catheter tip tends to advance further into the selected artery as the portion of the catheter distal to the elbow straightens out (Fig. 8). If the catheter is pushed slightly, it reforms by bending at the elbow and the catheter head prolapses into the ascending aorta. If the catheter is pushed too far, it will pull the catheter tip and the guidewire out of the artery. After cannulating the branch artery with a complex curve catheter, the selective carotid arteriogram can usually be performed with the catheter in that position. However, it is usually best to seed the catheter well. This is done by advancing the guidewire into the artery, removing redundancy from along the shaft of the catheter and adjusting the catheter position so that the secondary curve or elbow is wide open and hugging the inside curve of the artery as it comes off the arch.

If the catheter must be advanced further into the artery, it will require advancement on a stiff portion of guidewire. A lengthy segment of guidewire should be placed and may need to extend into the external carotid artery. A stiffer guidewire may also be used to help straighten the secondary curve of the catheter. The maneuvers discussed above may be particularly useful: having the patient hold a deep breath, turn the head, or cough may alter the conditions enough to permit catheter passage. A simpler approach may be to place the guidewire and exchange the complex curve catheter for a simple curve catheter that can be advanced more easily into the distal segment of the branch artery.

The Simmons type of complex curve catheter may also be reformed in the proximal descending aorta by using the subclavian artery (Fig. 7). The guidewire is directed into the left subclavian artery, usually with a simple curve catheter. The complex curve catheter is placed over the guidewire. The elbow of the complex curve catheter is placed in the origin of the subclavian artery. The guidewire is withdrawn enough to permit the elbow to begin to form. The catheter is advanced and rotated and the head is reformed as it passes proximally into the arch. The complex curve catheter is passed, tip down, into the ascending aorta. The catheter almost always tends to turn that way on its own. The catheter is then withdrawn and rotated, tip up, into the arch branch, as described above. The catheter is adjusted, usually with slight traction, to get it seeded well into the origin of the selected branch. Another option is to reform the catheter in the left subclavian artery and then advance the catheter with the tip up. This maneuver works well with the Vitek (Cook) catheter. The length of guidewire in the Vitek catheter head will also change its shape.

One of the challenging arch configurations that must be negotiated is the bovine arch, which is present in up to 27% of patients (Fig. 13) (3). This may take the form of a common trunk between the innominate artery and the left common carotid artery or the left common carotid artery may originate as a separate branch from the innominate artery. A JB2 catheter is particularly useful for this situation. The catheter is placed in the ascending aorta, then withdrawn with the tip pointed superiorly or angled anteriorly. If it is a common trunk or if a Simmons catheter is used, it is often best to rotate the catheter tip even more anteriorly. Another option is to place the catheter tip in the innominate artery, or even the right subclavian artery, then pull the catheter back while puffing contrast. The innominate and left common carotid artery can be roadmapped. The catheter tip is rotated into the left common carotid artery and the guidewire is advanced.

The complex curve catheters we use most commonly are shown in Fig. 4. They are the JB2, Simmons, and Vitek catheters. Each of these should be available in 5 Fr caliber and a 100-cm length. The Simmons catheters may be obtained in 4 Fr and the Vitek catheter can also be obtained in a 125-cm length. The JB2 catheter has a long,

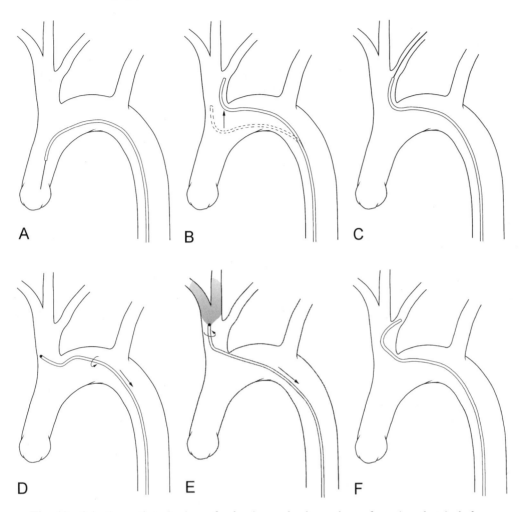

Fig. 13 Selective catheterization of a bovine arch. An arch configuration that includes a common trunk between the innominate artery and the left common carotid artery can be challenging. (A) The guidewire is passed into the ascending aorta and the selective cerebral catheter is passed over it. (B) The guidewire is withdrawn into the catheter. The JB2 catheter is steadily withdrawn with its tip up until it engages the artery. (C) The guidewire is advanced. (D) Another option is to rotate the catheter tip anteriorly to enter a common trunk. (E) An additional maneuver is to pass the catheter into the subclavian artery and road-map the innominate. The image intensifier is adjusted to achieve the optimal oblique view of the origin of the artery. The catheter is pulled back slowly and contrast is puffed until contrast refluxes into the left common carotid artery. (F) The catheter is rotated into the origin of the left common carotid artery.

gentle curve of its shaft and a hook-shaped tip. The Simmons catheters are doubly curved (Fig. 9). The Simmons 1 has a shorter tip and is simpler to reshape. The Simmons 2 and 3 have progressively longer tips and require more space to reshape. The longer the innominate artery, the more likely that a Simmons 3 catheter will be useful. The Vitek catheter is also doubly curved. It has a head about the size of a Simmons 1 catheter. The Vitek catheter tends to follow a guidewire into the carotid artery more readily than a Simmons catheter.

Choosing the Selective Cerebral Catheter

Whether using a simple or complex curve catheter, choosing the best catheter as the first choice will expedite the procedure and likely make it safer. In general, the simple curve catheter functions better for cannulation of the arch branches in segments I, IIa, and IIb. Segment III branches may be more challenging and often require reformed, complex curve catheters. Table 6 contains some general guidelines to assist in choosing a selective cerebral catheter. Different selective catheters may be required during the same case, since the innominate artery may originate in segment III while the left common carotid artery originates in segment I or II. The simplest shape is usually the best choice and most arch work, probably more than 90%, can be performed with simple curve catheters. However, for segment III arteries and occasionally for segment II, a complex curve catheter is required. Table 6 offers suggestions for first, second, and third choices, since it is frequently necessary to go to another choice if the initially selected catheter is not satisfactory. The authors advise that after a few attempts at cannulation, if the catheter does not pass, go on to another catheter.

Performing Selective Carotid Arteriography

After the selective cerebral catheter is advanced at least a few centimeters into the arch branch artery, the steerable guidewire is removed and the catheter is aspirated, assessed for microbubbles, and gently flushed with heparinized saline. Contrast is puffed into the artery to confirm correct positioning of the catheter tip. The catheter tip should not be placed into the sidewall of the artery or near a lesion. Power injection of contrast should not be performed until the position of the catheter is confirmed within the lumen of the origin of the branch artery. The catheter is aspirated, flushed with heparinized saline, and connected to the power injector tubing. The catheter is aspirated through the injector and the tubing is checked again for microbubbles. If contrast must be limited, a few milliliters of contrast may be infused with a simultaneous visual evaluation of the carotid bifurcation to help in choosing which projection is most likely to yield the best representation of the disease present. After beginning the study on one side, the protocol for lateral, anteroposterior, and oblique views is followed. When this is complete, the catheter is moved to the contralateral side. The protocol used by the authors is detailed below.

Carotid Arteriography Sequences

Some options for contrast injection rates and filming sequences are summarized in Table 5. When administering contrast through an end hole selective catheter, the rate of rise of pressure from the injector is adjusted to accommodate a smaller, lower flow artery. The rate of rise is set at 0.2 to 0.5 sec, indicating that the pressure will reach its maximum level over 0.2 to 0.5 sec from the start of the injection. Pressure in the injector may be set for 800 to 1200 psi for flush catheters as compared to 300 to 500 psi for selective catheters in cerebral arteries. Each catheter has a pressure limit stated on the package but these are rarely, if ever, approached. The lower pressure settings are meant to decrease the likelihood of artery damage or embolization from the contrast jet.

The administration of contrast into the innominate artery should be 5 to 8 mL/sec over 3 or 4 sec. An example sequence is 6 for 18, or 6 mL/sec for 3 sec. Image acquisition should be at 4 to 8 images per second until contrast washes out. Oblique views of the innominate artery, such as a right anterior oblique, are often required to open the innominate artery bifurcation to evaluate the origins of the right subclavian and right common carotid arteries. Injection into the common carotid artery is usually performed with 3 to 5 mL/sec over 2 or 3 sec. Example sequences include 4 for 8 (4 mL/sec for 2 sec), 3 for 9 (3 mL/sec for 3 sec) or 4 for 12 (4 mL/sec for 3 sec).

The rate and volume of contrast administration should be adjusted for the individual carotid anatomy. For example, if the preprocedure carotid duplex demonstrates an external carotid artery occlusion and a severe internal carotid artery stenosis, a lower rate and volume of contrast administration should be considered to evaluate the carotid bifurcation, such as 3 for 6. Delayed images of the bifurcation may reveal a standing column of contrast in the common carotid artery. To evaluate the intracranial circulation in the same patient, consider a longer injection, such as 3 for 12, to adequately opacify the distal internal carotid artery and its branches despite a flow restriction in the proximal artery. A lower rate may also be appropriate for a critical distal common carotid artery stenosis, but to fill the bifurcation distal the lesion, a longer injection may be useful (consider 3 for 9). If the rate and/or volume of contrast administration selected is too high, it could disrupt an unstable plaque. If it is too low, the images will not be complete and there will be flow streaming as the contrast mixes with unopacified blood as it passes through the artery of interest. In this case, the rate and/or volume is simply increased and the sequence repeated. Occasional situations are optimized with increased rate and volume of contrast administration. Any type of arteriovenous fistula to the internal or external carotid artery may dramatically increase flow. Likewise, contralateral to a carotid occlusion, flow rates are increased, and 5 for 10 or 5 for 15 may be required.

The carotid bifurcation is usually evaluated in the AP and lateral projections. Since the bifurcation and proximal internal carotid artery disease is worst along the posterior wall, additional oblique views are often required to demonstrate the most significant segment of the stenosis in profile (Fig. 14). During image acquisition the patient is coached to breath hold, stop swallowing, and to drop the shoulders and lengthen the neck.

Cerebral images are usually obtained with the selective catheter in the same place in the proximal common carotid artery. Anteroposterior and lateral views of the cerebral arteries are obtained. Images are acquired until contrast washes out of the venous phase. When highly selective intracerebral arteriography is required, the selective catheter is

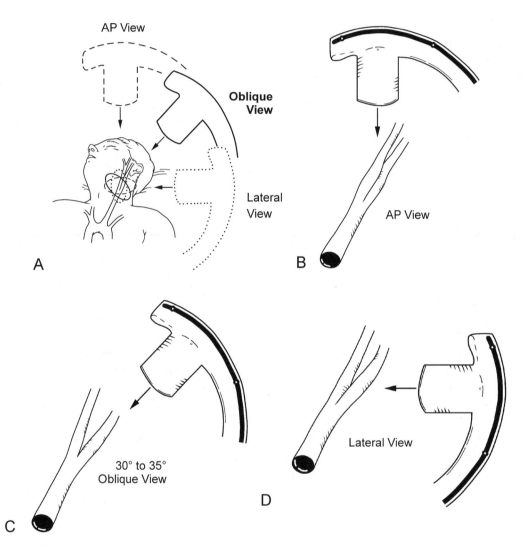

Fig. 14 Multiple obliques of the carotid bifurcation may be required. (A) The carotid artery is shown with its surrounding relationships. (B, C, D) The anteroposterior, oblique, and lateral views are presented, respectively, each demonstrating a different profile of the carotid bifurcation.

Table 7 Which Sequences Does a Carotid
Arteriogram Include?

Segment	Sequences
Arch aortogram (LAO)	1
Bilateral selective carotid arteriogram (AP, lateral, oblique of extracranial)	6
Bilateral cerebral runoff (AP, lateral)	4
Bilateral subclavian with vertebrals	2+

advanced into the proximal internal carotid artery. Without external carotid artery runoff, the amount of contrast injected may be less. Cerebral angiography is discussed in more detail in Chapter 5.

The sequences required to perform a complete carotid arteriogram are summarized in Table 7. In addition to the arch aortogram, each carotid artery is evaluated with an AP, lateral and oblique of the extracranial arteries, and an AP and lateral of the intracranial arteries. Occasionally, the extracranial or intracranial vasculature will require additional oblique views to fully define the anatomy. The posterior circulation may be evaluated on the arch study alone or specific selective catheterizations may be performed. This aspect of the procedure should be modified to suit the clinical situation. The proximal vertebral artery can usually be evaluated by contrast administration in the subclavian artery. Catheterization and contrast administration into the vertebral system should only be performed if there are specific indications. In addition, pressure should be decreased, rate of rise increased, and the patient should be well heparinized.

Protocol for Carotid and Cerebral Arteriography

There are several approaches to the order of events during carotid arteriography. Some surgeons start on the right side first since it is the most proximal arch branch, and often the most challenging. Another approach is to begin on whichever is the least diseased side. Some would advise starting on the most diseased side first and proceeding to the less diseased side with the idea that if problems develop, the procedure can be terminated with the most information available about the side in question. It probably does not matter. What matters is having a plan so that the procedure can progress in an orderly manner and that the information required is considered prior to the procedure. Included below is an example protocol for use during carotid arteriography.

1. Femoral access sheath.
2. Place starting guidewire into ascending aorta.
3. Advance pigtail catheter into ascending aorta.
4. Remove guidewire and flush catheter.
5. Connect to power injector.

6. Place image intensifier in left anterior oblique with widest arc.
7. Perform arch aortogram (15 for 30), mark origins of arch branches.
8. Assess arch, choose selective cerebral catheter.
9. Administer heparin.
10. Advance 0.035 steerable Glidewire, 180 or 260 cm, and remove pigtail.
11. Place 100-cm selective catheter into ascending aorta.
12. Simple curve catheter for segments I, IIa, IIb and complex curve for segment III.
13. Withdraw and rotate clockwise to enter innominate and advance guidewire.
14. Advance catheter into right common carotid artery.
15. Flush and connect to power injector.
16. Perform AP right carotid arteriogram (4 for 8, 0.5 rate of rise, 400 psi).
17. Perform AP right cerebral arteriogram (4 for 8, 0.5 rise, 10° craniocaudal).
18. Perform lateral right cerebral arteriogram (4 for 8, 0.5 rise).
19. Perform lateral right carotid arteriogram (4 for 8, 0.5 rise).
20. Perform oblique views of right carotid bifurcation as needed.
21. Withdraw selective catheter into the arch and place proximal to left common carotid artery (LCCA).
22. Rotate counterclockwise and withdraw to enter LCCA.
23. Advance catheter into left common carotid artery.
24. Repeat the sequence 16 through 20 for left carotid artery.
25. Selective either subclavian artery as needed.

Technical Tips for Carotid Arteriography

Table 8 includes technical tips that may assist the operator in planning and performing successful and uncomplicated carotid arteriography. A duplex evaluation of the carotid arteries prior to the arteriogram helps in several ways. It helps to plan the procedure since it provides information on the degree of stenosis. If there is a preocclusive lesion or other important findings, the pressure and volume of contrast administration can be adjusted accordingly. A duplex also helps the operator to plan ahead of time what the arteriogram should include. All the supplies should be assembled and multiple catheter choices available. Syringes are clearly labeled. Heparin administration may be of value in preventing thrombotic complications.

Using an access sheath helps catheter maneuverability by taking away a point of friction at the access site. It also makes catheter exchanges smoother. Each time the cerebral catheter is manipulated or flushed, there are potential sources of technical error that must be controlled. Catheters must be flushed every couple of minutes but a large volume of heparin–saline flush is not useful. Each time the catheter is flushed is another opportunity to create a problem. Bubbles must be prevented or meticulously removed from the system at every step. The catheter should be backbled before flushing. Guidewire removal should be steady and deliberate since whipping the guidewire creates suction and microbubbles in the catheter.

Table 8   Technical Tips for Carotid Arteriography

- Duplex prior to angiogram
- Clear bubbles from catheter
- Label syringes
- Use a sheath
- Administer heparin
- Don't pull guidewire too fast
- To help pass the catheter into the artery, consider;
  - Take a deep breath
  - Turn the patient's head
  - Cough
- Constant guidewire control is required
- Watch guidewire tip, prevent it from jumping forward
- If chosen selective catheter doesn't go, try another choice
- Backbleed catheter before flushing
- Puff contrast to confirm catheter position before performing pressure injection
- Adjust pressure and volume of contrast injection to the situation
- Don't flush too much
- Be specific about the information you need
- Keep it simple

Safe and effective selective catheter placement has its own nuances. Putting the patient through certain maneuvers, such as breath holding, head turning, or coughing, can help to pass a catheter that otherwise may not go. Vigilant guidewire control and careful observation of the catheter as pressure is applied to it also help to keep the patient out of trouble. Do not hesitate to exchange for another catheter if the first choice is not successful. This is where experience with a variety of catheters and an appropriate level of humility help to make the procedure successful. After the catheter is in place, its position should be confirmed with a puff of contrast before pressure injection.

Complications of Carotid Arteriography

Carotid arteriography may be complicated by access site, systemic, local arterial, or end organ complications (Table 9). End organ, or neurological complications, such as

Table 9   Complications of Carotid Arteriography

Access site	Systemic	Local arterial	Neurologic
Hematoma	Contract reaction	Dissection	TIA
Hemorrhage	Renal failure	Distal embolization	Stroke
Pseudoaneurysm	CHF		
AV fistula	MI		
Thrombosis			

transient ischemic attacks and stroke, are not common but are a major concern of all participating in carotid arteriography since they may be disabling or fatal. Carotid arteriography performed in patients with moderate to severe carotid stenosis produced a stroke rate of 1.0% to 1.2% (4,5). These carotid arteriograms were performed in approved institutions during the Asymptomatic Carotid Atherosclerosis Study (ACAS) and North American Symptomatic Carotid Endarterectomy Trial (NASCET) trials but were often more extensive than what may have been clinically necessary since multiple views and other maneuvers were required to fulfill the study requirements. In another study of cerebral arteriography for recent ischemic events due to all types of cerebral pathology, when all neurological deteriorations that occurred within 24 hr of arteriography were included, the periprocedural event rate was 5% (6). Risk factors for neurological events after carotid arteriography are listed in Table 10 (7).

The technique of carotid arteriography is designed to minimize the likelihood of stroke. Emboli to the brain during carotid arteriography may be comprised of thrombus, air bubbles, or atherosclerotic debris. Thrombus may be minimized by anticoagulation, judicious flushing of catheters, using only the contrast volume that is required for the study, and hydrating the patient adequately prior to the procedure. Thrombus may also be generated as a result of a local arterial dissection or lesion disruption. The guidewire should not be passed through a significant lesion or across a diseased carotid bifurcation unless it is necessary. The catheter tip location should be checked before high-pressure contrast administration is performed. The administration of air bubbles is a purely technical issue. The case should be kept as simple as possible. The more variables introduced, the more likely that unintended consequences will occur, such as cerebral air bubbles. Foster good communication with the support staff and be vigilant about checking every syringe and line for air. The embolization of atherosclerotic debris may occur with simple manipulation of the catheter tip. This

Table 10 Risk Factors for Stroke After Carotid Arteriography

Critical stenosis of carotid artery
Advanced age
Recent TIA or stroke
High-contrast volume
Lengthy procedure (>90 min)
Severe hypertension
Renal insufficiency or renal failure
Poorly controlled diabetes

Source: Modified from Morris P. Practical Neuroangiography. Philadelphia, PA: Lippincott, Williams & Wilkins, 1997:63.

problem can be minimized by picking the most functional catheter as the first choice for selective catheterization. Do not place the catheter tip too close to a significant atherosclerotic lesion and do not cross lesions that do not require crossing.

Access site and systemic complications are similar to those encountered with other types of arteriography. Access site complications, such as bleeding, ecchymosis, and pseudoaneurysm, are the most common complications. Systemic complications may include contrast reaction, exacerbation of congestive heart failure, renal failure, and others. Complications of carotid stent placement and their management are discussed in Chapter 19.

Completion Arteriography After Carotid Endarterectomy

Completion arteriography is a procedure with substantial value to any operator performing revascularization in any vascular bed. Completion arteriography is considered mandatory after any type of percutaneous revascularization. It provides a "last look" at the reconstruction and serves as (1) a point of reference for future care of the patient, (2) a quality control mechanism for the procedure, and (3) a method of assessing the quality of the reconstruction in the individual patient. The fact that many open vascular reconstructions have been performed in the past without standard completion assessments of some type does not mean that this approach is best for the patients. In fact, it is possible that we will take what we have learned in endovascular surgery, including better methods for imaging, and greatly expand our usage of completion arteriography after open surgery. There are two approaches for obtaining completion arteriography after carotid endarterectomy. One common method is to place a needle or small catheter into the proximal common carotid artery and perform an arteriogram of the immediate reconstruction and its runoff. Another option is to perform a transfemoral completion carotid arteriogram after carotid endarterectomy. The advantage of the transfemoral route is that an arch aortogram may be performed, along with selective catheterization of any area of the cerebral vasculature.

The femoral area is prepped at the beginning of the case. After carotid endarterectomy, a 5 Fr sheath is placed in the common femoral artery, and an arch aortogram is performed in the LAO projection. DSA using the portable fluoroscopy unit provides adequate imaging for this procedure. A power injector is required. Leads and cables must be moved out of the x-ray field. Occasionally, the arch aortogram clearly shows the endarterectomized segment and the operator may elect to conclude the arteriogram. When selective arteriography is required, the common carotid artery on the side of the endarterectomy is selectively catheterized. The catheter tip is maintained in the proximal common carotid artery and is not advanced near the endarterectomized segment. Projections of the carotid bifurcation and the intracranial runoff may be performed with the catheter in this position. Turning the patients head to the side may be helpful in obtaining the best views of the carotid bifurcation. Findings may include technical defects at the end points and along the endarterectomized surface, external carotid artery lesions, and arch or intracranial lesions. After images are evaluated, the catheter is removed and a sterile dressing is placed over the femoral sheath. The femoral sheath is removed later in the location where the patient is monitored postoperatively. Patients who are selected for surgery on the basis of duplex studies will not have had a previous arch aortogram or intracranial carotid arteriogram and these may be performed during the completion arteriogram.

Qualifications to Perform Carotid Arteriography

Privileges to perform carotid arteriography must be granted to the individual physician by the credentials committee of each hospital. Credentials committees consider many factors, including national standards, local practice patterns, the training and experience of the physician, and institutional and local politics. The physician must present qualifications to the committee and be able to demonstrate safe patient care. Privileges for carotid arteriography differ from those related to carotid angioplasty and stent placement since carotid arteriography is an established procedure. Some institutions have specific case number and even results requirements that must be fulfilled, while other hospitals might include carotid arteriography in combination with other types of arteriography as a general category. Most acute care hospitals include arteriography, at least as a general procedure type, somewhere in the list of commonly performed vascular procedures.

Carotid arteriography has been performed by vascular surgeons, neurosurgeons, neuroradiologists, general radiologists, vascular medicine specialists, interventional radiologists, interventional neuroradiologists, and others. The acknowledgment that many different specialties are involved in performing carotid arteriography is reflected in a guideline document for carotid arteriography, entitled "Quality Improvement Guidelines for Adult Diagnostic Neuroangiography" (8). This document was published jointly by the American Society of Interventional and Therapeutic Neuroradiology (ASITN), the American Society of Neuroradiology (ASNR), and the Society of Cardiovascular and Interventional Radiology (SCVIR, now SIR). These societies refer to the guideline paper as a credentialing instrument for cerebral angiography. No specific case numbers are required to achieve privileges or to maintain competence in carotid arteriography. This guidelines focus upon results: acceptability of indications for carotid arteriography; success rates in performing carotid arteriography; and complication rates, both neurological and non-neurological (Table 11). Vascular specialists are likely to agree with its principles: indications for carotid arteriography should be appropriate and the success of the procedure should be optimized while minimizing complications, and carotid arteriography is performed by multiple different specialties.

Carotid arteriography has never been the exclusive domain of any single discipline within medicine. The major societies, governing bodies, and institutions have in various

Table 11 Quality Improvement Guidelines for
Adult Diagnostic Neuroangiography

Threshold for appropriate indications:	99%[a]
Threshold for success of the case:	98%[b]
Threshold for complications:	
Permanent neurological deficit:	1.0%
Reversible neurological deficit	2.5%
Systemic complication	<1.0%
Puncture site/access complication	<1.0%

[a] Includes evaluation of extracranial cerebrovascular disease.
[b] Requisite information is obtained.
Source: Ref. 8.

ways acknowledged that many different specialties perform carotid arteriography. In addition, there are no published standards for the number of carotid arteriograms that must be performed during any fellowship or residency program to achieve competence in carotid arteriography. Fellowship requirements in interventional neuroradiology, for example, include a total of 100 cases and 12 months of training involving the treatment of brain aneurysms, AV malformations, tumors, intracranial vascular disease, trauma, and maxillofacial anomalies (9). Carotid arteriography would necessarily be required as part of most of these cases but there is no specific case requirement for carotid arteriography.

Carotid arteriography is a major conceptual and technical prerequisite to performing safe and effective carotid stent placement. The more experience one has with carotid arteriography, the more likely that the carotid stent learning curve will be shortened.

References

1. Amar AP, Larsen DW, Teitelbaum GP. Percutaneous carotid angioplasty and stenting with the use of gadolinium in lieu of iodinated contrast medium: technical case report and review of the literature. Neurosurgery 2001; 49:1265–1266.
2. Jacobs JM. Diagnostic neuroangiography: basic techniques. In: Osbourne A, ed. Diagnostic Cerebral Angiography. Philadelphia: Lippincott Williams & Wilkins, 1999:431–436.
3. Osbourne A. Aortic arch and great vessels. In: Osbourne A, ed. Diagnostic Cerebral Angiography. Philadelphia: Lippincott Williams & Wilkins, 1999:12–16.
4. Executive Committee for the Asymptomatic Carotid Atherosclerosis Study. Endarterectomy for asymptomatic carotid artery stenosis. JAMA 1995; 273:1421–1428.
5. North American Carotid Endarterectomy Trial Collaborators. Beneficial effect of carotid endarterectomy in symptomatic patients with high-grade stenosis. N Engl J Med 1991; 325:445–453.
6. Earnest F, Forbes G, Sandok BA, Piepgras DG, Faust RJ, Ilstrup DM, Amdt LJ. Com-

plications of cerebral angiography: prospective assessment of risk. Am J Radiol 1984; 142:247–253.

7. Morris P. Practical Neuroangiography. Philadelphia, PA: Lippincott, Williams & Wilkins, 1997:63.

8. Cooperative study between ASITN, ASNR, and SCVIR. Quality improvement guidelines for adult diagnostic neuroangiography. Am J Neuroradiol 2000; 21:146–150.

9. Higashida RT, Hopkins LN, Berenstein A, Hulback VV, Kerber C. Program requirements for residency/fellowship education in neuroendovascular surgery/interventional neuro-radiology: a special report on graduate medical education. Am J Neuroradiol 2000; 21:1153–1159.

5

Advanced Cerebrovascular Arteriography: Applications in Carotid Stenting

PETER A. SCHNEIDER

Hawaii Permanente Medical Group, Honolulu, Hawaii, U.S.A.

The purpose of this chapter is to provide addition detail about cerebral angiography as it applies to carotid stenting. This chapter focuses on four areas where increased knowledge will facilitate CAS. These include cerebral catheters, intracranial arteriography, managing intracranial pathology, and angiographic considerations for planning carotid stent placement.

More About Cerebral Catheters

The simple curve catheters have in common a single bend, or primary curve, at the tip (Chap. 4, Fig. 3). However, the length of the tip and the angle of the bend vary from one catheter to another. The simple curve catheters may have a straight shaft, such as the vertebral or the angled glide-cath, or the shaft may have a gentle curve such as an H1 or a JB1. These gentle curves along the shaft are meant to conform to aortic arch curvature. When the tip of the simple curve catheter is pointing superiorly, the shaft is passing from the patient's left to the patient's right as it ascends the aorta and crosses the aortic arch. After the catheter is seeded in the orifice of the innominate artery of left common carotid artery, the guidewire advancement tends to straighten the bend at the tip of the simple curve catheter and this sometimes makes the catheter pop out of the artery. Be prepared to probe the artery carefully and steer the guidewire into the artery.

Complex curve catheters have a primary and secondary curve and must be reshaped. The secondary curve redirects the tip in the opposite direction as the primary curve. Fig. 4 of Chap. 4 includes several complex curve catheters, such as the JB2, the Simmons, and the Vitek catheters. The JB2 has a long gentle curve along the shaft to conform to the curvature of the aortic arch and has a broad hook shape at the tip. The hook at the end is small enough that the catheter does not require much effort to reshape the head and it usually reshapes itself. This is an excellent catheter for use with a bovine arch (Chap. 4, Fig. 13).

The Simmons catheters (1, 2, and 3) vary with respect to the length of catheter distal to the secondary curve (Chap. 4, Fig. 9). The larger the catheter head, the more room is required to reshape the head. When the innominate artery is short, a Simmons 1 or 2 is used. The longer the innominate artery, the more likely that a Simmons 3 catheter will be useful. The length of catheter distal to the secondary curve is about twice as long in a Simmons 3 than in a Simmons 1. In Chap. 4, two different methods of reshaping a Simmons catheter are discussed (Figs. 6 and 7). Reshaping a Simmons catheter in the proximal descending aorta using the left subclavian artery may be safer since it avoids extra manipulations in the aortic arch. If a larger caliber and/or stiffer (6 Fr or nylon) Simmons catheter is used, the catheter can usually be reshaped in the proximal descending aorta without cannulating the left subclavian artery. After the guidewire is withdrawn, rotate the catheter 90–180° counterclockwise and advance the catheter. The tip usually catches the posterior aortic wall and the elbow forms as the shaft of the catheter is advanced. The catheter is then rotated so that the tip is pointed superiorly for catheterization of the arch branches.

The operator must get used to cannulation of the arch branches by either advancing the complex curve catheter from the descending aorta or withdrawing the catheter from the ascending aorta. Either approach to cannulation of the common carotid arteries may be used. One situation in which the advancement approach may be of value is in cannulating the left common carotid artery when the left common carotid artery and the innominate artery are very close together. In this case, the withdrawal technique tends to cause the catheter to jump from the innominate artery to the left subclavian artery, skipping over the left common carotid artery. In this case, try advancing the Simmons catheter or the Vitek catheter from the descending aorta. After the catheter head is reshaped, the catheter shaft is rotated so that the tip is pointing superiorly. As the catheter is advanced, the tip is rotated slightly anteriorly by rotating the catheter shaft counterclockwise. When the catheter tip is far enough across the arch to have gone past the left subclavian artery, the tip of the catheter is rotated clockwise so that it points superiorly and slightly posteriorly. The tip of the catheter usually catches the left common carotid artery.

The Simmons catheter may also be of value in cannulating the left common carotid artery when it originates from a bovine arch. To redirect the Simmons catheter tip into the left common carotid artery of a bovine arch, the following steps are required. (1) A Simmons catheter with a longer tip (Simmons 2 or 3) is required for a true bovine configuration (left common carotid artery originates from the innominate artery distal to its origin) since the tip of the catheter must reach from the arch, across the innominate artery, and far enough into the left common carotid artery so that it does not pop out. (2) The Simmons catheter is reshaped in the ascending or descending aorta and the innominate artery is catheterized (Chap. 4, Fig. 6). At this point, the tip of the catheter extends beyond the origin of the left common carotid artery in a bovine arch. (3) The catheter is rotated about 90° in the counterclockwise direction. The catheter is advanced slightly. This maneuver retracts the catheter tip slightly from the distal innominate artery and permits the tip of the catheter to be redirected. (4) The catheter is then withdrawn slightly and the tip is redirected into the left common carotid artery as the catheter is rotated clockwise, back to its original orientation.

The head of the Vitek catheter is very similar to that of the Simmons 1 catheter with an extra curve located proximal to the secondary curve. This "tertiary curve" creates a shape that is very well suited to cannulation of the arch branches by advancing the catheter from the proximal descending aorta (Fig. 1). Advancing the guidewire to the location of the secondary curve of the Vitek catheter makes it behave more like a Simmons catheter. The shape of the Vitek catheter is demonstrated in Fig. 4 of Chap. 4. A Vitek catheter is used to catheterize the great vessels in Fig. 4 of Chap. 11.

When a complex curve catheter is used for arteriography, the catheter is adjusted after the tip is used to catheterize the intended branch. By withdrawing the catheter a few millimeters, the secondary curve is fully open and hugging the origin of the artery. The complex curve cerebral catheter's appearance under fluoroscopy is similar to that of a hook-shaped catheter placed at the aortic flow divider when going up and over the aortic bifurcation. The maximum length of catheter distal to the secondary curve is unfolded in the common carotid artery. The arteriogram is usually performed from this position with little likelihood that the catheter will recoil so much that it will collapse into the arch with high-pressure administration of contrast. If the catheter must be advanced further into

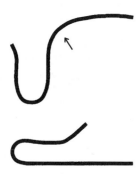

Fig. 1 Comparison of the Vitek catheter (top) and the Simmons catheter (bottom). The Vitek catheter has an extra curve.

the carotid artery, a significant length of guidewire must be advanced beyond the tip of the catheter, usually into the external carotid artery. The stiffer portion of the guidewire must pass through the secondary curve of the catheter. In order to advance the complex curve catheter, the secondary curve must be dislodged from the origin of the arch branch. After the secondary curve is straightened enough to advance the catheter, the advancement tends to flow more easily. Forward pressure on the catheter should be applied gently and persistently. When the catheter starts to advance, it may suddenly jump forward.

Most operators use 5-Fr catheters. These have a moderate amount of shaft strength. Some selective cerebral catheters can also be obtained that are 4 or 6 Fr. The smaller caliber 4-Fr catheters permit arteriography with a smaller caliber arteriotomy. Flow rates through the catheter are lower than 5-Fr catheters. These catheters are useful for patients with anatomically favorable arches, such as one may find with trauma patients. However, the shaft strength of the 4-Fr catheter is less and this makes the catheter less maneuverable. The responsiveness of the catheter head can be improved somewhat by placing the guidewire inside the catheter shaft during maneuvering. Larger 6-Fr catheters may also be used. They have higher flow rates and are easier to maneuver, even without a guidewire. However, they are also less gentle in encounters with the arterial wall and create a larger arteriotomy.

Most of the cerebral catheters are 100 cm in length. Some catheters are available in the 125-cm length; these include the angled glide-cath, H1, Simmons 2, and Vitek. When using the backloading method of carotid access for intervention, the longer cerebral catheter is required to catheterize the common carotid artery after the long carotid access sheath is placed in the arch. The disadvantage of the longer catheter is a little less control when manipulating the catheter head. In addition, guidewire length must also be adjusted accordingly to the longer catheter. Selective cerebral catheters are manufactured by numerous companies, an example of which is demonstrated in Fig. 2.

Intracranial Angiography

Carotid arteriography should include standard views of the intracranial arteries, such as anterior–posterior (AP) and lateral views. The AP and lateral views form the cornerstone of cerebral artery evaluation. Abnormalities or suspicious areas observed in these two views are usually investigated with additional maneuvers, including different views created by rotation of the image intensifier (side-to-side) or angulation (cranial or caudal), altering contrast injection technique or catheter position or the filming specifications.

The anterior–posterior view of the skull usually provides a good view of the distal portion of the internal carotid artery and the proximal segments of the anterior and

Fig. 2 Selective cerebral catheters. This is an example of one company's offerings in cerebral catheter shapes. There are other variable features, including caliber length, stiffness, radio-opacity of the shaft and tip, and construction material. (Courtesy of Cook, Inc.)

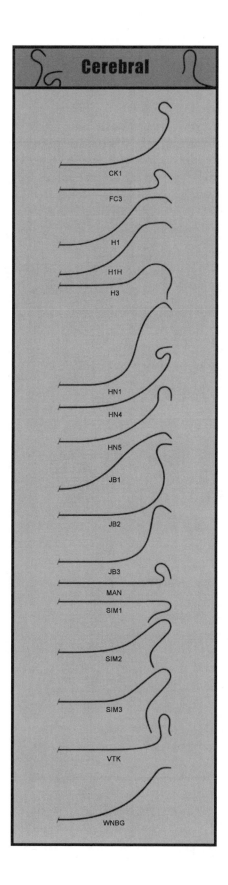

Cerebral

CK1

FC3

H1

H1H

H3

HN1

HN4

HN5

JB1

JB2

JB3

MAN

SIM1

SIM2

SIM3

VTK

WNBG

middle cerebral arteries. The skull is often evaluated with 5–10° of cranio-caudal angulation (Townes view). This maneuver superimposes the orbital rims upon the petrous ridges and improves the evaluation of the intracranial arteries by eliminating the usual subtraction artifact caused by the orbital rims (Fig. 3). Using fluoroscopy while angling the image intensifier demonstrates the best degree of cranio-caudal angulation as the impressions of the bones around the orbits and the skull base are superimposed. This usually provides the least obstructed view of the anterior cerebral and middle cerebral arteries (Fig. 4). The anterior–posterior projection is best for the middle cerebral artery (segments M1 through M4), the A1 segment of the anterior cerebral artery, the len-

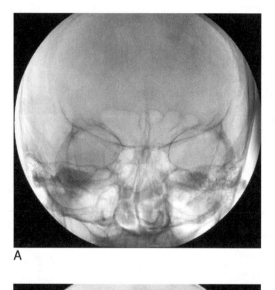

A

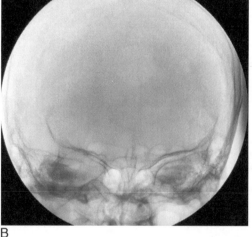

B

Fig. 3 AP versus Townes view. (A) In the AP view, the orbital rims project at a level superior to the petrous ridges. (B) By angulating the image intensifier into the cranio-caudal position, the orbital rims are superimposed upon the petrous ridges.

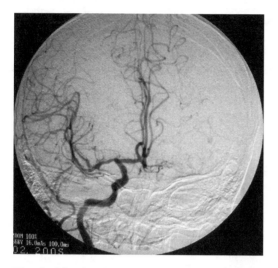

Fig. 4 The distal internal carotid artery, its bifurcation, and the proximal anterior and middle cerebral arteries are observed with less bony obstruction in the Townes view (cranio-caudal angulation).

ticulostriate branches from the M1 and sometimes A1 segments, and the anterior-communicating artery. The anterior–posterior view of the skull is usually performed with a 9- or 12-in. field of view. An effort is made to fill the entire field of view with skull so that the dispersion of the x-ray beam is uniform in distribution.

A lateral view of the skull is achieved by superimposing the auditory canals using fluoroscopy. The lateral view of the intracranial circulation is best for the anterior cerebral artery distal to the A1 segment, the distal internal carotid artery, the ophthalmic artery, and the posterior cerebral artery if there is flow from anterior to posterior (Fig. 5). The lateral view of the skull is performed with a 9- or 12-in. field of view. The distance between the image intensifier and the skull is adjusted to fill the field of view with bone. Placing the image intensifier close to the skull reduces scatter.

The AP and Townes views tend to superimpose the supraclinoid and horizontal portions of the internal carotid artery. The lateral view of the distal internal carotid artery usually demonstrates the siphon well but will not delineate the internal carotid artery bifurcation. If there is disease suspected in the distal internal carotid artery that requires further evaluation, a 15–45° oblique is useful to help "unfold" the multiple curves of the carotid siphon and demonstrate the internal carotid artery bifurcation (transorbital oblique, Fig. 6). The cavernous internal carotid artery may also be interrogated using a paraorbital oblique (55° oblique). An anterior–posterior projection with caudo-cranial angulation (Caldwell view) also provides information about the distal internal carotid artery and will permit its various curves to be separated (Fig. 7). Further caudo-cranial angulation (Waters view) places the petrous ridges in the inferior part of the field of view. This approach is useful for evaluation of siphon aneurysms or basilar artery aneurysms, especially when combined with side-to-side rotation of the image intensifier. In patients

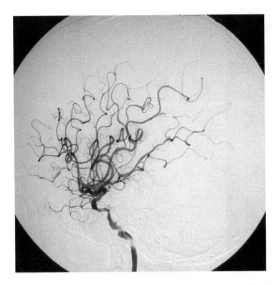

Fig. 5 The lateral cerebral arteriogram is useful for a profile view of the intracranial internal carotid artery, the anterior cerebral artery distal to the A1 segment, and the major middle cerebral artery branches. In this case, there is a critical bifurcation stenosis and severe intracranial internal carotid artery disease. The anterior cerebral artery is not seen because it fills from the contralateral side.

with substantial cross-filling to the contralateral hemisphere through a patent anterior communication artery, the bilateral anterior cerebral arteries will be superimposed in the lateral projection. An oblique is useful in this situation.

Standard views of the vertebral arteries also include the AP and lateral. The AP view is performed with cranio-caudal angulation. This permits a look through the foramen magnum and demonstrates the laterally traveling branches of the posterior circulation. The disadvantage of this view is that the basilar artery appears shortened. A Caldwells view (caudo-cranial angulation) shows the length of the basilar artery.

Table 1 summarizes some of the choices for the evaluation of suspected pathology in various arteries. In the sections below, there is additional information about appropriate views to obtain when intracranial aneurysms or stenoses are encountered.

Catheter placement for intracranial arteriography is usually in the common carotid artery, well proximal to the bifurcation, when extracranial cerebrovascular disease is the indication for the procedure. The advantage of this position is that it avoids crossing the carotid bifurcation with the guidewire and catheter. The disadvantage is that there is usually substantial runoff into the external carotid artery, depriving the intracranial arteries of the administered contrast and obscuring the same arteries by superimposed external carotid artery branches. After placement of the catheter, observe it using fluoroscopy as the guidewire is withdrawn to ensure that the catheter does not move when the support is removed. When the guidewire is removed, be certain there is free backbleeding from the catheter before proceeding. A long, single end hole, selective

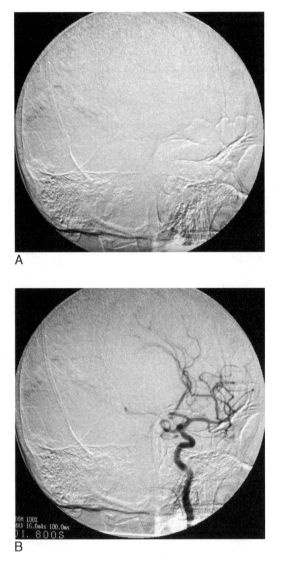

Fig. 6 A transorbital view. (A) The transorbital view is performed with 15–45° of rotation and 5–10° of cranio-caudal angulation. (B) The internal carotid artery branches and the proximal anterior and middle cerebral arteries are visualized within the orbital rim.

cerebral catheter may have its tip against the arterial wall and suction will be created when the guidewire is removed. This likelihood increases as smaller and more distal arteries are catheterized. Remove the guidewire steadily and avoid whipping it. If there is concern that suction may develop, hold the catheter hub upright and drip heparin saline into the hub as the guidewire is removed. If there is no backbleeding from the catheter, withdraw the catheter slowly until backbleeding occurs. Puff contrast by hand before using the high-pressure injector to be certain that the catheter tip is in the correct place in the correct artery and that there is no spasm or occlusive lesion near the catheter tip.

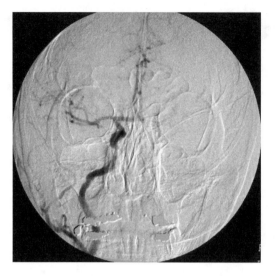

Fig. 7 Caldwells view of the distal internal carotid artery is performed with no rotation and 5–10° of caudal angulation. In this case, a distal internal carotid artery stenosis is present (arrow).

Table 1 Image Intensifier Position for the Evaluation of Intracranial Pathology

Artery for evaluation	View	Rotation (side-to-side)	Angulation (cranio-caudal)	Comment
Internal carotid artery	Paraorbital oblique	55°	5–10° cranial	Cavernous segment
	Haughton view	90°	45° cranial	Cavernous segment
	Transorbital oblique	15–45°	5–10° cranial	Ophthalmic segment
	Caldwells oblique	15–45°	5–10° caudal	Ophthalmic segment
Bifurcation of ICA	Transorbital oblique	15–45°	5–10° cranial	Through the orbit
	Submentovertex	0	90° cranial	Top-down view
	Caldwells view	0	5–10° caudal	
Anterior-communicating artery	Transorbital oblique	15–45°	5–10° cranial	Lateral view if aneurysm projects anteriorly
	Caldwells oblique	15–45°	5–10° caudal	
Middle cerebral artery	Transorbital oblique	15–45°	5–10° cranial	M1 and M2 segments
	Submentovertex	0	90° cranial	
Posterior-communicating artery	Transorbital oblique	15–45°	5–10° cranial	Often well visualized on lateral view
	Paraorbital oblique	55°	5–10° cranial	
	Haughton view	90°	45° cranial	
Distal vertebral/basilar	Townes oblique	10–30°	25–30° cranial or caudal	Basilar tip

The more severe the extracranial carotid bifurcation disease, the more challenging it is to obtain excellent images of the circulation distal to the lesion. The pressure and volume of contrast administration for intracranial arteriography are summarized in Table 5 of Chap. 4. In order to opacify the arteries and avoid flow streaming, the flow of contrast must exceed that of the blood. However, the shear stress generated by the rapidly flowing contrast may cause plaque disruption or injure the arterial wall. A longer injection time under lower pressure should be considered. When a preocclusive carotid lesion is present, a 3 for 9 or 3 for 12 contrast administration may be required (3- or 4-sec injection). If a critical stenosis is present, lower pressure is safer (300 psi). When carotid arteriography is performed with the catheter tip in the internal carotid artery, a lower volume and pressure are required (3 for 6 or even 2 for 4 may be adequate). Since the distal internal carotid artery is prone to spasm, a higher rate of rise should also be considered (0.5) to avoid injury to the arterial wall. If the catheter is placed in the internal carotid artery, complete systemic anticoagulation should be utilized. If multiple injections of contrast are anticipated, consider moving the catheter tip after every 2 or 3 runs to help prevent spasm.

Image acquisition may be achieved at 4 frames per second at the carotid bifurcation, but a higher frame rate, such as 8 frames per second, should be used for the intracranial circulation. Contrast administered in the common carotid artery may be somewhat dilute when it reaches the intracranial arteries. In addition, if there is any significant collateral inflow from the posterior communication artery (lateral view), the anterior communication artery (AP view), or the external carotid artery, some "to and fro" contrast flow may be observed with higher frame rates. This is quite common in hemispheres that are distal to a critical carotid bifurcation stenosis. Consideration of collaterals and anatomic variants is discussed in more detail later in this section.

The intracranial arteries are the only ones in the body that are completely surrounded by bone, making the acquisition of clean images more challenging. When contrast administered in the common carotid artery is imaged in the cerebral circulation, a slight delay between injection and image acquisition (0.5–1 sec) will provide images with less artifact. This avoids the acquisition of nonmask images that do not contain contrast. If there is even the slightest movement during these images, it deteriorates the final result because of the irregular surface of the overlying bone. A little longer delay (2–3 sec) may be appropriate if the carotid bifurcation lesion is preocclusive since contrast will be delayed at the bifurcation. If there is doubt about the timing, perform a contrast injection and observe the time to reaching the distal internal carotid artery. The patient must be absolutely still during intracranial imaging; patients are coached to avoid moving or swallowing. Sometimes even breathing causes too much movement and the patient must hold breath. Imaging is continued into the venous phase to observe for signs of venous malformations and tumors.

Collaterals of clinical importance are listed in Table 2. The Circle of Willis is highly variable, not just in terms of anatomic presence of specific collateral, but also their degree of development in terms of flow and physiological contribution in ischemic states. Patients with long standing extracranial cerebrovascular disease may develop lush col-

Table 2 Collateral Pathways in Cerebral Arteriography

Extracranial to intracranial
  Occipital artery to distal vertebral artery
  Ascending pharyngeal to petrous branches of internal carotid artery
  Facial artery to ophthalmic artery
  Superficial temporal artery to ophthalmic artery
  Internal maxillary artery to carotid siphon
Hemisphere to hemisphere
  Anterior-communicating artery
Anterior–posterior
  Posterior-communicating artery: Internal carotid artery to posterior cerebral artery
   Variants: Fetal origin of posterior cerebral artery (PCA arises directly from ICA)
    Infundibulum (dilatation of ICA at origin of PCOA)
Primitive trigeminal artery: Cavernous internal carotid artery to vertebral artery
Persistent otic artery: Petrous internal carotid artery to vertebral artery
Persistent hypoglossal artery: Distal cervical ICA (C1 or C2 level) to vertebral
Proatlantal intersegmental artery: Cervical ICA (C2 or C3 level) to vertebral

ICA = internal carotid artery.
PCOA = posterior communicating artery.
PCA = posterior cerebral artery.

lateral networks. The primary intracranial collaterals of interest are the anterior-communicating artery, the posterior-communicating artery, and collaterals from the external carotid to the internal carotid systems. If the anterior cerebral artery is not observed on the AP view, it is usually patent but supplied by the contralateral hemisphere through the anterior-communicating artery. A contralateral contrast injection may be required or an ipsilateral injection with contralateral manual carotid compression. The posterior-communicating artery may be visualized on the lateral view carrying contrast from the anterior to the posterior circulations. However, if there is significant inflow from the posterior-communicating artery to a poorly perfused hemisphere, the posterior-communicating artery may not be well visualized. The external carotid artery, via the occipital artery, often supplies collateral flow to the distal vertebral artery, which may then provide additional cerebral perfusion or may serve the upper extremity in subclavian steal syndrome. Arteriography provides mostly anatomical information. Failure to visualize a collateral does not necessarily mean that the collateral is not functional.

Normal variants and congenital anomalies are numerous in the cerebral circulation. The angiographer must be able to rapidly interpret these findings so that they are not considered pathological findings. Although this is not an exhaustive list, some clinically important variants and anomalies are summarized in Table 3.

What To Do When Intracranial Pathology is Present

Much of successful vascular practice is the development of pattern recognition: normal versus normal variant versus abnormal. Identifying and evaluating intracranial vascular

Table 3 Anatomical Variants and Anomalies in Cerebral Arteriography

Arch
    Innominate and left common carotid artery share common trunk (20%)
    Left common carotid artery originates from innominate artery (7%)
    Left common carotid artery and left subclavian artery form common trunk (1%)
    Left vertebral artery originates from arch (0.5%)
    Aberrant right subclavian artery (originates from left side of the arch and passes posterior to esophagus, <0.5%)
Internal carotid artery
    Location of carotid bifurcation may be T2 to C1
    Absence of internal carotid artery
    Anomalous origin of the internal carotid artery (directly from the arch)
    Hypoplasia of the internal carotid artery
    Duplication of the internal carotid artery
    Anomalous branches of the internal carotid artery (ascending pharyngeal, occipital)
    Aberrant petrous internal carotid artery (course through middle ear)
    Persistent stapedial artery
    Isolated internal carotid artery (fetal origin of the PCA and absent A1 segment)
    Early bifurcation of the middle cerebral artery

pathology is no different. The more familiar the surgeon is with the normal anatomy and its variants, the more rapidly and thoroughly that an abnormality will be identified and the more likely that the appropriate arteriographic maneuvers will be performed. The anatomy of the intracranial arteries is reviewed in Chap. 1. Repetition and experience enhance the process of developing good pattern recognition skills for the intracranial vasculature.

During intracranial arteriography, focus upon any areas that appear "abnormal" and consider the following (Fig. 8). Is it normal or not? There are a limited number of possible pathologies, but the lesion may be obscured by the numerous and circuitous cerebral arteries and their branches and collateral pathways. If it is abnormal, was it caused by the current procedure (acute occlusion, dissection, spasm) or is it a more chronic condition (aneurysm, stenosis, arteriovenous malformation (AVM), tumor)? If acute pathology, such as a vessel occlusion or filling defect, is present, has there been a change in the patient's condition? Is the lesion, whether acute or chronic, something likely to require treatment? Will the presence of this incidentally identified lesion affect the management of the carotid bifurcation disease? If the lesion requires treatment, what additional information is needed? The more likely it is to require treatment, the more information is usually required. Is it high flow or low flow? Adjust the technique to fit the pathology. Which major cerebral artery serves the lesion? Use rotation (from side to side) of the image intensifier and angulation (cranial or caudal) to tease out the anatomy.

Patient assessment and management during carotid interventions is discussed in Chap. 8 and the treatment of neurological complications is discussed in Chap. 14. Complications of carotid interventions are discussed in more detail in Chap. 19. If an acute abnormality such as an arterial filling defect or an apparently acute occlusion is

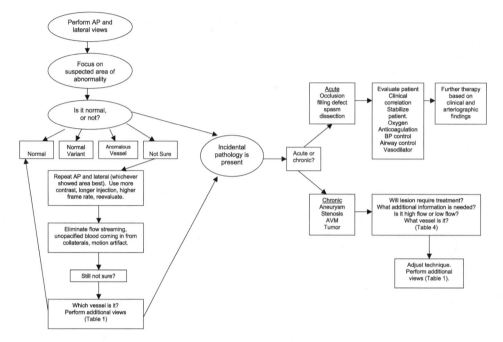

Fig. 8 What to do when incidental intracranial pathology is present.

seen during arteriography, the following maneuvers are required. (1) Assess the patient clinically. Administer oxygen and control blood pressure. (2) Administer more anticoagulation and check an activated clotting time (ACT) to ensure it is in the appropriate range. (3) Obtain a magnified view at the best angle and rotation with more contrast.

Thrombus may form that is related to the presence of the catheter or guidewire or be caused by spasm or arterial injury. Sometimes, unopacified blood flowing into the opacified blood stream through a collateral will cause flow streaming that mimics the appearance of an intraluminal filling defect. If thrombus is present, anticoagulation, aspiration, and catheter-directed thrombolytic administration should be performed (Chap. 14).

Spasm may result from guidewire or catheter encounters with the arterial wall or the shear generated by contrast administration. This does not occur very often when the catheter tip is in the common carotid artery. However, the internal carotid artery and the vertebral artery are much more prone to spasm. Multiple, full-strength administrations of contrast into an isolated cerebral hemisphere may also cause spasm or even challenge the blood/brain barrier. If this is a concern, it may be beneficial to pause between runs for a few minutes and consider using half-strength contrast.

When spasm occurs, it is usually located around the catheter tip or just distal to the catheter tip. It is not possible to predict how long it will last. If the spasm has created a critical stenosis, be sure and check the patient's anticoagulation status and administer heparin as needed to achieve systemic anticoagulation. Before removing the catheter, aspirate vigorously to remove any thrombus that may have formed when spasm occurred. Administer nitroglycerine through the catheter in 100-µg doses. The catheter may also be aspirated as it is being pulled back from the location of the spasm. Additional nitroglycerine is administered to flow through the area from which the catheter was removed. Spasm or arterial injury may also be avoided by altering the catheter tip position slightly between runs whenever multiple contrast runs are required from a single catheter position. In addition, it also helps to rotate and adjust the catheter tip so that its curvature is in line with the general configuration of the artery. The most common cause of cerebral artery spasm is subarachnoid or intracranial hemorrhage. This type of spasm is usually prolonged and requires other types of treatment, such as careful blood pressure control, intracranial catheter-directed vasodilator therapy, or balloon angioplasty.

In the next sections, the various incidental "chronic" pathologies that may be encountered are discussed, such as cerebral aneurysms, intracranial occlusive disease, arteriovenous malformations, and tumors (Table 4).

Cerebral Aneurysm

Among patients who present with extracranial cerebrovascular disease, a previously undiagnosed, and usually asymptomatic, cerebral aneurysm will occasionally be identified. Although the presence of the cerebral aneurysm rarely influences whether and how the carotid bifurcation lesion should be treated, aneurysms require treatment based upon their own merit.

Most patients presenting with subarachnoid hemorrhage as a result of cerebral aneurysms or with symptomatic but unruptured aneurysms will be evaluated first with CT or MRI scanning. CT scan is more sensitive for signs of acute hemorrhage, while MRI is more sensitive for identifying (down to about 3 mm) and sizing aneurysms. As with many other types of aneurysms, when the lesion is asymptomatic, its diameter is what seems to correlate best with rupture risk. Patients who present with symptomatic aneurysms require cerebral arteriography to better define the anatomy and assist in planning treatment. The angiographic appearance of an aneurysm is often used to help determine whether the lesion should be coil-embolized or clipped.

When an aneurysm is encountered, several important pieces of arteriographic information are required. (1) From which artery does the aneurysm originate? (2) What is the relationship between the aneurysm and its vessel of origin? (Does it have a neck? What is the configuration of the neck? In which view is it best demonstrated?) (3) Does the aneurysmal segment have any branches that also require clipping or embolization during aneurysm treatment? (4) What is the configuration of the aneurysms? (In which direction does it point? Does it have multiple lobes? Does it have intraluminal thrombus?)

The prevalence of cerebral aneurysms in the general population is estimated to be less than 1% (1). Unsuspected aneurysms are encountered in less than 3% of routine

Table 4 Evaluation of Incidentally Identified Intracranial Pathology

Pathology	Will lesion require treatment?	Will lesion affect treatment of carotid stenosis?	What additional information is needed to evaluate lesion?	Flow in lesion	Technique adjustments	Which vessel feeds the lesion?
Aneurysm	Depends on size and symptoms	Only if very large or symptomatic	Arteriogram—parent artery, neck location, neck size, and configuration; MRI—size of aneurysm	Low	Increase contrast volume, magnify field, longer injection, lower pressure, limit anticoagulation	Check AP and lateral; Check Table 1; Perform additional views with appropriate degrees of side-to-side rotation and cranio-caudal angulation
Stenosis	Probably medical—antiplatelet, anticoagulation	Probably not. Only if symptomatic or if more severe than carotid bifurcation stenosis	Arteriogram—degree of stenosis, location and length of stenosis, and adjacent arterial branches	Very low	Decrease pressure, longer injection, more anticoagulation	Check AP and lateral; Check Table 1; Perform additional views with appropriate degrees of side-to-side rotation and cranio-caudal angulation
AVM	Only if lesion is large and patient symptomatic or young and healthy	Produces false elevation of duplex velocity, may harbor aneurysms	Arteriogram—location of origin feeder arteries and overall flow; Venous component? MRI—size of AVM	High	Increase volume and injection time, increase frame rates limit anticoagulation	Check AP and lateral; Check Table 1; Perform additional views with appropriate degrees of side-to-side rotation and cranio-caudal angulation
Tumor	Highly likely	Yes. May require tumor management before carotid repair	Arteriogram—vessel of origin, rapidity of flow	Variable	Limit anticoagulation; Perform delayed filming at lower frame rate	Check AP and lateral; Check Table 1; Perform additional views with appropriate degrees of side-to-side rotation and cranio-caudal angulation

cerebral arteriographic studies (2). More than 80% of cerebral aneurysms occur in the anterior circulation. Most cerebral aneurysms are saccular, and ruptured saccular aneurysms may be responsible for up to 15% of strokes (1). Smoking and hypertension, which are prevalent among patients with carotid bifurcation stenosis, are also associated with aneurysm formation. Other conditions that are associated with aneurysms include polycystic kidney disease, sickle cell anemia, assorted collagen vascular diseases, fibromuscular dysplasia, and moyamoya disease. The most common locations for aneurysms are the anterior-communicating artery, the distal internal carotid artery, the posterior-communicating artery, and the middle cerebral artery. Most aneurysms occur at the point where an artery branches. This can make the arteriographic evaluation of aneurysms more challenging since the neck of the aneurysm must be visualized, as well as its relationship to the parent artery and branches, without obscuring it with superimposition of these same arteries. Aneurysms are best measured in size using magnetic resonance imaging. Two or more aneurysms are present in 15–20% of patients with aneurysms (3,4). Therefore when one is identified, a complete study is warranted.

Current recommendations include the treatment of all ruptured aneurysms and those causing symptoms (1). However, there is some uncertainty about the appropriate level of aggressiveness in the treatment of asymptomatic aneurysms, such as those that may be encountered as incidental findings in the arteriographic evaluation of carotid bifurcation occlusive disease. The annual risk of rupture in followed asymptomatic aneurysms in retrospective studies has ranged from 1.4% to 2.3% (5,6). A large, multicenter natural history study demonstrated that the annual rupture risk for aneurysms less than 10 mm in size in patients without a history of previous subarachnoid hemorrhage was only 0.05% (7). When a patient had a previous subarachnoid hemorrhage from an aneurysm in another location, the annual rupture risk for an identified but asymptomatic aneurysm was 0.5%. Aneurysms of 10–20 mm had a 1% annual rupture risk, while lesions larger than 20 mm had a 6% annual rupture risk. Therefore asymptomatic aneurysms of 10 mm or more are usually considered for repair, especially if there has been a previous subarachnoid hemorrhage (1). Some experts advise that aneurysms of 6 mm or larger may be appropriate for treatment in young, good risk patients. In elderly patients, mechanical treatment is usually only recommended for large aneurysms in otherwise healthy patients (8).

When an aneurysm is considered for treatment, the arteriographic appearance helps the clinician decide which form of treatment is appropriate, whether it is medical management and observation, coil embolization, parent artery occlusion, or surgical clipping. In treating asymptomatic aneurysms throughout the vasculature, the less invasive the procedure, the more applicability it has to patients with varying levels of health. Coil embolization is less invasive than surgical clipping, has a low morbidity rate, and can be accomplished in most well selected cases. A large meta-analysis demonstrated a perioperative complication rate of less than 4% for coil embolization (9). A small neck from the parent vessel without encroachment of other structures is the best situation. Unfortunately, the late recanalization rate for coiled cerebral aneurysms can be as high as 40–50% for large aneurysms (≥20mm) and 5–10% for small aneurysms (10,11).

Table 1 lists some of the views that should be considered for aneurysm interrogation. Table 4 provides a framework for evaluation of a cerebral aneurysm. If an artery is suspicious in contour for aneurysmal dilatation, obtain the standard AP and lateral views and examine both runs from start to finish with the focus on the area of concern. Although it is not always possible on the basis of these views to know whether there is an aneurysm or the artery from which it originates, the next maneuver should be based upon the highest likelihood.

Depending upon the most likely artery of origin, a view is selected. If an extended catheter in-dwelling time is anticipated, consider additional heparin administration. The best images are obtained when the catheter is advanced to the proximal internal carotid artery and the overlying external carotid artery branches remain nonopacified. This is only possible, however, when there is no carotid bifurcation stenosis. Internal carotid artery catheter placement is usually satisfactory at the mid-cervical level (C3). It is usually a straight segment and the likelihood of reflux of contrast is low.

The contrast administration pressure is decreased, and a longer injection time with higher volume is used with a magnified field of view (usually 6 in.). In planning views to assess aneurysms, especially when the artery of origin is not yet clear, it is often useful to perform a roadmap of the circulation, and then rotate (toward one side or the other) and angle (cranial or caudal) the image intensifier to unfold the lesion. When the best view is chosen, magnify the view with a 6-in. field of view. Puff contrast to see if the desired structures are included. Careful records must be kept of the angle and rotation of the gantry and also the patient's head position. This will facilitate finding the best position for the image intensifier for any later treatment that is required.

Anterior-communicating artery aneurysms tend to project along the same horizontal line as seen in the AP projection of the A1 segment. An ipsilateral anterior oblique projection at 15–45° (transorbital oblique) should be obtained. This view usually places the A1 segment and the anterior-communicating artery within the projection of the ipsilateral orbit. This may be required at a few different degrees of rotation to tease out the junction of the A1 and A2 segments. Contralateral carotid compression may be required to fully opacify an anterior-communicating artery. If there is a lobe of aneurysm projecting anteriorly or posteriorly, a 15–45° rotation with caudo-cranial angulation may be helpful (Caldwells oblique).

Posterior-communicating artery aneurysms are usually visualized best with a steep anterior ipsilateral oblique of 55° (paraorbital oblique) and an injection of contrast into the vertebral artery. The dominant vertebral artery should be selected. Vertebral artery flow can be augmented by inflating bilateral brachial blood pressure cuffs. Flow from posterior to anterior in the posterior-communicating artery can also be enhanced by manual ipsilateral carotid artery compression during the vertebral artery injection.

Middle cerebral artery aneurysms are best evaluated with the Townes and transorbital oblique since these views move the petrous bone out of the field. Another helpful view is obtained by placing the image intensifier at close to 90° in the caudo-cranial direction, looking nearly straight through the skull from top to bottom (submentovertex view).

Occasionally during intracranial arteriography, an infundibulum will be observed. This is a small dilatation of the main artery at a location where a branch originates. This is sometimes seen on the lateral view at the origin of the posterior-communicating artery.

Intracranial Occlusive Disease

Intracranial atherosclerotic occlusive disease is much more likely to be encountered during routine arteriography in patients with carotid bifurcation occlusive disease. The incidence appears to be close to 20% (12). Approximately 5–10% of strokes are caused by intracranial atherosclerosis (13,14). Risk factors for the development of intracranial atherosclerosis are diabetes, hypertension, and advanced age (15,16). Although lesions may occur in any artery, the anterior circulation locations that are likely to be clinically significant in patients with carotid bifurcation disease are the distal intracranial internal carotid artery and the M1 segment of the middle cerebral artery. The annual stroke rate for significant stenosis of a major intracranial cerebral artery (siphon, MCA, etc.) is approximately 7–8% (17). Among patients with significant extracranial carotid bifurcation stenosis, the presence of intracranial disease was an independent predictor of stroke (18).

Most intracranial occlusive disease is managed medically at the present. Available data suggest that coumadin is better than clopidogrel and that it is also better than aspirin (17,19,20). When a patient fails medical therapy, balloon angioplasty may be considered. The results of intracranial balloon angioplasty in several small series depend upon the size of the artery, the length and morphology of the lesion, its location, and the adjacent structures. The initial technical success rates vary from 70% to 90% (21–23). At 1 year, lesions of 5 mm or less in length fare substantially better than those that are longer than 10 mm. Periprocedural stroke and death rates were approximately 10%. Deaths have resulted from vessel rupture, stroke, and guidewire perforation. Recommended technique is to use an undersized balloon, dilated slowly, in a favorable lesion. Since the technique is determined by sizing and anatomy, the arteriographic evaluation must be complete. Views for evaluation of intracranial stenosis are listed in Table 1.

The presence of significant intracranial atherosclerosis, even if it is not treated, may influence blood pressure management and the use of anticoagulation and antiplatelet agents in the perioperative period for carotid stenting and over the long term. It may be more appropriate to liberalize rather than to tighten control of blood pressure. Systemic anticoagulation should be administered during carotid arteriography. Glycoprotein IIb/IIIa inhibitors should be considered during carotid stent placement. The overall risk of any procedure, whether it be an arteriogram, a carotid stent, or an endarterectomy, is probably increased by the presence of intracranial occlusive disease. In order to assess the degree of stenosis, the same views may be used as are employed during evaluation of an aneurysm. The distal internal carotid artery may be evaluated in the lateral, Caldwell,

Waters, or transorbital oblique. The middle cerebral artery may be evaluated in the AP, lateral, transorbital oblique, and submentovertex views.

Arteriovenous Malformations

Undiagnosed arteriovenous malformations are rare, especially in the population in which atherosclerosis is prevalent. Duplex evaluation of the carotid arteries may yield elevated velocities throughout the carotid system and higher than expected for the sonographic appearance of the bifurcation lesion. In this case, a CT or MRI scan should be obtained prior to proceeding with arteriography.

Since arteriovenous malformations are high flow lesions, higher frame rates and contrast volumes are required to evaluate them. Arteriovenous malformations frequently have associated aneurysms that also require treatment. Each major artery that could potentially be feeding an arteriovenous malformation should be interrogated. In general, the larger the lesion and the faster the flow, the more challenging it is to treat these lesions.

Brain Tumors

Tumors may appear as mass areas of differential perfusion, either more than or less than the surrounding normal brain tissue. Usually, an AP and lateral view are appropriate. The primary cerebral artery that serves the area in which the tumor arises should be injected with contrast. Excessive anticoagulation should be avoided since some tumors are more likely to result in intracranial hemorrhage.

Angiographic Considerations for Planning Carotid Stent Placement

At some point in the future, it is likely that preoperative magnetic resonance arteriography will be the only required study prior to carotid stent placement. Technique and devices will probably improve to the point where almost any arch and any carotid lesion can be crossed. However, at the present time, carotid arteriogram is the most appropriate and safest pathway to carotid stent placement.

Information required from a carotid arteriogram to help plan stent placement is summarized in Table 5. The surgeon must get the "feel" of the arch in a given case. To assist in planning catheterization of the carotid arteries, the arch is divided into segments as described in Chap. 2. Chap. 4 provides an introduction to the use of cerebral catheters. As mentioned previously, if the carotid artery can be selectively catheterized with a simple curve catheter, it avoids the challenge of attempting to exchange the complex curve catheter or advancing the complex curve catheter past its secondary curve or

Table 5   What Do You Need to Know from a Carotid Arteriogram that Helps in Planning Carotid Stent Placement?

- Get the "feel" of the arch and its branch origins.
- Assess the level of challenge of catheterization of the carotid artery, estimate the likelihood of success of sheath access, and make a plan for carotid sheath placement.
- Identify unfavorable anatomical arch configurations and arch pathology.
- Identify lesions at the origin of the innominate or common carotid arteries that may require treatment or prevent safe access.
- Evaluate external carotid artery anatomy (Is there a place to anchor an exchange guidewire?).
- Are there kinks or coils in the common carotid artery or the internal carotid artery that could be worsened by the stent? Visualize the bifurcation with the stent in place. What will the new configuration look like? Will some relative straightening at the location of the stent cause worsening of a kink at some other location?
- Are there bifurcation or lesion issues that increase risk, such as preocclusive stenosis, long stenosis, large ulcer, mobile plaque, intraluminal thrombus, or heavy calcification?
- Is the internal carotid artery distal to the lesion of adequate size?
- Is there a cerebral protection device available that will safely cross the lesion and be deployable in the internal carotid artery distal to the bifurcation?
- Is there intracranial occlusive disease that will affect the conduct of the case and influence the overall risk?
- Is there any incidental intracranial pathology that must be investigated and managed prior to treatment of the carotid bifurcation stenosis?

elbow into the distal external carotid artery. Simple curve catheters do not require reshaping the catheter head as do complex curve catheters. Unfavorable arch configurations and pathology and lesions at the origin of the branch arteries are identified. The integrity of the external carotid artery for functioning as a location to anchor the guidewire is assessed. Chap. 6 provides information about how the arch segment classification system can be used to help make a plan for carotid sheath placement. Kinks and coils in the common carotid and the internal carotid arteries are assessed. The bifurcation and the lesion must be evaluated for features that increase risk, such as preocclusive or lengthy stenosis, complex ulcer, mobile plaque, intraluminal thrombus, or heavy calcification. The internal carotid artery distal to the lesion must be of adequate size. The whole configuration must be able to accept a cerebral protection device safely. Intracranial pathology must also be identified.

Many vascular specialists feel a moral dilemma about whether it is appropriate to subject patients to carotid arteriography when duplex scanning followed by carotid endarterectomy have been shown to be efficacious. This is certainly a reasonable concern. Each vascular specialist must decide which approach is best. However, consider the fact that refusal to participate in carotid arteriography denies selected current patients the opportunity to benefit from carotid stent placement and denies the practitioner an opportunity to participate in the future treatment of carotid disease. Patients who develop carotid disease in the future will be necessarily managed by nonvascular physicians if the vascular physicians, those who have the most experience in the management of carotid disease, are not capable of providing treatment.

References

1. Bederson JB, Awad IA, Wiebers DO, et al. Recommendations for the management of patients with unruptured intracranial aneurysms. A statement for healthcare professionals from the Stroke Council of the American Heart Association. Stroke 2000; 31:2742–2750.

2. Atkinson JL, Sundt TL, Houser OW, et al. Angiographic frequency of anterior circulation intracranial aneurysms. J Neurosurg 1989; 70:551–555.

3. Bjorkesten G, Halonen V. Incidence of intracranial vascular lesions in patients with subarachnoid hemorrhage investigated by four-vessel angiography. J Neurosurg 1965; 23:29–32.

4. Jacobs JM. Angiography in intracranial hemorrhage. Neuroimag Clin North Am 1992; 2:89–106.

5. Wiebers DO, Whisnant JP, Sundt TM, et al. The significance of unruptured saccular intracranial aneurysms. J Neurosurg 1987; 66:23–29.

6. Yasui N, Suzuki A, Nishimura H, et al. Long term follow-up study of unruptured intracranial aneurysms. Neurosurgery 1997; 40:1155–1159.

7. The ISUIA Investigators. Unruptured intracranial aneurysms: risks of rupture and risks of surgical intervention. N Engl J Med 1998; 339:1725–1733.

8. Stoodley MA, Weir BKA. Intracranial aneurysms: Overview. In: Marks MP, Do HM, eds. Endovascular and Percutaneous Therapy of the Brain and Spine. Philadelphia: Lippincott Williams & Wilkins, 2002:119–140.

9. Brilstra EH, Rinkel GJ, van der Graaf Y, van Rooij WJ, Algra A. Treatment of intracranial aneurysms by embolization with coils: a systematic review. Stroke 1999; 30:470–476.

10. Vinuela F, Duckwiler G, Mawad M. Guglielmi detachable coil embolization of acute intracranial aneurysm: perioperative, anatomical, and clinical outcomes in 403 patients. J Neurosurg 1997; 86:475–482.

11. Byrne JV, Sohn MJ, Molyneux AJ, et al. Five-year experience in using coil embolization for ruptured intracranial aneurysms: outcomes and incidence of late rebleeding. J Neurosurg 1999; 90:656–663.

12. Hass WK, Fields WS, North RR, et al. Joint study of extracranial arterial occlusion II: arteriography, techniques, sites and complications. JAMA 1968; 203:961–968.

13. Sacco RL, Kargman DE, Qiong G, et al. Race-ethnicity and determinants of intracranial atherosclerotic cerebral infarction. Stroke 1995; 26:14–20.

14. Benesch CG, Chimowitz MI. Best treatment for intracranial arterial stenosis? 50 years of uncertainty. Neurology 2000; 55:465–466.

15. Yoo KM, Shin HK, Chang HM, et al. Middle cerebral artery occlusive disease. J Stroke Cerebrovasc Dis 1998; 7:344–351.

16. Gorelick PB, Caplan LR, Langenberg P, et al. Clinical and angiographic comparison of asymptomatic occlusive disease. Neurology 1988; 38:852–858.

17. EC/IC Bypass Study Group. Failure of extracranial–intracranial arterial bypass to reduce the risk of ischemic stroke. N Engl J Med 1985; 313:1191–1200.

18. Kapelle LJ, Eliasziw M, Fox AJ, et al. Importance of intracranial atherosclerotic disease in

patients with symptomatic stenosis of the internal carotid artery. Stroke 1999; 30:282–286.

19. CAPRIE Steering Committee. A randomized, blinded trial of clopidogrel versus aspirin in patients at risk of ischemic events. Lancet 1996; 348:1329–1339.

20. Chimowitz MI, Kokkinos J, Strong J, et al. The warfarin–aspirin intracranial disease study. Neurology 1995; 45:1488–1493.

21. Connors JJ, Wojak JC. Percutaneous transluminal angioplasty for intracranial atherosclerotic lesions: evolution of technique and short term results. J Neurosurg 1999; 91:415–423.

22. Mori T, Fukuoka M, Kazita K, et al. Follow-up study after intracranial percutaneous transluminal cerebral balloon angioplasty. Am J Neuroradiol 1998; 19:1525–1533.

23. Marks MP, Marcellus M, Norbash AM, et al. Outcome of angioplasty for atherosclerotic intracranial stenosis. Stroke 1999; 30:1065–1069.

6

Access for Carotid Interventions

PETER A. SCHNEIDER

Hawaii Permanente Medical Group, Honolulu, Hawaii, U.S.A.

The purpose of this chapter is to provide a step-by-step approach to obtaining secure and adequate caliber access to be used as a conduit for intervention in the carotid artery. This chapter discusses how to assess the anatomy, assemble supplies for access, place the access sheath, and troubleshoot the access. General approaches to sheath placement and tips for dealing with access challenges are also discussed. Gaining safe and direct access to the common carotid artery is the cornerstone of carotid angioplasty and stent placement.

Assess the Anatomy

Arch anatomy and its variations have been reviewed in Chap. 1 and the classification for arch anatomy segments was discussed in Chap. 2. Arch aortography, selective arch branch catheterization, and carotid arteriography have been presented in Chap. 4. The next step is sheath placement into the appropriate arch branch to secure access for intervention. Sheath placement for carotid intervention begins with an assessment of the anatomy. Table 1 contains a list of anatomical features that should be considered when planning sheath placement.

The segment of the arch in which the branch originates influences the level of difficulty encountered in selective catheterization of the carotid artery (Chap. 4), and this feature plays a significant role in sheath placement. Access of an arch branch for intervention becomes more challenging in the progression from segment I to segment III (Fig. 1, Chap. 2). There is more about this later in the section "Approach to the Arch."

Table 1   Anatomical Features Which Influence Sheath Placement

Arch anatomy variations (e.g., bovine arch)
Location of origin of arch vessel (see "Segmental Arch Anatomy Classification" in Chap. 2)
General shape of the arch (tortuosity, angulation)
Atherosclerotic plaque within the arch
Occlusive disease at the orifice or within the proximal portion of the branch artery
Angulation of the arch branches after takeoff
Occlusion of external carotid artery origin
Branches of the external carotid artery

Other anatomical factors must also be considered. The general shape of the arch may be gently rounded or it may be elongated, tortuous, or angulated (Fig. 1). Patients with long standing hypertension or arterial enlargement tend to have elongated arches that accentuate the acute angle turn of the arch. Each additional turn or angle that is added to the femoral-carotid route adds to the level of difficulty. Distal to the origin of each branch, angulation or tortuosity of the innominate or common carotid artery may also work against smooth sheath placement. Plaque in the arch or occlusive disease at the branch origin or in the proximal artery is a relative contraindication to sheath placement. An external carotid artery that is occluded or lacks adequate branches cannot be used for anchoring the stiff guidewire over which the sheath is passed.

Supplies for Arch Access

Supplies for standard carotid and cerebral arteriography are listed in Table 3 of Chap. 4. Catheters for selective catheterization of the carotid arteries are discussed at length in Chap. 4. After selective cannulation of the appropriate common carotid artery, the

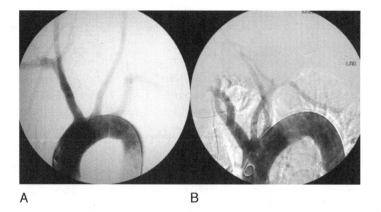

A   B

Fig. 1   Variations in arch anatomy. (A) Arch anatomy may be gently rounded with branches originating from the "top" of the arch. (B) The arch may also be elongated with its branch vessel origins shifted toward the patient's right and inferiorly.

Table 2 Supplies for Arch Access

Guidewires
    Angled tip, 0.035-in. steerable Glidewire, 260 cm
    Superstiff Amplatz, 0.035, variable length floppy tip (1 or 6 cm), 260 cm
    Optional: Microvena, Stiff Nitinol, 260 cm
Catheters
    Angled tip, simple curve, 5-Fr selective catheter, 100 cm
    Complex curve, 5-Fr selective catheter, 100 cm
    Straight, exchange, 100 cm
Sheaths
    Straight 90-cm shuttle sheath, 6 and 7 Fr, radiopaque tip, dilator, Tuohy–Borst
        or hemostatic valve
Guiding catheters
    Various shapes, 8 and 9 Fr, 80–100 cm length

selective catheter is placed in the external carotid artery. A stiff guidewire is placed, the selective catheter is removed, and the access sheath or guiding catheter is placed over the stiff guidewire. Supplies for arch access are listed in Table 2.

Whether to use a guiding sheath or a guiding catheter is an important consideration and the two are compared in Table 3. Use of a guiding sheath is simpler. A guiding sheath has its own tapered dilator, and it does not require an additional femoral access sheath to introduce it or secure it. Sizing is simple since it is described by its inside diameter, or "what will pass through it." The main disadvantage of the guiding sheath is the limitation to a straight tip since special shapes are not yet available as they are with guiding catheters. Guiding catheters offer a variety of tip shapes, which include several types of simple curves. These multipurpose tip variations may be used to help direct the guiding catheter into the common carotid artery when working with a difficult arch or to direct the therapeutic catheter into the internal carotid artery when the bifurcation is angulated. Guiding catheter tips are soft and atraumatic. If the guiding catheter becomes dislodged or needs to be advanced slightly or adjusted during the case, it can usually be done without inserting an obturator or dilator. Beyond the shape feature and the flexibility, guiding catheters present several disadvantages. There is no prefitted dilator to assist with passage, and they are usually placed over a selective catheter that does not

Table 3 Guiding Sheath or Guiding Catheter?

Guiding sheath	Guiding catheter
Straight tip	Different tip shapes
Has its own dilator	No dilator
Sizing is simple	Sizing is complex
Does not require additional sheath	Requires femoral access sheath
Hemostasis by Tuohy–Borst or standard valve	Use Tuohy–Borst for hemostasis
Provides excellent support	Can be advanced without dilators

Table 4   Properties of the Guiding Sheath

Name: Shuttle Sheath
Manufacturer: Cook Inc., Indianapolis, IN
Caliber: 6 Fr (ID=0.088 in.), 7 Fr (ID=0.100 in.)
Length: 90 cm
Surface: Hydrophilic coating
Dilator tip: Tapered, smooth transition
Sheath tip: Straight, soft, flexible, radiopaque band
Hemostatic valve: Tuohy–Borst or access adapter

provide a smooth transition from one catheter caliber to the next. They require a femoral access sheath that increases the size of the femoral arteriotomy. This is because they are too soft and flexible to pass through the access site. Guiding catheters are sized by their outside diameter. The operator must check the inside diameter specification to ensure that the delivery catheter is of the correct profile to pass through the guiding catheter.

Many carotid stenting systems are available that can be delivered through a 6-Fr guiding sheath or an 8-Fr guiding catheter. In these relative sizes (6 Fr ID=2 mm, 7 Fr ID=2.3 mm), each step smaller in catheter caliber introduces greater flexibility and trackability and enhances the ease with which the sheath may be advanced into the common carotid artery. Properties of the guiding sheath used most commonly by the author are listed in Table 4. There is a smooth transition from the tapered dilator to the soft, flexible sheath tip (Fig. 2). The rate-limiting factor on the profile of the system is usually the outside diameter of the delivery catheter for the self-expanding stent. Outside diameters and sheath sizes for some stents used in carotid interventions are listed in Table 5. It is highly likely that many systems will be 5-Fr compatible in the near future.

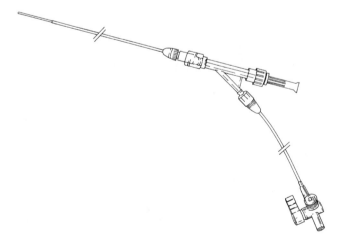

Fig. 2   Guiding sheath. The Shuttle Sheath (Cook Inc.) offers a smooth transition from dilator tip to the shaft of the sheath.

Table 5 Outside Diameters of Some Stent Delivery Catheters

Stent	Stent expanded diameter (mm)	Outside diameter delivery catheter	Sheath Size (Fr)	Platform
Precise (Cordis)	6–7	5.5 Fr (1.85 mm)	6	0.018
	8–10	6.0 Fr (2.0 mm)	6	0.018
PreciseRx (Cordis)	6–7	5.0 Fr (1.65 mm)	5	0.014
	8–10	6.0 Fr (2.0 mm)	6	0.014
Dynalink (Guidant)	6–10	5.9 Fr (1.96 mm)	6	0.018
Wallstent (Medi-tech)	6–8	4.8 Fr (1.67 mm)	5	0.014
	10	5.9 Fr (1.96 mm)	6	0.014

Placement of Access for Carotid Intervention

1. After femoral guidewire placement, use vessel dilators to enlarge the arteriotomy and place a 6- or 7-Fr standard access sheath, appropriately sized to the intended guiding sheath. Administer heparin. IIb/IIIa inhibitors may also be administered if desired (more on this in Chap. 8). Perform selective catheterization of the common carotid artery using the simplest selective cerebral catheter possible.

2. Administer contrast through the selective catheter to road-map the carotid bifurcation. The image intensifier should be angled to achieve the best projection of the bifurcation based upon the previous arteriogram. Ipsilateral, steep anterior oblique, or near lateral projections are often the most useful. Advance a 0.035-in. steerable Glidewire into the external carotid artery. Although the external carotid artery origin is usually located anteromedially, its branches often cross posteriorly making it difficult to discern without a road map, at least initially, whether the guidewire is advancing into the internal or external carotid artery.

3. In general, simple curve selective catheters, such as the H1 Headhunter, the angled taper Glidecath, and the Vert catheter, track more easily into the external carotid artery than the complex curve catheters such as the Simmons and the Vitek. The complex curve catheters have a secondary curve or elbow that must be straightened inside the common carotid artery before tracking becomes easier.

4. After advancing the catheter into the external carotid artery, perform a digital run or road map to see where the longest and largest branches are located for placing the guidewire to get the best anchor. Contrast usually refluxes out of the external carotid artery and into the internal carotid artery, so do not inject too forcefully. The catheter tip must be far enough into the external carotid artery (≥ 2 cm), so that a cough, turn of the head, or minor movement does not pop the catheter out of the external carotid artery and into the bifurcation where its tip could cause damage.

5. After advancing the catheter into the proximal a few centimeters of the external carotid artery and road mapping, advance the Glidewire into a distal-most branch of the external carotid artery. Advance the selective catheter over the Glidewire as far as it will go. Remove the Glidewire. Make sure the catheter backbleeds before placing the Amplatz exchange guidewire. If the catheter tip is against the wall of the external carotid artery branch and there is no back flow, pulling the guidewire will create suction and bubbles. When the exchange guidewire is introduced to fill the lumen, air will be pushed into the system. After backbleeding the selective catheter, place an Amplatz superstiff guidewire. The Amplatz guidewire is 260 cm in length and has a short, floppy segment at the tip. Perform fluoroscopy of the catheter tip in the distal external carotid artery as the Amplatz guidewire is advanced. If the catheter tip begins to withdraw, stop advancing the Amplatz superstiff guidewire. This is usually a sign that the catheter is not anchored well enough in the external carotid artery and the Amplatz superstiff guidewire is about to pull the catheter out of the external carotid artery. The catheter may require better seeding in the external carotid artery (see "Trouble Shooting the Access"). If the selective catheter seems that it is being pulled out of the external carotid artery by the guidewire, consider exchanging for a stiffer selective cerebral catheter, such as a vertebral catheter. The Amplatz superstiff guidewire should be advanced as far into the external carotid artery branches as possible. Do not force the guidewire, however, as perforation of the small branch artery may occur and cause significant problems in an anticoagulated patient. The patient may complain of facial, jaw, or ear pain as the Amplatz guidewire tip is reaching its destination.

6. After the Amplatz guidewire is in place in the distal external carotid artery, remove the selective catheter. Ensure that the guidewire tip remains in the distal external carotid artery using spot fluoroscopy. Remove the femoral sheath. Place the guiding sheath through the femoral access. Prior to advancing the sheath into the common carotid artery, open and prepare the guidewire, distal protection device, and balloons intended for usage so that the procedure may proceed expeditiously once the sheath is in the common carotid artery.

7. Briefly survey the course of the guidewire using fluoroscopy before advancing the sheath. There may be slack in the Amplatz superstiff guidewire in the descending aorta or arch, and this should be carefully and gently removed without withdrawing the tip of the guidewire. This may be done by focusing the fluoroscopic image on the guidewire tip and slowly withdrawing the guidewire until some sign of movement is seen in the guidewire tip. The sheath is more likely to advance smoothly if the guidewire is in its straightest possible course.

8. Advance the guiding sheath into the common carotid artery. The image intensifier should be positioned so that field of view includes the tip of the

Amplatz guidewire in the distal external carotid artery on the upper part of the field, while the arch branch origin is visible in the lower part of the field. This can be performed by placing the image intensifier close to the patient and using a 14- or 16-in. field. This permits observation of the exchange guidewire tip as the sheath turns superiorly into the arch branch. The guidewire should be pinned carefully. If the guidewire is pushed forward, it may perforate the external carotid artery branch. As the dilator comes into view and approaches the turn into the common carotid artery, carefully observe the shape of the dilator and sheath to see that it is tracking over the guidewire. If the turn into the artery is too tight, the sheath may prolapse into the proximal arch and pull the guidewire out of the external carotid artery. Sheath passage around a turn may be facilitated by having the patient take a deep breath or turn their head to help straighten this segment slightly as the sheath passes by.

9. The sheath is advanced with a steady, even, forward force while the Amplatz superstiff guidewire is pinned and the tip of the guidewire is observed under fluoroscopy. The sheath progress cannot be observed along its entire course since the image intensifier is stationary to observe the guidewire tip. If excessive resistance is met, stop pushing and pan inferiorly to see the location, angles, and course of the guidewire and the sheath. Occasionally, slack has built up along the guidewire that must be removed. Occasionally, there is too much tortuosity for the chosen access device to cross (see "Trouble Shooting the Access"). If there is excessive tortuosity in the abdominal aorta and iliac arteries, consider passing a larger sheath that is 45 cm in length. If the intended carotid sheath is 6 Fr, for example, pass a 7- or 8-Fr sheath that will help to straighten some of the tortuosity and pass the 6-Fr carotid sheath through it.

10. The tip of the dilator does not have a radiopaque marker as the end of the sheath does. However, the tip of the dilator does extend for several centimeters beyond the end of the sheath. Care must be taken to avoid mechanical dilatation of the carotid lesion with the tip of the dilator. This is especially true for focal lesions in the common carotid artery or bifurcation lesions that begin in the common carotid artery. The dilator must be withdrawn slightly so that it extends only 1 or 2 cm beyond the tip of the sheath. The silhouette of the dilator tip can often be visualized on the magnified fluoroscopic image (small field of view).

11. Advance the sheath until the radiopaque tip is a few centimeters or more inside the common carotid artery. This is often at the level of the clavicle or just superior. A mental note of this location should be made at the time of the arch study. If the operator is uncertain of where the relative landmarks are located to identify the origin of the artery and the bifurcation for safe sheath tip placement, review the arch study. The tip of the sheath must be far enough inside the artery that it does not pop out and back into the arch, but not so far into the artery that it crosses or butts up against the lesion. The

sheath tip should be placed a few centimeters or more proximal to the lesion so there is working room for the intervention.

12. The dilator is removed. The sheath is backbled and then flushed gently, taking care to avoid bubbles. Prior to removing the Amplatz guidewire, perform a selective carotid arteriogram through the sidearm of the sheath to check sheath position, locate the lesion, and ensure that there has been no damage to the common carotid artery during sheath passage. If the sheath must be advanced further, maintaining the stiff guidewire in place is necessary until this is completed. With each maneuver, such as sheath placement or removal of the dilator, the anatomical relationships of the carotid artery may change and tortuosity may disappear or be introduced.

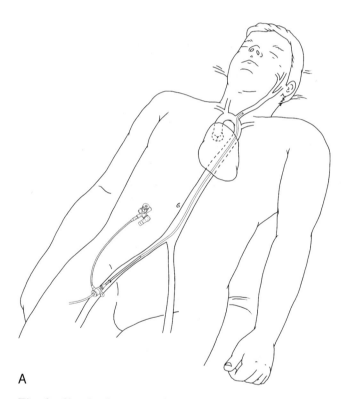

A

Fig. 3 Sheath placement. (A) The common carotid artery is catheterized with a selective catheter. (B) A road map of the carotid bifurcation is obtained. Care is taken to position the image intensifier so that the bifurcation is "opened up." (C) A steerable guidewire is advanced into the external carotid artery and the selective catheter is advanced. (D) The selective catheter is used to perform a road map of the external carotid artery. A long branch of the external carotid artery is selected to anchor the guidewire. (E) The selective catheter is advanced into the distal portion of the selected external carotid artery branch. The Amplatz Superstiff exchange guidewire is advanced into the distal external carotid artery. (F) After placement of the stiff exchange guidewire, the femoral access sheath is removed. The long carotid guiding sheath is advanced into the common carotid artery.

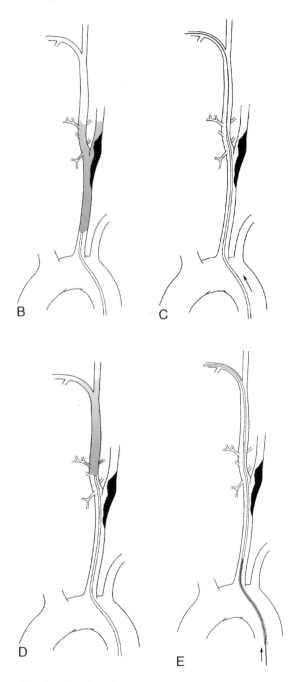

Fig. 3 Continued.

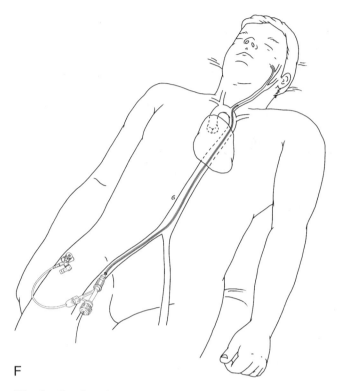

F

Fig. 3 Continued.

13.   Remove the Amplatz guidewire from the external carotid artery. The carotid
        bifurcation is road-mapped by administering contrast through the sidearm
        of the sheath. The guidewire intended for crossing the carotid lesion is
        advanced. When there is severe angulation at the origin of the internal
        carotid artery, it is useful to leave the Amplatz guidewire in place to occupy
        the origin of the external carotid artery while the lower profile treatment
        guidewire is advanced into the internal carotid artery. If sheath position is
        tenuous or the arch anatomy was particularly challenging, the sheath may
        become unstable when the stiff guidewire is removed. In this case, leave the
        Amplatz guidewire in place as a support until the treatment guidewire is
        advanced into place (buddy wire technique). When the Amplatz guidewire is
        removed, observe with fluoroscopy to ensure that the sheath does not back
        out of the common carotid artery (Fig. 3).

Alternate Methods of Sheath Placement

In general, the stiff guidewire is placed in the external carotid artery and a long guiding
sheath or guiding catheter is placed over it, following the sequence of events described
above. Variations of this approach are described.

1. Backloading Method. Occasionally, it may be appropriate to advance the guiding sheath into the distal aortic arch or proximal descending aorta before the common carotid artery has been cannulated. This may be useful in situations where the distal arch or more distal aorta or iliac arteries are tortuous enough to complicate access. After the guiding sheath is placed in the distal arch, a long selective cerebral catheter (120 or 125 cm) is used to cannulate the common carotid artery that is only a few centimeters beyond the tip of the sheath. The H1, Vert, and Vitek are examples of simple and complex curve cerebral catheters that come in these longer lengths. The longer cerebral catheters are required to extend beyond the 90-cm carotid guiding sheath. With a Tuohy–Borst adaptor, this sheath is nearly 100 cm, almost the same length as standard cerebral catheters. The selective catheter is advanced into the external carotid artery, the Amplatz superstiff guidewire is placed, and the sheath is advanced the rest of the way into the proximal common carotid artery directly over the cerebral catheter. The advantage of this approach is that the sheath has already crossed most of the distance from the femoral access site before the arch branch is engaged. The guiding sheath can be used to support the selective cerebral catheter as it initially enters the common carotid artery. The disadvantage of this approach is that the transition from catheter to guiding sheath is not smooth and could cause damage to the roof of the arch or the origin of the branch when passed. Using a 6-Fr cerebral catheter (only limited shapes are available in this caliber) inside a 6-Fr guiding sheath will help to provide a smoother transition.

2. Guiding Catheter. Another method of obtaining access is to place a guiding catheter directly over a selective cerebral catheter. If this method is used, the longer cerebral catheter, usually 5 Fr OD, must be preloaded into the guiding catheter (8 Fr OD). Both the guiding catheter and the selective cerebral catheter are advanced together through an 8-Fr femoral access sheath. The selective cerebral catheter must be long enough that it extends about 20–30 cm beyond the end of the guiding catheter. The guiding catheter is advanced far enough to permit the cerebral catheter to reach and cannulate the common carotid artery. After the cerebral catheter is placed in the external carotid artery, the guiding catheter is advanced directly over the cerebral catheter so that the selective cerebral catheter is used as the dilator or obturator. There is a size mismatch between the two catheters, and there is potential that the tip of the guiding catheter will scrape the arterial wall when it is advanced.

3. Some specialists recommend use of the Arrow guiding sheath (Arrow, Reading, PA) when standard access sheaths kink during passage (1). The arrow sheath is straight but flexible and is wrapped on the outside with corrugated metal rings that articulate. The advantage of this sheath is that it provides very good support to the procedure without kinking. The disadvantage of this sheath is that there is concern that the corrugated metal rings on the surface of the shaft may damage the artery wall, especially at the branch origin at the location of the turn superiorly into the common carotid artery.

4. When the lesion is located in the distal common carotid artery or the external carotid artery is occluded, the external carotid artery may not be available to anchor the guidewire. In this case, consider the following option. Place an Amplatz superstiff guidewire with a 1-cm floppy tip in the distal common carotid artery. Identify the location of the lesion so that the guidewire is not permitted to cross it. Advance the sheath over the guidewire in this location. Use breath holding and a head turn and gradual steady forward pressure on the sheath. Carefully control the guidewire to make sure it does not jump forward or prolapse into the aorta.

Approach to the Arch

Success at sheath placement depends upon anatomy. Once the sheath is safely placed, the likelihood of success of the procedure is significantly enhanced. During the initial arch aortogram, much is learned about a specific arch and what will be required to treat it. During selective catheterization of the arch branches, the maneuvers required are noted so that later intervention can be performed with this knowledge. The selective catheter type used (whether simple curve or complex curve) and knowledge of the amount of effort required to cannulate the common carotid artery both facilitate an in-depth assessment. In general, if the common carotid artery is difficult to cannulate or if a complex curve catheter, such as a Simmons or a Vitek, is required, the curves that the sheath must traverse will be challenging. The branches of the external carotid artery are also evaluated with consideration toward anchoring the stiff guidewire in the longest branch available. The straightest external carotid artery branch is not always the best since the guidewire will anchor better if there is some curvature at its tip. In addition, be on the lookout for major collaterals between the occipital artery and the vertebral system. If this communication is present, use a different external carotid artery branch. The path between femoral access and the carotid lesion is about curves in opposing directions. The sheath must cross any aortoiliac tortuosity that is present. There is a major turn from the patient's left side to the right side as the sheath enters the arch. The degree of curvature required for the final turn superiorly into the common carotid artery often determines whether the access is possible. There will be stress on the system because of turns already made. A simple turn superiorly is easier to cross than a major switchback from right to left.

Arch anatomy is divided into segments that correlate with the level of difficulty of access placement (Fig. 1 of Chap. 2). The peak of the inner curve of the aortic arch acts as a fulcrum over which the sheath must be placed to enter all arteries in segment III and some arteries in segment II, such as arteries originating in segment IIb (Fig. 4). This fulcrum point tends to be higher in the patient's chest when the arch is elongated and tends to be lower in normals and patients with a slightly wider arch caliber. This fulcrum is significant in negotiating turns for arteries that have their origins in segments II and III.

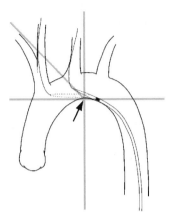

Fig. 4 The inner curve of the arch acts as a fulcrum (arrow). The guiding sheath must pass over the inner curve or "floor" of the arch of the aorta. Gaining access to arch branches which are in segments II or III require sheath passage over this fulcrum.

Sheath placement usually follows a fairly straight pathway for arteries that originate in segment I (Table 6). The left subclavian artery usually originates in segment I and the left common carotid artery sometimes does. Segment II is more challenging than segment I. Factors that influence access in segment II include the width of the arch of the aorta and the distance to the right of the midline of the arch. When the left common carotid artery or the innominate artery originates in segment II, the further toward the patient's right side and the narrower the arch, the more difficult it may be to place the sheath. The deep part of segment II to the patient's right side and inferiorly is denoted IIb. The vertical distance between the peak of the inner curve of the arch and the origin of the artery for treatment becomes an important working feature. This distance can be increased temporarily by having the patient take a deep breath at a crucial time, such as during sheath passage. As discussed above, the more pronounced these anatomic features are, the more the approaching sheath must corner two oppositely oriented

Table 6 Considerations for Different Arch Segments

	Anatomy	Catheter	Considerations
Segment I	Superior to fulcrum Left side of arch	Simple curve	Straightest path to carotid Easiest to maneuver
Segment II	Superior to fulcrum Right side of arch	Simple curve	Distance to right is important Width of arch is important Work against fulcrum More challenging than segment 1
Segment III	Inferior to fulcrum Right side of arch	Complex curve	Distance to right is important Distance inferior to fulcrum Work over fulcrum Most challenging, may be impossible

turns, one to the patients right (to get over the arch) and one superiorly or even back toward the patient's left (to get up the common carotid artery). The higher the fulcrum, or the inner curve of the aortic arch, the tighter the turning radius the sheath must make. With each turn, the radial force applied to the guidewire by the advancing sheath tends to withdraw the guidewire from the external carotid artery. Arteries that have their origins in segment III may be very difficult or impossible to access with a sheath. In segment III, the origin of the artery is inferior to the fulcrum of the aortic arch. The further into segment III a vessel originates, the more the course of the sheath approximates two successive 180° hairpin turns. Some arch anatomy or disease is severe enough that access is contraindicated due to the risk of arterial injury or embolization. Descriptions of alternative access methods for the carotid artery are described (2–5).

Troubleshooting the Access

1. The selective catheter pulls out of external carotid artery when the Amplatz superstiff guidewire is advanced. Remove the Amplatz guidewire. Replace the steerable Glidewire and advance the selective catheter back into the external carotid artery. Road-map the external carotid artery and find the best branch for anchoring the guidewire. It is not always the longest branch. Sometimes it is better to place the catheter in a curved branch so that its end is somewhat coiled. Advance the catheter as far into the branch as it will go. Place the Amplatz guidewire again. If no success, exchange the selective cerebral catheter for a stiffer catheter. For example, if an angled taper Glidecath was used to select the carotid, consider exchanging out for a stiffer nylon catheter.

2. Advancement of the sheath pulls the Amplatz guidewire out of the external carotid artery. Back the sheath off if it is not already into the common carotid artery. Replace the Amplatz guidewire in the external carotid artery and bury the guidewire as far as possible into the external carotid artery. Consider using a superstiff guidewire with a very short floppy tip. Survey the course of the guidewire. Take the slack out of the Amplatz superstiff guidewire before advancing the sheath again. Find the segment of the Amplatz guidewire with the tightest radius of curvature. This is usually the turn from the arch into the innominate or common carotid artery, and this is usually the turn which the sheath cannot make and which causes the guidewire to be withdrawn from the external carotid artery. Turn the patient's head to the side to see if this maneuver helps to straighten the guidewire. If not, turn to the other side. Rotating the neck toward one side or the other will often favorably alter the anatomy. Have the patient take a deep breath and observe the guidewire to see if this maneuver helps to straighten the guidewire. This tends to elongate and straighten the arch branches and makes some angles less acute while depressing the arch of the aorta inferiorly in the chest. A combination of these maneuvers can then be used as the sheath is advanced again. The potential benefits of these maneuvers at straightening the course for sheath placement can be estimated by surveying the guidewire with fluoroscopy. Another ma-

neuver to consider in this situation is to exchange the Amplatz guidewire for a Nitinol guidewire (Microvena) which is smooth but almost impossible to kink once it reaches body temperature. As a last resort, palpate the location of the guidewire on the patient's scalp or face and manually compress the tissue at this location to pin the guidewire in place as the sheath is being advanced.

3. The sheath meets with high resistance during advancement. Do not push against high resistance. Stop and reevaluate. Check the guidewire for kinks. Look for the possibility of any anatomic obstruction. If there is concern that

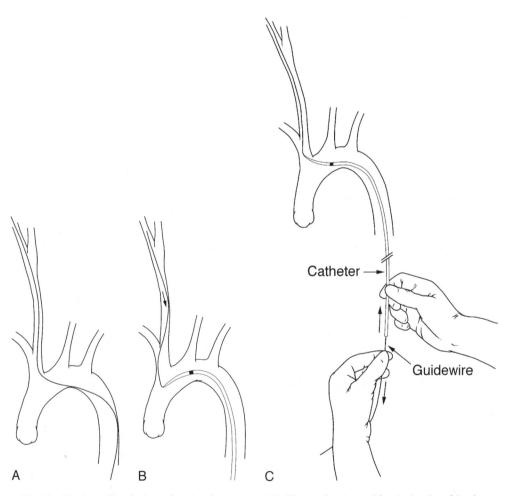

Fig. 5 Push–pull technique for sheath passage. (A) The anchoring guidewire is placed in the external carotid artery. (B) The tip of the sheath tends to prolapse into the ascending aorta and pull the guidewire out of the carotid artery since the turn superiorly is too tight. (C) The sheath is backed off slightly and the guidewire is straightened. As the sheath is pushed again, traction on the guidewire is increased just a little. This permits the guidewire to be well pinned but also pulls the guidewire out just a little bit. This seems to help the sheath slide along the guidewire the few extra centimeters required to make it into the carotid artery.

the tip of the sheath is catching on a plaque or an atherosclerotic ledge, place a catheter over the guidewire and pass it through the area to see if it catches. Make sure the guidewire is in the right place before the larger access sheath is placed over it. Reevaluate tortuosity of the iliac arteries and infrarenal aorta. If there is a lot of tortuosity in this area, by the time these turns are made, the turns in the arch are more difficult to make because of the torque on the whole system. If this is the case, place a 30–45 cm sheath across this area and into the infrarenal aorta that is 1- or 2-Fr sizes larger than the carotid access sheath. Then place the carotid access sheath through it.

4.   The sheath tip is within a few centimeters of the vessel origin but will not advance. This is usually because the overall torque in the system is high after too many turns. Some of the maneuvers mentioned above can be used. Consider pulling the guidewire back steadily and slowly for a few centimeters as the sheath is simultaneously advanced. This is the push–pull technique and it may help to smooth out the crucial curve in the guidewire enough to allow sheath passage (Fig. 5). Be careful not to lose guidewire access.

Tips for Carotid Artery Access for Intervention

1.   Line everything up ahead of time.
2.   Make sure everything fits through the sheath you plan to use.
3.   Make sure the guidewire, balloon catheters, and stent deployment catheters are long enough to accommodate the length of the sheath you selected.
4.   Assess the arch by analyzing the anatomy during the planning phase of the case. Anticipate the likely level of challenge posed by the anatomy (especially the arch) in each case and be ready to perform maneuvers to enhance your likelihood of success.
5.   Use the lowest profile sheath possible (usually either 6 or 7 Fr).
6.   Put the sheath in warm saline bath to improve its flexibility. (Be sure that your assistant does not put the Nitinol stent in the same warm saline bath.)
7.   Use the external carotid artery to anchor the guidewire for sheath placement and place the Amplatz guidewire as far into the artery as possible, but do not perforate a distal branch.
8.   Use special maneuvers to help with sheath delivery when they are needed. These include the following; have the patient take a deep breath, turn the patient's head, take slack out of the guidewire, compress the guidewire tip along the face or scalp, use a very short floppy tip on the superstiff guidewire, and use the push–pull technique.
9.   Do not perform mechanical dilation of the carotid lesion with the tip of the dilator when the sheath is advanced. Withdraw the dilator slightly if needed.
10.   Do not force the sheath.
11.   Watch the guidewire tip as the sheath is advanced so the sheath is not permitted to pull the guidewire out of the external carotid artery.

References

1. Myla S. Carotid access techniques: An algorithmic approach. Carotid Interv 2001; 3:2–12.
2. Dietrich EB. Techniques of carotid artery stenting. In: Criado FJ, ed. Endovascular Intervention: Basic Concepts and Techniques. Armonk, NY: Futura Publishing, 1999:145–161.
3. Al-Mubarak N, Vitek JJ, Iyer SS, et al. Carotid stenting with distal balloon protection via the transbrachial approach. J Endovasc Ther 2001; 8:571–575.
4. Houdart E, Mounayer C, Chapot R, et al. Catheter modication for easier cannulation of the common carotid artery during angioplasty and stenting. J Endovasc Ther 2001; 8:579–582.
5. Dangas G, Laird JR, Mehran R, et al. Carotid artery stenting in patients with high-risk anatomy for carotid endarterectomy. J Endovasc Ther 2001; 8:44–45.

7

Patient Selection for Carotid Interventions: Anatomical and Comorbid Factors

ROBERT B. McLAFFERTY and KIM J. HODGSON

Southern Illinois University School of Medicine, Springfield, Illinois, U.S.A.

The purpose of this chapter is to provide guidelines for selecting patients best suited to carotid angioplasty and stent placement. Optimal patient selection remains paramount to a beneficial outcome during carotid intervention by endovascular methods, as it may be the best means of preventing complications in the first place. Meticulous technique and attention to detail are deserved for all endoluminal interventions, but for carotid intervention particularly, breaches in technique or pushing the "anatomical envelope" risks neurological disaster. While the technical challenges may be commensurate with those of other vessels, the unforgiving nature of the brain compared to other end organs mandates a choreographed procedure meticulously performed. Although endoluminal rescue procedures to ameliorate neurological sequelae from a carotid intervention can be employed, these options are extremely limited and outcomes less reliable when compared to those available to correct endovascular complications in the peripheral vascular tree.

Increasing knowledge as to what types of patients are most safely suited for carotid intervention will minimize complications. While some patient-selection criteria are unique to endoluminal intervention, other conditions make the patient high risk whether undergoing an endoluminal or operative intervention. Herein, four fundamental areas are addressed to familiarize the endovascular specialist with optimal patient selection for carotid angioplasty and stent placement. These include patient comorbidities, local arterial access issues, aortic arch anatomy and pathology, and carotid artery anatomy and pathology.

Patient Comorbidities

Several medical conditions may preclude a patient from undergoing a safe endovascular carotid intervention. None of these conditions are absolute and, depending on the clinical scenario, any of them may be mitigated by other circumstances. First and foremost, patients being assessed for carotid intervention need to be neurologically stable. Patients with stroke in evolution, somnolence, or depressed mental status, who are unable to follow commands or cannot lie still due to agitation or confusion, should not undergo endovascular carotid intervention. The use of intravenous sedation or narcotics should be minimized during carotid intervention to allow close monitoring for focal and nonfocal neurological symptoms. Additionally, the patient must follow commands in order to optimize fluoroscopic technique. These include keeping the head still in certain positions, refraining from swallowing, and holding respiration during digital subtraction arteriography. These maneuvers allow for detailed visualization of the aortic arch and carotid arteries—an absolute necessity in performing safe carotid intervention.

Patients with severely compromised pulmonary status, whether acute or chronic, who cannot lie flat on the fluoroscopy table due to shortness of breath will not tolerate carotid intervention. After maximizing pulmonary toilet, patients thought to be borderline can undergo simple bedside testing in a fully supine position for 30 min. The development of anxiety, increased respiratory rate, and oxygen desaturation may be harbingers of difficulty in completing a carotid intervention.

Severe chronic renal insufficiency may proscribe a patient from undergoing carotid intervention. Although most patients with only a mild elevation of serum creatinine will tolerate carotid intervention, patients with levels greater than 3.0 mg/dL are at risk of temporary or permanent contrast nephropathy. Intravenous hydration, in advance of the intervention, remains the mainstay of prevention (1). Nonionic contrast load can be further limited by performing a diagnostic carotid arteriogram as a separate procedure prior to carotid intervention. The standard preintervention carotid arteriogram, which functions as a confirmatory study to a previous duplex scan or MRA, includes defining aortic arch anatomy with nonselective catheterization in the left anterior oblique projection combined with selective catheterization of both common carotid arteries viewed in multiple projections. In the absence of renal insufficiency, however, intervention can be carried out at the time of the diagnostic angiogram. Other measures to prevent contrast nephropathy may include the oral administration of *n*-acetylcysteine (mucomyst) prior to intervention, or intravenous fenoldepam during and following intervention (2,3). Present studies proposing the use of fenoldepam for the prevention of contrast nephropathy have not demonstrated any benefits (3).

Patients known to develop severe hypertension recalcitrant to medical therapy may be at very high risk for complications during and after endovascular carotid intervention. The development of coronary, pulmonary, and neurological sequelae from persistent malignant hypertension may hamper safe completion of the procedure. Some have noted that the combination of severe hypertension in women with aortic arch tortuosity and a heavily calcified carotid artery bifurcation carries a prohibitive risk of carotid intervention (4). Although patients with severe hypertension are also at high risk during operative intervention, control of pulmonary and circulatory status during general anesthesia in the operating room is usually simpler than with a conscious patient in a catheterization laboratory.

Patients who are allergic to antiplatelet agents or at high risk of hemorrhagic complications from prolonged antiplatelet therapy should not undergo endovascular carotid intervention. These drugs include aspirin, ADP receptor blocking agents such as Ticlid or Plavix, and glycoprotein IIb/IIIa inhibitors such as Abciximab. Most often patients are pretreated with aspirin and Plavix prior to carotid intervention, and this combination therapy is continued for an additional 3 to 6 months following the procedure. Examples of medical conditions rendering the patient at high risk for hemorrhage during dual antiplatelet therapy include intracranial hemorrhage within one year of the intervention, active peptic ulcer disease, or other recent problems causing gastrointestinal hemorrhage.

Local Arterial Access

The overwhelming majority of carotid interventions are performed through common femoral artery access, with the brachial artery approach being utilized for most others. Technical challenges with the former relate primarily to long working distances, ranging between 70 and 100 cm from the site of access to the target lesion. Significant iliac artery tortuosity, with or without stenosis, compromises the responsive movement of guidewires and catheters and the precise placement of angioplasty balloons and stents. Recently developed monorail balloon/stent designs (rapid exchange systems) promise to minimize movement of guidewires and antiembolic filters during the intervention, which can be problematic because of the short working distances from the carotid bifurcation to the carotid artery siphon. Giving due consideration to local access and related issues will facilitate a safe carotid intervention.

Patients who are morbidly obese or have a large abdominal pannus may present a formidable challenge, even after successful common femoral artery access. Guidewire and catheter torque response can be hampered in these patients. Additionally, these patients are at high risk of local bleeding complications (hematoma and/or pseudo-aneurysm formation) secondary to increased difficulties in compressing the arterial puncture site in these patients who are also on maximal antiplatelet therapy. When common femoral artery bleeding does occur in a morbidly obese patient, the hematoma is often much larger due to delayed identification of the problem because of difficulties in detection. In combination with a fragile cardiopulmonary status, significant blood loss from the common femoral artery can be catastrophic. In cases with highly unfavorable iliofemoral access opportunities, the brachial approach may be considered. Access via the brachial artery presents technical challenges for even the experienced endovascular specialist. Optimal patient selection depends on whether arterial branch angles of the aortic arch and great vessels can be safely negotiated. Generally, brachial artery access contralateral to the carotid artery intended for intervention provides for the minimal amount of acute branch angles.

Aortic Arch Anatomy and Pathology

Whereas traversing a diseased iliac system has its risks and challenges, the pathway to the carotid via the aortic arch is where the risks begin to include stroke, the very condition the intervention is intended to prevent. Assessing the suitability of the aortic arch and brachiocephalic vessels requires evaluation of the shape and curvature of the arch, position of origin of the great vessels on the arch, identification of aberrant anatomy, and evaluation of the degree of great vessel atherosclerotic disease, calcification, and tortuosity. All of these factors must be taken into account to maximize safe and stable negotiation of guidewires and catheters into the desired position in the common carotid arteries and their branches. At this stage of carotid intervention, the experience of the endovascular specialist plays an important role in determining which patients are safe to dilate from the standpoint of the difficulty imposed by the aortic arch anatomy and pathology.

Shape, curvature, and origin of the great vessels originating from the aortic arch can be categorized into one of three levels of difficulty. Determining the level of the aortic arch depends on the position of the left subclavian artery. This vessel becomes an anchor as the aortic arch elongates from increasing age, hypertension, and/or disease of the aortic valve. The general shape of the arch can be determined from a high-quality nonselective arteriogram of the aortic arch viewed in the left anterior oblique position. A horizontal line is drawn through the highest point of the aortic arch. Each level of aortic arch difficulty depends on the position of the innominate artery and left common carotid artery in relation to the horizontal line. In a Level I aortic arch, the great vessels arise along the horizontal line. A Level II aortic arch is present if the origin of the great vessel that must be traversed for carotid intervention lies within three common carotid artery diameters below the horizontal line. Likewise, a great vessel lying greater than three common carotid artery diameters below the horizontal line designates a Level III aortic arch. This general categorization of aortic arch shape is reviewed in Chap. 2. Fig. 1 shows Level I, II, and III aortic arches. With each increase in aortic arch level comes escalating technical challenges and risk of complications, as the coaxial transfer of energy during catheter direction and exchange becomes increasingly difficult. Complications and their inherent sequelae include arterial embolization, perforation, dissection, occlusion, stroke, and intracranial hemorrhage.

Some variations in the anatomic configuration of the arch and the origins of the great vessels are relatively common. A (pure) bovine arch, whereby the origin of the left common carotid artery arises from the innominate artery, occurs in 8–10% of indi-

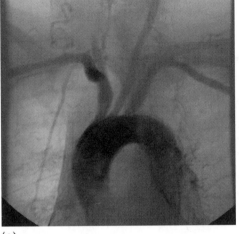

(a)

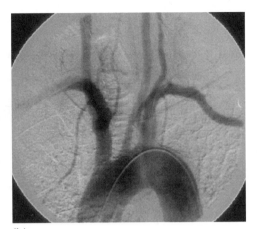

(b)

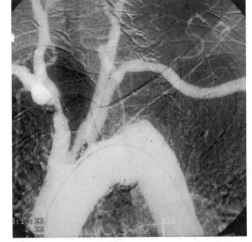

(c)

Fig. 1 The three arteriograms illustrate Level I, II, and III aortic arches. Each increasing level represents more difficulty in accessing the great vessels and maintaining catheter stability by endovascular means. This information is of value for assessing the overall shape of the aortic arch and may be supplemented by using the "surf and turf" classification for segmental arch anatomy described in Chapter 2.

viduals. The anatomic configuration in which the innominate artery and left common carotid artery share a common origin occurs in approximately 15% of individuals. Pure bovine arches present more technical challenges and difficulty gaining and maintaining stable access. If the angle of the left common carotid artery is severely acute to the aortic arch, a right brachial artery access may be warranted. Although many anatomic variations of the great vessels may be accessible, accomplishing this safely and expeditiously is heavily dependent on the experience and skill of the endovascular specialist. Thus, patient selection is dependent on a consistent and realistic impression of one's skills coupled with an understanding of the incremental difficulties that various anatomic features will impart to the procedure.

Other factors involving the aortic arch that may limit patient selection for carotid intervention include the presence of severe aortic calcification ("eggshell aorta"), evidence of extensive diffuse aortic wall irregularity ("shaggy aorta"), and ostial stenosis of innominate or left common carotid arteries. An eggshell aorta presents risks for intimal disruption and embolism because of the lack of compliance while directing guidewires and catheters. This inability of the vessels to move in line also decreases the "torque ability" of catheters and guidewires used to gain access and perform an intervention. A patient with a shaggy aorta is at very high risk of massive atheroembolism, often from locations that put the cerebrum at risk. Although this type of atherosclerotic disease in the aorta remains rare, the presence of loose feathery atherosclerotic debris can cause catastrophic distal embolism to the viscera and lower extremities, often leading to death.

Patients with atherosclerotic ostial stenosis of the innominate right common carotid and left common carotid arteries will require endovascular angioplasty and possible stenting prior to their carotid bifurcation intervention. Occasionally, the extent of proximal disease may preclude a safe carotid intervention. Examples may include stenotic lesions with atherosclerotic disease that appears soft or pedunculated, severe calcified stenotic lesions not responsive to angioplasty and stenting, and long diffuse stenoses involving the entire length of the common carotid artery.

Carotid Artery Anatomy and Pathology

A variety of anatomical and pathological conditions of the carotid bifurcation influence the technical challenges, risks, and overall efficacy of the procedure. Emphasis should be placed on the specific performance characteristics of the guidewires, angioplasty catheters, stent delivery systems, and embolization protection systems utilized. In combination, the particular mix of factors composing each intervention dictates that each procedure is unique, although common challenges and issues prevail. Just as features of the aortic arch anatomy and disease impact on establishing a stable catheter position in the common carotid artery, bifurcation issues significantly impact on lesion crossing, need for predilatation, and ability to use one of the embolic protection devices.

Particularly problematic is tortuosity of the internal carotid artery (Fig. 2), which, if severe enough, may limit the ability to effectively perform carotid intervention. Marked acute angulation and ectasia, particularly within several centimeters distal to the stenotic lesion, leave little working distance between an embolic carotid protection device and deployment of a stent. Additionally, some embolic carotid protection devices may not have complete arterial wall apposition when opened across a guidewire whose position in the vessel deviates from the center coaxial line, as is often the case in tortuous segments. Kinks are often seen at the distal terminus of a carotid plaque, with or without

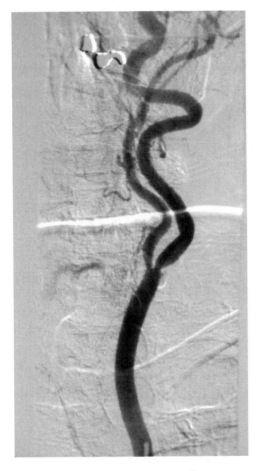

Fig. 2 The carotid arteriogram illustrates a very tortuous internal carotid artery (arrow). Depending on the proximity of the tortuous segment to the carotid stenosis, this may preclude a patient from having a carotid stent placed.

tortuosity. Predicting the conformational change that the stented lesion will undergo can be exceedingly problematic, as kinks can easily be translated to other segments of a tortuous artery in the process of treating the primary lesion.

Other conditions that may preclude patients from being selected for carotid intervention are related to their inherently high risk for embolism or thrombosis. These include the presence of an internal carotid artery "string sign," a carotid artery luminal filling defect on arteriogram indicating the possibility of acute thrombus, a soft, pedunculated-appearing stenotic lesion, severe carotid artery bifurcation calcification, and occlusion of the external carotid artery (which requires large unprotected guidewire crossing of the internal carotid lesion in order to obtain sheath position in the common carotid artery). These types of lesions may be more safely treated by carotid endarterectomy, where embolization is minimized by clamping the arteries proximally and distally prior to disrupting the plaque. Stenoses so severe that they impede passage of an embolization protection device require unprotected predilatation so that subsequent passage can occur with the least possible plaque resistance. This predilatation is usually only to 3 mm in diameter, just enough to clear a pathway for the filter device, yet not so much as to likely produce a large embolic shower. Similarly, discrete tandem lesions in both the common and internal carotid arteries that require separate dilatation and stents are at increase risk of embolization.

Summary

Minimizing complications and improving outcome during endovascular carotid intervention remains heavily dependent on how patients are selected to undergo the procedure. Addressing the four fundamental topics covered in this chapter in a comprehensive manner will provide the endovascular specialist with a basic foundation upon which to build. The learning curve in carotid intervention begins after guidewire and catheter skills are mastered in other parts of the arterial-venous tree. After that point, patient selection for the beginner in carotid intervention may be vastly different from that of the expert. Patients with minimal complicating features, as outlined in this chapter, are best suited for the beginner, while more complex patient scenarios are better suited for the endovascular specialist who has performed a large number of carotid interventions. The combination of the patient's clinical resume and the physician's experience truly dictate how a patient is selected. Knowing when not to perform an endovascular carotid intervention may be one of the greatest signs of experience.

References

1. Solomon R, Werner C, Mann D, D'Elia J, Silva P. Effects of saline, mannitol, and furosemide in renal function induced by radiocontrast agents. N Engl J Med 1994; 331(21): 1416–1420.
2. Tepel M, van der Giet M, Schwarzfeld C, Laufer U, Liermann D, Zidek W. Prevention of radiographic-contrast-induced-agent reductions in renal function by acetylcysteine. N Engl J Med 2000; 343(3):180–184.
3. Chu VL, Cheng JW. Fenodepam in the prevention of contrast media-induced acute renal failure. Ann Pharmacother 2001; 35(10):1278–1282.
4. Case selection for carotid stenting. In: Subbarao M, ed. Carotid Stent: Train the Teacher Program Manual. Hoag Heart and Vascular Institute, 2003.

8

Periprocedural Management of Patients Undergoing Carotid Interventions

W. TODD BOHANNON

Texas Tech University, Lubbock, Texas, U.S.A.

PETER A. SCHNEIDER

Hawaii Permanente Medical Group, Honolulu, Hawaii, U.S.A.

The purpose of this chapter is to discuss the perioperative management of patients undergoing carotid stent placement and other brachiocephalic interventions. The strategies for anticoagulation, treatment of procedural hemodynamic changes, and access management are described. Follow-up care and surveillance are discussed. The setup of the endovascular operating room for carotid stent placement is described in Chap. 3. The technical aspects of the carotid stenting procedure are outlined in Chaps. 9, 10, and 11. The preferences of these surgeons for perioperative management techniques are detailed in these chapters. The strategy and pharmacology of managing peri-procedural neurological complications are detailed in Chap. 14. As with most vascular procedures, if the patient is well selected and the procedure planned and conducted appropriately, the perioperative course is usually smooth and the outcome acceptable. Nevertheless, carotid stenting can be made safer and less stressful with a commonsense approach to patient care at the time of the procedure.

Before the Case

We prefer to perform an arch aortogram and selective carotid arteriogram as a separate procedure before the carotid stent operation. This study is essential in assessing and planning carotid access and evaluating the lesion and the cervical internal carotid artery and the intracranial vascular anatomy. Arch assessment is presented in Chap. 2. This approach permits the opportunity to study the case and its nuances before the day of the carotid stent placement. Patient selection is discussed in Chap. 7. Arteriography is an essential tool in patient selection for carotid stenting. This requirement may decrease later as experience is gained, but at present, it is useful. A thorough and documented neurological exam is essential, especially if an untoward cerebral event occurs in the perioperative period. Specific practice guidelines for carotid stenting in your vascular department helps to make the indications for the new procedure clear to all involved. Informed consent for a new procedure is likewise a sensitive issue. The opportunity to do this with as much information available as possible is desirable.

Strategy for Anticoagulation and Antiplatelet Agents

ORAL ANTIPLATELET AGENTS

The periprocedural administration of antiplatelet agents is an essential component of the carotid stenting procedure. When clopidogrel was compared with aspirin in patients at risk of ischemic events (CAPRIE), an 8% to 10% relative risk reduction of ischemic stroke, myocardial infarction, or vascular death was demonstrated in patients taking 75 mg of clopidogrel daily (1). Clopidogrel has a slower onset of action compared to aspirin, and patients should take clopidogrel for an appropriate period before angioplasty and stenting. Clopidogrel, or Plavix (75 mg by mouth per day), is administered for 5 days before the procedure, and then for 4 to 6 weeks afterward.

Most data accumulated for adjunctive antiplatelet therapy and angioplasty and stenting have been associated with the treatment of coronary occlusive disease. Combined antiplatelet therapy with aspirin and clopidogrel has been associated with a low rate of ischemic events (2). However, few practitioners advise both aspirin and Plavix for carotid stent placement. In additional, there may be some disadvantage as aspirin has been found in some studies to inhibit the actions of thrombolytic agents (3). Ticlopidine (Ticlid) is an alternative for those who cannot take clopidogel. If patients were not treated with Plavix for several days prior to the procedure, administer 300 mg in a single dose before the procedure.

HEPARIN

Heparin is administered prior to catheterizing the common carotid artery, usually after access is obtained. The usual dose is 100 units per kilogram. Some surgeons prefer a set dose, such as 5000 or 10,000 units. The activated coagulation time (ACT) is used to guide heparin administration. A goal ACT of 250 to 300 sec is achieved prior to intervention. The dosage of heparin should be reduced (75 units per kilogram) when glycoprotein IIb/IIIa receptor inhibitors are used. Heparin doses are repeated through the procedure as necessary. However, it has been our experience that with a half-life of 90 min, the case is completed before the anticoagulant effect of the first dose has substantially diminished. The distal protection device has usually been retrieved within 1 hr of administering the initial heparin bolus. Heparin is usually not continued after the procedure.

Angiomax (bivalirudin) is preferred by some surgeons and it is a reasonable alternative in patients that cannot tolerate heparin. Angiomax is a direct thrombin inhibitor with a half-life of 25 min. Angiomax is monitored with the ACT. A bolus of 1 mg/kg is given intravenously followed by an infusion of 0.2 mg/kg per hour. The effect of Angiomax is prolonged in patients with renal insufficiency.

IIB/IIIA INHIBITORS

Platelet aggregation is mediated by the binding of fibrinogen to the platelet glycoprotein integrin IIb/IIIa. Platelet glycoprotein IIb/IIIa receptor inhibitors have been successful in reducing ischemic complications in coronary artery angioplasty and stenting (4–8). The antiplatelet effects of abciximab (ReoPro, Centocor, Malvern, PA), tirofiban (Aggrastat, Merck & Co., Whitehouse Station, NJ) and eptifibatide (Integrilin, COR Therapeutics, San Francisco, CA) are similar at the currently recommended dosages for treatment of coronary artery disease with coronary stenting (9). These agents are administered intravenously as a bolus followed by a constant infusion.

While some reports have supported the routine use of glycoprotein IIb/IIIa inhibitors to reduce ischemic complications associated with carotid angioplasty and stenting (10–12), others have found either no benefit or higher complication rates associated with IIb/IIIa use (13–15). Wholey et al. reviewed 550 patients who underwent carotid angioplasty and stent placement and compared those who received IIb/IIIa inhibitors and those receiving heparin alone (15). The stroke and death rate was significantly higher in those receiving glycoprotein IIb/IIIa inhibitors compared to heparin alone (6.0% vs. 2.4%; $p = 0.04$). Two of the four neurologic deaths were due to intracerebral hemorrhage. Hofmann and colleagues demonstrated no reduction in ischemic complications with bolus Abciximab administered before carotid artery angioplasty and stenting (13). In another study comparing abciximab and heparin during carotid stent placement, 5% of abciximab patients developed intracerebral hemorrhage vs. none in the heparin group (14).

Routine use of glycoprotein IIb/IIIa inhibitors does not appear to be necessary, and may increase the risk of cerebral or access sites hemorrhagic events. IIb/IIIa inhibitors may be a useful adjunct in selected patients. Perioperative intravenous administration of glycoprotein IIb/IIIa inhibitors should be considered in the following circumstances: patients who are actively having symptoms from their carotid lesion, patients who did not have an appropriate preoperative loading of clopidogrel, patients with severe intracranial occlusive disease, and patients with highly ulcerated carotid bifurcation lesions. When IIb/IIIa inhibitors are administered, the dose of heparin should be decreased (75 units/kg).

Intraoperative glycoprotein IIb/IIIa inhibitors have also been administered intra-arterially in the same manner that a thrombolytic agent might be. Situations where thrombus formation is developing within the stent or the patient has sustained a distal embolus have been treated by some experts using a direct catheter infusion of Reopro (16,17).

Strategy for Procedure-Related Hemodynamic Changes

GENERAL HEMODYNAMIC CONSIDERATIONS

During balloon dilatation, and occasionally with passage of the cerebral protection device, it is quite common for abrupt hemodynamic changes to occur (18–20). Monitoring by anesthesia personnel is absolutely essential to successful carotid stenting. An arterial monitoring line is used on every case. Many of the patients currently considered candidates for carotid stent placement have underlying cardiac problems with limited tolerance for profound hemodynamic changes, especially if hemodynamic alterations are not reversed immediately. Because of the possibility of hypotension and bradycardia, underlying hypertension during the early part of the case is usually not treated too aggressively. Mild sedation often improves severe hypertension. If treatment of hypertension is required, it is better to treat with short-acting vasodilators than with beta-blockers. If a distal occlusion balloon is intended for cerebral protection, maintaining the blood pressure above 140 mm Hg may be desirable. Filter usage also depends on brisk forward flow since the filter may fill with debris. Therefore, induced hypotension prior to cerebral protection device deployment and balloon dilatation and stent placement should be avoided. Once the stent has been placed and there is continuous stretching of the carotid bulb, it is less common for hypertension to persist that requires treatment. In this sense, hemodynamic management of the carotid stent patient is quite a bit different than a carotid endarterectomy patient.

HEART RATE

The most common sudden change in hemodynamics is bradycardia due to stimulation of the carotid bulb. During endarterectomy, it is not unusual for some bradycardia to occur during manipulation of the bifurcation, causing the surgeon to pause intermittently during the dissection or to administer lidocaine into the area around the bulb. By the time the bifurcation is opened, the bulb has usually been denervated. It is rare for carotid endarterectomy to induce profound or sustained bradycardia. In the case of carotid stenting, the innervation to the carotid bulb remains intact. Bradycardia is common and may be severe or prolonged. Hypotension occurs as a result of the bradycardia. Dilatation of the carotid bifurcation may also cause a sinus pause so lengthy that the patient is functionally asystolic.

During the early era of carotid stent placement, many advocated pacemaker placement prior to the procedure. When temporary venous pacemakers were implanted in a series of patients prior to carotid stent placement, 62% of patients experienced some pacer firing at the time of stent placement (19). This approach has its own set of complications and in one series was responsible for a death due to pacer wire perforation of the myocardium (21). Pacemaker capability should be immediately available, either transvenous or external, but pacemaker insertion should be reserved for special cases. If bradycardia is treated promptly, it is rare for pacing of the myocardium to be required. The administration of atropine (0.5 to 1.0 mg) prior to balloon dilatation usually prevents or at least blunts the bradycardia. Since tachycardia may also cause problems, we usually administer the smaller dose (0.5 mg) and usually give it within 1 min of the inflation of the balloon. Among patients with baseline bradycardia or who are on beta-blockers or digoxin, a dramatic tachycardia in response to atropine is rarely observed. In addition, the bradycardic response to balloon dilatation may be more profound than that observed in other patients. Therefore, in these patients, we usually administer the larger dose of atropine (1.0 mg). Patients who have recurrent stenosis have had the carotid bifurcation denervated during the previous carotid operation. In our experience, it is uncommon for these patients to develop severe bradycardia. Therefore, we do not usually treat these patients with atropine prior to balloon angioplasty, but the atropine is drawn up and is ready for administration if needed. Patients with indwelling pacemakers obviously do not need a vagolytic agent so atropine is not given. However these patients do occasionally develop hypotension that requires treatment.

BLOOD PRESSURE

Sometimes with balloon angioplasty, and especially after the stent is placed, hypotension occurs that is more severe than can be accounted for by the bradycardia alone. The bradycardia is treated first, usually with atropine. A fluid bolus should be considered since dehydration tends to make all the hemodynamic swings a little worse than they otherwise would be. Not uncommonly, a vasopressor is required for a time during the case and in the immediate postoperative period. We usually use Neosynephrine to maintain a systolic pressure of 100 mm Hg or higher. If the patient is symptomatic at this level of blood pressure (due to lack of cerebral or myocardial perfusion), then higher blood pressures are induced. After the case it is unusual for pressors to be required for more than a few hours. Rarely, a patient will require vasopressors for 24 hr or more (18). Occasionally, some of the patient's antihypertensive medications must be discontinued and the patient discharged home on a lesser antihypertension regimen. The blood pressure usually returns to preoperative levels within the first couple of weeks after stent placement.

Dramatic and continued hypertension, like that commonly seen around the time of carotid endarterectomy, is less common. When this occurs, however, it should be treated aggressively since carotid stent placement is associated with a higher rate of intracranial hemorrhage in the postoperative period than what is usually seen with carotid endarterectomy. A systolic blood pressure less than 150 mm Hg is desirable. If bradycardia and/or hypotension are going to occur as a result of carotid stent placement, they develop during the procedure. After the procedure, if hypertension is present, it should be treated in a manner similar to that for carotid endarterectomy. Patients with severely elevated baseline blood pressure prior to the procedure are at higher risk for a perioperative neurological event (20).

Neurological Monitoring

Many surgeons prefer that the patient honk a horn intermittently using the hand on the side opposite the carotid stenosis being treated. This provides evidence that the patient is conscious, able to follow commands, and has gross motor function in the upper extremity. It is reasonable to use this tool, but keep in mind that it is only a gross assessment of neurological function. It is quite possible to be evolving a fairly severe stroke and still be able to perform these activities.

Transcranial Doppler has been performed during carotid stenting, and it is known that cerebral emboli do occur and that they correlate with certain events during the procedure (22–25). Emboli occur when the lesion is traversed initially, when predilatation is performed, when the stent is placed, and when the poststent balloon angioplasty is performed. This method of monitoring may be useful for the operator to assess the consequences of certain maneuvers by quantifying TCD "hits." However, TCD does not correlate with clinical findings since most of these emboli are not clinically significant, at least at the time of the case (23,24).

Strategy for Management of Arterial Access Sites

The arterial system can almost always be accessed through the femoral arteries. Most of the time, a right-handed surgeon will access the right common femoral artery and work forehand during the case. However, for the purposes of carotid access, there is probably no difference between the right and left femoral access sites if the pathway is clear. If there is aortic occlusion or bilateral iliac artery occlusion, brachial artery access should be considered. We also do our best to avoid using femoral access when the patient has a significant aortic aneurysm. Use of an exchange guidewire and a large sheath without outflow control is a setup for lower extremity embolization. Aortic and iliac artery tortuosity may also severely compromise the ability to maneuver the catheters and guidewires in the arch. In this case, it is sometimes helpful to use a sheath-within-a-sheath technique to help minimize the affect of the tortuosity. This is done by estimating the distance from the groin that must be crossed to get past the areas of severe tortuosity in the aortoiliac system. Place a larger straight sheath through area (e.g., 45-cm length, 7 or 8 Fr sheath). Then place the carotid access guiding sheath or guiding catheter through the straight sheath already in place.

Brachial access has been used with success for carotid stent placement (26). The distance is shorter, but the angle of approach is usually less favorable. The arch aortogram must be carefully studied to evaluate the potential pathways from the brachial artery to the target carotid artery. Whichever one provides the least acute angle is usually chosen. When treating a right carotid bifurcation stenosis, it may be best to access the left brachial artery and "bounce" the guidewire off the upper inner curve of the aortic arch and then superiorly into the carotid artery. There is usually at least a few centimeters or more of distance along the arch between where the catheter enters the arch from the left subclavian and then exits the arch into the innominate artery. A complex curve catheter is usually required since a complete change in direction at the arch results from this approach. A 65-cm length, C2 cobra or Sos Omni 2 (Angiodynamics) may be useful. A short exchange guidewire, such as Amplatz or Rosen (180-cm length) may be used. Always use graduated dilators at the brachial artery access to avoid tearing the artery. Sheath access may be gained using a Raabe sheath (Cook), either 50 or 70 cm, an up and over sheath (Cook) or a Destination sheath (Medi-Tech). Left carotid stenosis may be approached through either brachial artery using the same techniques. The arch aortogram is studied to pick the route with the least acute angle of approach. The distance between the left common carotid artery and the innominate artery or the left subclavian along the arch may be very short. This makes the approach to the left common carotid artery a 180° hairpin turn. A bovine arch (left common carotid artery origin from the innominate artery) should probably be approached through the right brachial artery.

After the stent is placed and the completion runs of the carotid bifurcation and the intracranial arteries are performed and reviewed, the long carotid access sheath is exchanged for a short, standard-length hemostatic access sheath of the same caliber. After the procedure, some surgeons use a closure device at the femoral access site, such as Perclose (Abbott). When we use a closure device, we prefer to re-prep and drape over the same field using betadine and a new layer of sterile towels. Patients have already received intravenous antibiotics. Others prefer to permit the anticoagulation to dissipate and remove the sheath later, and hold manual pressure at the site. Percutaneous brachial access with a 6 Fr sheath can usually be done safely. If the person is small (such that the brachial artery may be less than 4–5 mm in diameter) or a larger sheath is used, it may be safer to cut down on the artery after the case and stitch it closed. We have not used closure devices on the brachial artery. Complications of access sites are discussed in Chap. 19.

After the Case

The patient is monitored after the procedure, usually until the following day. This permits treatment of hemodynamic changes and neurological monitoring. Intracranial hemorrhage is an uncommon but devastating complication that occurs more frequently after carotid stent placement (3.8% to 5.0%) than after carotid endarterectomy (0.6%) (14,27). This may reflect a hyperperfusion phenomenon and appears to be related to blood pressure changes and use of antithrombotic agents (14,28). In a report of seven patients, five experienced neurologic deterioration within an hour of the procedure (29).

Postprocedure hemodynamic instability due to hypotension, bradycardia, or hypertension is common, and may affect more than three quarters of the patients (18). Some have advocated outpatient carotid stenting (21,30,31). This may be appropriate at some future time. There may be a subset of patients, recurrent stenosis, for example, who have little or no central hemodynamic effect from the procedure and who could be considered for outpatient status in the perioperative period. Most of the time, however, carotid stent recipients are patients with multiple comorbidities who were not good candidates for endarterectomy. In the setting of an investigational procedure, it is probably best to monitor the patients for 24 hr each until more is known.

Blood pressure management is discussed above. Rarely, a longer hospital stay is required because the patient requires continued administration of vasopressors to maintain adequate blood pressure. This resolves on its own with the appropriate level of support. Often, the preoperative antihypertensive regimen must be decreased for discharge. In this case, the patient should be seen within a few days to a week for a blood pressure check.

Plavix (75 mg/day) is continued for 4 to 6 weeks after stent placement. Duplex surveillance is performed in the perioperative period. One option is to perform duplex of the carotid arteries prior to discharge. This is especially useful if the patient lives a long distance from the hospital. The likelihood of demonstrating something on duplex that would require intervention is very low, especially if the patient is stable/asymptomatic from a neurological standpoint and the completion arteriograms were satisfactory. We usually perform duplex within the first 2 weeks of stent placement, then at 6 and 12 months, and then annually. If there is evidence of recurrent stenosis, the frequency of the surveillance studies is increased. This is the same protocol for surveillance we use after carotid endarterectomy. Preliminary data suggest that the rate of recurrent stenosis after carotid stent placement is similar to that which occurs after carotid endarterectomy, ranging from 3% at 12 months to 8% at 18 months (32–34).

The duplex follow-up of arterial stents is complicated by a change in compliance of the artery that is caused by the stent. Some velocity elevation appears to accompany this phenomenon, often without apparent stenosis (35,36). We have observed velocities up to 150 cm/sec without any carotid stenosis, and up to 200 cm/sec with mild stenosis. Although the velocity standards for stenosis associated with a stent have not been completely worked out, the trend in velocity during the follow-up period has some value in guiding the clinician. Our threshold for arteriography includes new neurological symptoms consistent with the side of the stent, progressive elevation of velocity during the surveillance period, demonstration of mobile plaque or thrombus associated with the stent, or an absolute velocity above 300 cm/sec.

Technical Tips

1. Perform an arteriogram as a separate procedure prior to carotid stent placement.
2. Plavix should be taken preprocedure for 5 days if possible.

3. A high-dose load should be considered in patients preprocedure who have not been taking Plavix.

4. IIb/IIIa inhibitors should be used in those patients who cannot or have not taken Plavix.

5. Plavix should be given for at least 4 weeks following stent placement, and aspirin should be taken lifelong.

6. Heparin should be administered to achieve an ACT of >250 sec.

7. IIb/IIIa inhibitors should be reserved for certain high-risk patients, but the heparin dose is usually decreased.

8. Atropine should be given prior to angioplasty of native carotid stenoses to prevent severe bradycardia or even asystole.

9. If hypertension requires treatment during the case, use short-acting vaso-dilators, rather than beta-blockers.

10. A closure device may be considered in CAS patients, particularly when IIb/IIIa inhibitors are used.

References

1. A randomised, blinded, trial of clopidogrel versus aspirin in patients at risk of ischaemic events (CAPRIE). CAPRIE Steering Committee. Lancet 1996; 348:1329–1339.

2. Bhatt DL, Kapadia SR, Bajzer CT, Chew DP, Ziada KM, Mukherjee D, Roffi M, Topol EJ, Yadav JS. Dual antiplatelet therapy with clopidogrel and aspirin after carotid artery stenting. J Invasive Cardiol 2001; 13:767–771.

3. Thomas GR, Thibodeaux H, Erret CJ, Bednar MM, Gross CE, Bennett WF. Intravenous aspirin causes a paradoxical attenuation of cerebrovascular thrombolysis. Stroke 1995; 26:1039–1046.

4. Use of a monoclonal antibody directed against the platelet glycoprotein IIb/IIIa receptor in high-risk coronary angioplasty. The EPIC Investigation. N Engl J Med 1994; 330:956–961.

5. Platelet glycoprotein IIb/IIIa receptor blockade and low-dose heparin during percutaneous coronary revascularization. The EPILOG Investigators. N Engl J Med 1997; 336:1689–1696.

6. Randomised placebo-controlled trial of abciximab before and during coronary intervention in refractory unstable angina: the CAPTURE Study. Lancet 1997; 349:1429–1435.

7. Randomised placebo-controlled and balloon-angioplasty-controlled trial to assess safety of coronary stenting with use of platelet glycoprotein-IIb/IIIa blockade. The EPISTENT Investigators. Evaluation of Platelet IIb/IIIa Inhibitor for Stenting. Lancet 1998; 352:87–92.

8. O'Shea JC, Tcheng JE. Eptifibatide in percutaneous coronary intervention: the ESPRIT Trial results. Curr Interv Cardiol Rep 2001; 3:62–68.

9. Neumann FJ, Hochholzer W, Pogatsa-Murray G, Schomig A, Gawaz M. Antiplatelet effects of abciximab, tirofiban and eptifibatide in patients undergoing coronary stenting. J Am Coll Cardiol 2001; 37:1323–1328.

10. Kapadia SR, Bajzer CT, Ziada KM, Bhatt DL, Wazni OM, Silver MJ, Beven EG, Ouriel K, Yadav JS. Initial experience of platelet glycoprotein IIb/IIIa inhibition with

abciximab during carotid stenting: a safe and effective adjunctive therapy. Stroke 2001; 32:2328–2332.

11. Qureshi AI, Ali Z, Suri MF, Kim SH, Fessler RD, Ringer AJ, Guterman LR, Hopkins LN. Open-label phase I clinical study to assess the safety of intravenous eptifibatide in patients undergoing internal carotid artery angioplasty and stent placement. Neurosurgery 2001; 48:998–1004.

12. Schneiderman J, Morag B, Gerniak A, Rimon U, Varon D, Seligsohn U, Shotan A, Adar R. Abciximab in carotid stenting for postsurgical carotid restenosis: intermediate results. J Endovasc Ther 2000; 7:263–272.

13. Hofmann R, Kerschner K, Steinwender C, Kypta A, Bibl D, Leisch F. Abciximab bolus injection does not reduce cerebral ischemic complications of elective carotid artery stenting: a randomized study. Stroke 2002; 33:725–727.

14. Qureshi AI, Suri MF, Ali Z, Kim SH, Lanzino G, Fessler RD, Ringer AJ, Guterman LR, Hopkins LN. Carotid angioplasty and stent placement: a prospective analysis of peri-operative complications and impact of intravenously administered abciximab. Neuro-surgery 2002; 50:466–473.

15. Wholey MH, Wholey MH, Eles G, Toursakissian B, Bailey S, Jarmolowski C, Tan WA. Evaluation of glycoprotein IIb/IIIa inhibitors in carotid angioplasty and stenting. J Endovasc Ther 2003; 10:33–41.

16. Ho DS, Wang Y, Chui M, Wang Y, Ho SL, Cheung RT. Intracarotid abciximab injection to abort impending ischemic stroke during carotid angioplasty. Cerebrovasc Dis 2001; 11:300–304.

17. Lee KY, Heo JH, Lee SI, Yoon PH. Rescue treatment with abciximab in acute ischemic stroke. Neurology 2001; 56:1585–1587.

18. Qureshi AI, Luft AR, Sharma M, Janardhan V, Lopes DK, Khan J, Guterman LR, Hopkins LN. Frequency and determinants of postprocedural hemodynamic instability after carotid angioplasty and stenting. Stroke 1999; 30:2086–2093.

19. Harrop JS, Sharan AD, Benitez RP, Armonda R, Thomas J, Rosenwasser RH. Prevention of carotid angioplasty-induced bradycardia and hypotension with temporary venous pacemakers. Neurosurgery 2001; 49:814–820.

20. Howell M, Krajcer Z, Dougherty K, Strickman N, Skolkin M, Toombs B, Paniagua D. Correlation of periprocedural systolic blood pressure changes with neurologic events in high-risk carotid stent patients. J Endovasc Ther 2002; 9:810–816.

21. Tan KT, Cleveland TJ, Berczi V, Mckevitt FM, Venables GS, Gaines PA. Timing and frequency of complications after carotid artery stenting: what is the optimal period of observation? J Vasc Surg 2003; 38:236–243.

22. Al-Mubarak N, Roubin GS, Vitek OR, Iyer SS, New G, Leon MB. Effect of distal-balloon protection system on microembolization during carotid stenting. Circulation 2001; 104:1999–2002.

23. Van Heesewijk HP, Vos JA, Louwerse ES, Van Den Berg JC, Overtoom TT, Ernst SM, Mauser HW, Moll FL Ackerstaff RG. New brain lesions at MR imaging after carotid angioplasty and stent placement. Radiology 2002; 224:361–365.

24. Rapp JH, Pan XM, Sharp FR, Shah DM, Wille GA, Velez PM, Troyer A, Higashida RT, Saloner D. Atheroemboli to the brain: size threshold for causing acute neuronal cell death. J Vasc Surg 2000; 32:68–76.

25. Orlandi G, Fanucchi S, Fioretti C, Acerbi G, Puglioli M, Padolecchia R, Sartucci F, Murri L. Characteristics of cerebral microemboli during carotid stenting and angioplasty alone. Arch Neurol 2001; 58:1410–1413.

26. Al-Mubarak N, Vitek JJ, Iyer SS, New G, Roubin GS. Carotid stenting with distal balloon protection via the transbrachial approach. J Endovasc Ther 2001; 8:571–575.

27. Morrish W, Grahovac S, Douen A, Cheung G, Hu W, Farb R, Kalapos P, Wee R, Hudon M, Agbi C, Richard M. Intracranial hemorrhage after stenting and angioplasty of extra-cranial carotid stenosis. Am J Neuroradiol 2000; 21:1911–1916.

28. Pfefferkorn T, Mayer T, Von Struckrad-Barre S, Covi M, Hamman GF. Hyperfusion-induced intracerebral hemorrhage after carotid stenting documented bt TCD. Neurology 2001; 57:1933–1935.

29. Qureshi AI, Saad M, Zaidat OO, Suarez JI, Alexander MJ, Fareed M, Suri K, Ali Z, Hopkins LN. Intracerebral hemorrhages associated with neurointerventional procedures using a combination of antithrombotic agents including abciximab. Stroke 2002; 33:1916–1919.

30. New G, Roubin GS, Iyer SS, Lawrence EJ, Octgen M, Al-Mubarak N, Monssa I, Maser JN, Vitek JJ. Outpatient carotid artery stenting: a case report. J Endovasc Surg 1999; 6:316–318.

31. Zarins CK. Outpatient carotid stenting: feasible, yes, but advisable? J Endovasc Surg 1999; 6:319–320.

32. Chakhtoura EY, Hobson RW, Goldstein J, Simonian GT, Lal BK, Haser PB, Silva MB Jr, Padberg FT Jr, Pappas PJ, Jamil Z. In-stent restenosis after carotid angioplasty-stenting: incidence and management. J Vasc Surg 2001; 33:220–225.

33. Gable DR, Bergamini T, Garrett WV, Hise J, Smith BL, Shutze WP, Pearl G, Grimsley BR. Intermediate follow-up of carotid artery stent placement. Am J Surg 2003; 185:183–187.

34. Willfort-Ehringer A, Ahmadi R, Geschwandtner ME, Haumer M, Lang W, Minar E. Single-center experience with carotid stent restenosis. J Endovasc Ther 2002; 9:299–307.

35. Ringer AJ, German JW, Guterman LR, Hopkins LN. Follow-up of stented carotid arteries by Doppler ultrasound. Neurosurgery 2002; 51:639–643.

36. Lu CJ, Kao HL, Sun Y, Liu HM, Jeng JS, Yip PK, Lee YT. The hemodynamic effects of internal carotid artery stenting: a study with color-coded duplex sonography. Cerebrovasc Dis 2003; 15:264–269.

9

Technique of Carotid Bifurcation Angioplasty and Stent Placement: How We Do It

W. TODD BOHANNON and MICHAEL B. SILVA, JR.

Texas Tech University, Lubbock, Texas, U.S.A.

The purpose of this chapter is to describe, in a stepwise fashion, our technique of carotid angioplasty and stenting (Table 1). Carotid angioplasty and stenting (CAS) requires careful patient selection, counseling, and procedural planning. The potential for devastating neurological complications with CAS makes the treatment of carotid artery stenoses more challenging than angioplasty in other areas of the body (1–9). However, the basic principles of angioplasty and stenting in these arterial beds also apply in the carotid system. Secure arterial access, careful guidewire traversal of the target lesion, and appropriate balloon and stent selection is essential for successful endovascular treatment of all arterial stenoses including those in the extracranial cerebrovasculature.

Sheath Access and Guidewire Positioning

The first challenge in carotid artery interventions is gaining secure assess to the common carotid artery. Depending on the arch anatomy, the positioning of a sheath into the common carotid artery may be the most technically difficult aspect of the procedure.

Table 1 Carotid Angioplasty and Stent Procedure

a. Retrograde CFA puncture with Cournand needle or micropuncture set.
b. Sequential dilation to 7 Fr.
c. Intravenous heparin (70 units/kg).
d. Consider IIb/IIIa inhibitor in high embolic risk patients.
    i. Integrilin: 65 μg/kg IV bolus then 0.25 μg/kg/hr.
    ii. Aggrastat: 0.2 μg/kg IV bolus over 30 min then 0.05 μg/kg/hr.
e. Cannulate aortic arch branch vessels.
    i. With or without arch aortogram (20–30° LAO).
    ii. Angled glide catheter (simple curve) or Simmons (complex curve).
f. Guidewire and angled glide catheter placed in external carotid artery.
g. Exchange length Amplatz superstiff guidewire placed in external carotid artery.
h. Guide sheath (90 cm) in proximal common carotid artery (Shuttle sheath).
    i. Above clavicle.
i. Guidewire crossing of target lesion.
    i. 0.018- or 0.014-inch guidewire with tip of wire in distal ICA.
    ii. Alternatively, position filter wire or occlusion balloon wire.
j. Remove Amplatz guidewire.
k. Carotid angiogram through guide sheath to delineate stenosis.
l. Atropine 0.5 to 1.0 mg IV before PTA.
m. PTA with 3- or 4-mm balloon.
    i. Aspirate sheath with 30-mL syringe as balloon deflates.
n. Carotid angiogram to assess PTA results.
o. Stent placement.
p. Assess need for poststent dilatation.
q. Remove sheath once ACT < 150.

Fr, French; IV, intravenous; LAO, left anterior oblique; PTA, percutaneous transluminal angioplasty; ACT, activated clotting time.

PATIENT PREPARATION AND POSITIONING

Diagnostic and therapeutic cerebral vascular procedures are done in the angiography suite. Generally, a formal diagnostic carotid and cerebral angiogram has been previously performed. Satisfactory baseline images in multiple plains of the extracranial and intracranial cerebral circulation are important prior to intervention. The intracerebral images are necessary as a reference for comparison to the cerebral runoff after CAS. Following successful femoral sheath insertion, the patient is systemically anticoagulated with intravenous heparin (70 units per kilogram). Additionally, in patients at higher risk for emboli, a IIb/IIIa inhibitor, such as eptifibatide (Integrilin) or tirofiban (Aggrastat) is administered at relatively lower doses than typically used in the coronary system.

SHEATH ACCESS OF THE COMMON CAROTID ARTERY

The image intensifier is positioned so the aortic arch can be viewed in an oblique projection at approximately 25–30°. If the proximal branch artery anatomy is relatively straightforward, an arch aortogram is not necessary. An angled glide catheter (Medi-Tech) is the initial catheter of choice and can be used in conjunction with a 0.035-in.

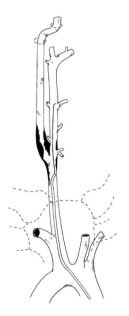

Fig. 1 Common carotid access. The selective catheter is used to cannulate the common carotid artery. The steerable guidewire is advanced into the external carotid artery.

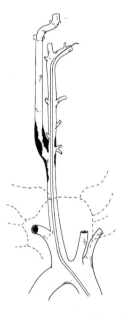

Fig. 2 External carotid artery access with guidewire position in the distal external carotid artery. After the steerable guidewire is advanced well into the external carotid artery, the selective cerebral catheter is advanced into the external carotid artery. Road-mapping the external carotid artery is useful for locating and selecting the largest and/or longest external carotid artery branch that is most suitable for anchoring the guidewire.

Glidewire (Medi-Tech) to cannulate the innominate artery and right common carotid arteries, as well as the left common carotid artery (Fig. 1). If an angle glide catheter is not successful, other shaped catheters, such as a Simmons catheter, may be used. The position of the glidewire must be monitored closely, and the carotid lesion should not be inadvertently crossed. The angled glide catheter is positioned in the proximal common carotid artery, and the initial carotid and intracranial angiograms are obtained in both AP and lateral projections. Next, the image intensifier of the C-Arm is positioned so that the carotid bifurcation can be best demonstrated. The glide catheter, over the angled Glidewire, is positioned as far into the external carotid artery as possible (Fig. 2). This glidewire is then exchanged for a 0.035-in. Amplatz exchange length guidewire. Over the Amplatz guidewire, a 90-cm 6 Fr Shuttle sheath (Cook) is positioned in the common carotid artery (Fig. 3). The tip of the shuttle sheath should be securely placed within the common carotid artery above the patient's clavicle.

A neurological assessment should be performed after sheath access. A horn or other noise-making device placed in the contralateral hand can be squeezed throughout the procedure to assess the patient's motor function and capacity to follow commands. A standard series of questions can be asked to evaluate speech and cognitive abilities.

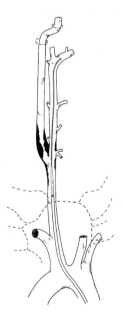

Fig. 3 Sheath access in the common carotid artery. After the stiff exchange guidewire is placed in the external carotid artery, the carotid access sheath is advanced over the stiff exchange guidewire. The tip of the sheath has a radiopaque marker and it is advanced to the level of the clavicle if possible.

Carotid Angioplasty and Stent Placement

PREPARATION FOR ANGIOPLASTY

A 0.018- or 0.014-in. guidewire (depending on the stent to be deployed) is advanced across the internal carotid stenosis with the tip of the guidewire placed within the distal internal carotid artery (Fig. 4). In reality, a 0.014-in. guidewire is almost exclusively used since both the 0.014- and 0.018-in. angioplasty balloons and stent systems can track over this caliber guidewire. If the Amplatz guidewire is left in the external carotid artery, the 0.014-in. guidewire will often preferentially cross the internal carotid stenosis without the need for a catheter (buddy wire technique). When a catheter is needed, the 4 Fr 120-cm length glide catheter is used rather than the standard 100-cm catheter. Once the long guiding sheath is placed, the added length of the glide catheter is necessary for any further catheter manipulations or guidewire exchanges.

Alternatively, if a distal occlusion balloon or filter-wire cerebral protection device is used, this would be placed instead of the 0.014-in. guidewire. Each of these cerebral protection devices has specific procedures for placement and removal that should be reviewed prior to their placement.

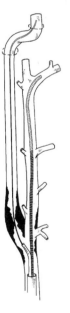

Fig. 4   Internal carotid artery access. The dilator for the sheath is removed. The low-profile 0.014- or 0.018-in. guidewire for the balloon angioplasty and stent placement is advanced across the lesion and into the distal internal carotid artery. The exchange guidewire may be removed prior to passage of the internal carotid artery guidewire. However, in this example, it is maintained in place to assist in straightening the artery and enhance the cannulation of the internal carotid artery. The internal carotid artery guidewire is advanced to the base of the skull.

CAROTID ANGIOPLASTY

Because it is not uncommon for patients to have bradycardia and hypotension with carotid angioplasty, hemodynamic assessments are made continuously throughout the procedure. To limit the bradycardia associated with angioplasty of native arterial lesions, the patient is given 0.5 to 1 mg of intravenous atropine. In addition, in preparation for percutaneous transluminal angioplasty (PTA), a cerebral angiogram is performed in the anterior–posterior and lateral projections. A carotid angiogram is performed through the guiding sheath to further delineate the carotid bifurcation and the stenosis. The image intensifier is placed in an optimal position to separate the origins of the internal and external carotid arteries. PTA of the carotid stenosis is carefully performed with a 3- or 4-mm angioplasty balloon (Fig. 5). During balloon deflation, a 30-mL syringe is used to aspirate blood from the common carotid artery and sheath to reduce the particulate debris that may have entered the bloodstream with the PTA. The results of the PTA are assessed with an angiogram performed through the guide sheath.

STENT PLACEMENT

The size of the predilatation angioplasty balloon in relation to the native artery is taken into account when deciding what size of stent to use. Both the internal carotid artery and the common carotid artery diameters are important considerations when selecting the stent. A self-expanding stent, such as a Precise stent (Cordis) or Wallstent (Medi-Tech) is used following angioplasty of the carotid stenosis (Fig. 6). Once the stent is deployed, an angiogram is performed to access the stent placement. Following deployment, a difficult

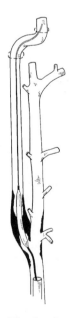

Fig. 5   Carotid angioplasty. A low-profile 3- or 4-mm angioplasty balloon is used to predilate the lesion at the carotid bifurcation.

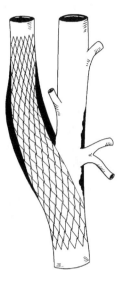

Fig. 6 Carotid stent placement. A self-expanding stent, sized appropriately for the common carotid artery, has been deployed across the carotid bifurcation to cover the lesion.

decision is then required—whether or not to perform post-stent dilation. If necessary, expedient balloon inflation to profile and rapid deflation is performed. Again, if a cerebral protection device is not used, a 30-mL syringe is used to aspirate the sheath during balloon deflation. In contrast to angioplasty or stenting in other arterial beds, the assessment of the post-stent angiographic result in the carotid arteries is different. It is common to accept a mild to moderate residual carotid artery stenosis and avoid potential complications of emboli or rupture with repeated angioplasty or overdilatation. We do not usually perform post-stent angioplasty unless there is a significant residual stenosis.

Completion

A completion angiogram is performed following stent deployment. This should include an AP and lateral view of the cervical region, as well as AP and lateral views of the intracranial anatomy. The preprocedure cerebral angiogram is used as a comparison. A neurological assessment is performed following angioplasty and stent placement. Any deficit on the exam should prompt additional review of the completion angiogram and possibly a repeat completion study of the stent site and the cerebral runoff. If there are no neurological or technical issues, the catheters and guidewires are removed. The sheath is then exchanged for a standard 6 Fr short sheath. This sheath is removed once the activated clotting time (ACT) is less than 150. Hypotension should be treated accordingly, and often requires a temporary infusion of vasopressors.

Technical Tips

1. Always obtain a thorough baseline neurological exam and good-quality cerebral runoff images prior to carotid intervention. Both will be important for comparison following angioplasty and stenting if any neurological issues arise.
2. Place an Amplatz or similar stiff guidewire as far as possible into the external carotid artery, but be very conscious of the tip of the wire during the sheath placement. Arterial perforation is possible with inadvertent guidewire advancement.
3. Do not hesitate in placing the guiding sheath well into the common carotid artery. However, remain aware of the length of the sheath's introducer tip. During advancement of the sheath, the additional length of introducer beyond the sheath may be difficult to visualize and could disrupt an unstable carotid plaque.
4. Predilate with a relatively small balloon to limit plaque disruption. An image of the contrast filled balloon is saved to compare its size to the native internal and common carotid arteries.
5. A mild residual stenosis is usually acceptable. If postdilation of the stent is required, avoid repeated angioplasty. Also, do not overdilate and risk rupture of the carotid artery.

Conclusion

The basic principles of endovascular interventions are the same with carotid artery interventions. Stable and secure access to the carotid lesion is the essential first step and is followed by guidewire crossing of the carotid artery lesion. These steps require a technical familiarity with the arteries in the cervical region. The remainder of the procedure requires precise judgment in balloon and stent selection as well as technical ability. The potential for neurological and cardiovascular complications when performing percutaneous carotid artery stenting necessitate meticulous preparation and planning.

References

1. Chakhtoura EY, Hobson RW, Goldstein J, Simonian GT, Lal BK, Haser PB, Silva MB Jr, Padberg FT Jr, Pappas PJ, Jamil Z. In-stent restenosis after carotid angioplasty-stenting: incidence and management. J Vasc Surg 2001; 33(2):220–225.
2. Criado FJ, Lingelbach JM, Ledesma DF, Lucas PR. Carotid artery stenting in a vascular surgery practice. J Vasc Surg 2002; 35(3):430–434.
3. Diethrich EB, Ndiaye M, Reid DB. Stenting in the carotid artery: initial experience in 110 patients. J Endovasc Surg 1996; 3(1):42–62.

4. Hobson RW, Goldstein JE, Jamil Z, Lee BC, Padberg FT Jr, Hanna AK, Gwertzman GA, Pappas PJ, Silva MB Jr. Carotid restenosis: operative and endovascular management. J Vasc Surg 1999; 29(2):228–235.

5. Mathur A, Roubin GS, Iyer SS, Piamsonboon C, Liu MW, Gomez CR, Yadav JS, Chastain HD, Fox LM, Dean LS, Vitek JJ. Predictors of stroke complicating carotid artery stenting. Circulation 1998; 97(13):1239–1245.

6. Qureshi AI, Luft AR, Janardhan V, Suri MF, Sharma M, Lanzino G, Wakhloo AK, Guterman LR, Hopkins LN. Identication of patients at risk for periprocedural neurological decits associated with carotid angioplasty and stenting. Stroke 2000; 31(2):376–382.

7. Roubin GS, New G, Iyer SS, Vitek JJ, Al Mubarak N, Liu MW, Yadav J, Gomez C, Kuntz RE. Immediate and late clinical outcomes of carotid artery stenting in patients with symptomatic and asymptomatic carotid artery stenosis: a 5-year prospective analysis. Circulation 2001; 103(4):532–537.

8. Shawl F, Kadro W, Domanski MJ, Lapetina FL, Iqbal AA, Dougherty KG, Weisher DD, Marquez JF, Shahab ST. Safety and efcacy of elective carotid artery stenting in high-risk patients. J Am Coll Cardiol 2000; 35(7):1721–1728.

9. Wholey MH, Wholey MH, Jarmolowski CR, Eles G, Levy D, Buecthel J. Endovascular stents for carotid artery occlusive disease. J Endovasc Surg 1997; 4(4):326–338.

10

Technique of Carotid Bifurcation Angioplasty and Stent Placement: How I Do It

TIMOTHY M. SULLIVAN

Mayo Clinic, Rochester, Minnesota, U.S.A.

The purpose of this chapter is to describe one vascular surgeon's approach to carotid angioplasty and stent placement (CAS). Carotid angioplasty and stent placement is an evolving technique in the treatment of patients with carotid occlusive disease. As the procedure becomes more standardized and as novel stents and embolic protection devices become more widely available, it may supplant carotid endarterectomy (CEA) in the treatment of many patients with both symptomatic and asymptomatic high-grade stenosis of the carotid bifurcation. Therefore it is imperative that vascular surgeons become facile with carotid angiography and intervention.

There is currently a paucity of well-controlled data regarding the safety and efficacy of CAS; as such, my practice has been limited to treating those patients deemed "high-risk" for CEA, accounting for 10–20% of all patients treated. Symptomatic patients with greater than 50% angiographic stenosis and asymptomatic patients with greater than 80% angiographic stenosis are considered for intervention, either surgical or percutaneous. Table 1 suggests what I think are reasonable criteria for patients at increased risk for CEA, and may serve as a general guide for those embarking on a program of carotid stenting. Relative contraindications to CAS are also included. In my opinion, these procedures should be performed by physicians with a thorough knowledge of the pathophysiology and natural history of carotid disease, and by those with current expertise in peripheral interventional procedures. For those unable to

Table 1 Possible Indications for Carotid
Angioplasty in "High-Risk" Patients

1. Severe cardiac disease:
   a. requiring coronary PTA or CABG
   b. history of congestive heart failure
2. Severe chronic obstructive pulmonary disease
   a. requiring home oxygen
   b. FEV-1 <20% predicted
3. Severe chronic renal insufficiency
   a. Serum creatinine >3.0 mg%
   b. Currently on dialysis
4. Prior carotid endarterectomy (restenosis)
   a. contralateral vocal cord paralysis
5. Surgically inaccessible lesions
   a. at or above the 2nd cervical vertebra
   b. inferior to the clavicle
6. Radiation-induced carotid stenosis
7. Prior ipsilateral radical neck dissection
8. Contralateral internal carotid occlusion

participate in Food and Drug Administration (FDA)-approved trials, the procedure
should be performed as part of a local Institutional Review Board (IRB)-approved
protocol with dispassionate oversight, independent pre- and postprocedure neurological examination, and prospective case review. In addition, development of a "Carotid
Stenting Program" may help facilitate cooperation among those specialties with a desire
to participate in this high-profile arena. A team of experienced personnel should be
assembled (including one or two physicians and a technician) to ensure patient safety,
maximize exposure in a small cadre of operators, and avoid duplication of effort. All
patients considered for CAS should have informed consent and counseling regarding
the risks/benefits vis-à-vis CEA and "best medical therapy," and a clear understanding

Table 2 Limitations of and Contraindications
to Carotid Angioplasty/ Stenting

Inability to obtain femoral artery access
Unfavorable aortic arch anatomy
Severe tortuosity of the common carotid artery
Severely calcified/undilatable stenoses
Lesions containing fresh thrombus
Extensive stenoses (longer than 2 cm)
Critical (99+%) stenoses ("string sign")
Lesions adjacent to carotid artery aneurysms
Contrast-related issues:
   Chronic renal insufficiency
   Previous life-threatening contrast reaction

as to the investigational nature of the procedure. In addition, they must agree to regular and careful follow-up examinations. Factors that limit the utility of stents or that may pose a contraindication to stent placement in some cases are listed in Table 2.

Preprocedure Preparation

For those with limited experience in carotid intervention, I believe that a diagnostic arch, carotid, and cerebral angiogram (performed well in advance of the proposed intervention) is mandatory; a high-quality magnetic resonance angiogram (MRA) that includes the aortic arch may substitute. This allows for careful, unhurried evaluation of the aortic arch and brachiocephalic origins, which is imperative in determining the ease (or lack thereof) of sheath/guide access to the common carotid arteries (CCA), which is an absolute key to procedural success. If the brachiocephalic trunk (innominate) or left common carotid arteries originate in a location more than two "CCA diameters" (approximately 2 cm) below the dome of the aortic arch, one should anticipate difficulty with access. In addition, measurements of lesion length, maximum percent stenosis, and CCA and internal carotid artery (ICA) diameter can be determined by placing a radiopaque marker of known diameter in the field of view (Fig. 1). Ball bearings of progressively increasing diameter (2 through 7 mm) are ideal; alternatively, a quarter can be

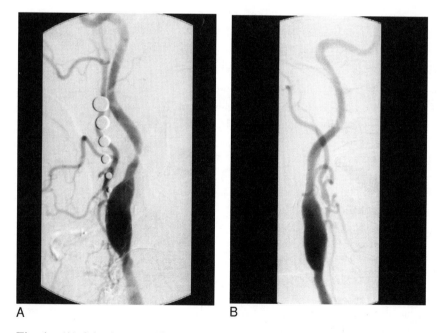

A   B

Fig. 1 (A) Selective carotid arteriogram-high-grade symptomatic recurrent stenosis. Note ball bearings (2–7-mm diameter) to assist with vessel sizing. (B) Following angioplasty and nitinol stent placement.

utilized (24.4-mm diameter). These measurements allow for preprocedure selection of balloons and stents, and facilitate a smoother, more efficient procedure, which ultimately accomplishes the main goal: patient safety and exemplary results.

All patients should have a careful history and physical examination, paying close attention to comorbid medical conditions and femoral pulses (which impacts access). In addition to the preprocedure arteriogram/MRA, a duplex ultrasound should be performed in an accredited vascular laboratory, ideally by the same laboratory that will be performing the follow-up examinations. I prefer to treat patients with aspirin (ASA) 81 mg daily for at least 1 week before their procedure, in addition to clopidogrel (Plavix) 75 mg daily for at least 3 days before. All patients receive antibiotics (typically 1 g of cefazolin IV) just before their procedure.

Procedural Details

Regardless of the exact physical location of the procedure, access to high-quality imaging equipment is mandatory; in my opinion, portable C-arms are probably inadequate for this purpose. I currently work in the neuroradiology suite (which has the advantage of a biplane unit), and have developed an excellent working relationship with my neuroradiology colleagues. This arrangement avoids duplication of effort and equipment, and the room is staffed by knowledgeable personnel and by a CRNA, who continuously monitors the patient with EKG, blood pressure, and pulse oximetry. Patients are placed in a supine position; both groins are routinely prepared. The head is placed in a cradle and gently secured to decrease patient motion during critical portions of the procedure. The procedure is performed with the patient awake, although minimal sedation is acceptable in particularly anxious subjects.

The procedure is performed in the following steps, with a few exceptions. Although one must, of course, be able to make adjustments to unanticipated situations, I would encourage the operator to standardize the procedure as much as possible.

1. Retrograde femoral access with a 5-Fr sheath.
2. Full heparin anticoagulation (typically 100 mg/kg body mass) after arterial access is gained and before manipulation of catheters in the aortic arch and brachiocephalic vessels.
3. Following selective catheterization of the ipsilateral mid to distal common carotid artery, a selective arteriogram of the carotid bifurcation is performed, paying careful attention to choose a view that provides minimal overlap of the internal and external carotid arteries and provides maximum visualization of the target lesion.
4. I have utilized two techniques for advancing a sheath into the common carotid artery: (1) The preferred technique is to place an exchange-length guidewire into the terminal branches of the external carotid artery (ECA); my personal favorite is a stiff, angled Glidewire (realizing that sheath exchange

over this guidewire, given its lubricious nature, can be tricky). The diagnostic catheter and 5-Fr sheath are removed (while maintaining constant visualization of the guidewire in the ECA during this process) and a long (70–90 cm, depending on patient body habitus) 6-Fr sheath is advanced, with its dilator, into the common carotid artery. Care must be taken to identify the tip of the dilator, which is not radiopaque, as it may extend a significant distance from the end of the sheath, depending on the brand of sheath utilized. Inadvertently advancing the dilator into the carotid bulb could have disastrous consequences. In patients with short CCAs or low bifurcations, the sheath can be advanced over the dilator once the sheath edge (radiopaque marker) is past the origin of the CCA. (2) Alternatively, the long sheath can be advanced into the transverse arch over a guidewire. The dilator is removed, and an appropriate selective diagnostic catheter is advanced into the common carotid artery; a stiff guidewire is then advanced into the ECA. Using the guidewire and catheter for support (by pinning both at the groin), the sheath (without dilator) is advanced into the CCA. This technique may be advantageous in "hostile" arches, in that the catheter and guidewire provide more support than a guidewire alone, but risks "snowplowing" the edge of the sheath at the junction of the aortic arch and the innominate or left common carotid artery (without the protection of the sheath dilator), causing dissection or distal embolization. One should not underestimate the importance of gaining and maintaining sheath access to the distal CCA: Once the 0.035-in. guidewire is removed (and ultimately exchanged for a 0.014-in. wire), "support" for angioplasty and stent placement is solely provided by the sheath. If the sheath backs up into the aortic arch during the interventional procedure, it is virtually impossible to advance into the CCA over a 0.014-in. guidewire or protection device. Patient selection and recognition of which arches to avoid are paramount to success. In particularly difficult arches, deep inspiration or expiration may occasionally facilitate sheath advancement by subtly changing the configuration of the brachiocephalic origins once guidewire access has been obtained.

5. For patients with occluded ECA, sheath access to the common carotid may be difficult. I have utilized two techniques to overcome this challenge: (1) A stiff 0.035-in. wire with a preshaped "J" can be placed into the distal CCA, taking care to avoid the bulb and bifurcation. The "J" configuration prevents guidewire traversal of the lesion. A stiff guidewire with a shapeable tip can be used to the same end. (2) Alternatively, a guidewire with variable diameter (TAD wire, 0.018-in. tip, enlarging to 0.035 in. more proximally) can be used to cross the internal carotid lesion, giving additional guidewire support to facilitate sheath advancement. While a reasonable option, this technique ultimately necessitates crossing the target lesion twice.

6. Once the sheath is in place, the guidewire and dilator are removed. I prefer to attach the sheath sidearm to a slow, continuous infusion of heparinized saline solution to avoid stagnation of blood in the sheath. A selective angiogram of

the carotid bifurcation is then performed through the sheath, again demonstrating the area of maximal stenosis, the extent of the lesion, and normal ICA and CCA above and below the lesion. Road-mapping, if available, is helpful in crossing the lesion with an embolic protection device or guidewire.

7. It is wise to have determined an Activated Clotting Time (ACT) before crossing the lesion and performing CAS. For patients in whom balloon-occlusion of the ICA is being utilized for embolic protection, an ACT maintained at >300 sec is desired. If a filter-type device or standard guidewire is employed, an ACT >250 sec is sufficient. The interventional team should discuss in detail the steps that will subsequently be performed, so that all members are "on the same page." Balloons should be flushed and prepped (with special care to remove all air from the system in the unlikely event of balloon rupture), the stent opened and on the table, and the crossing guidewire/embolic protection device prepped. For de novo lesions, I typically administer atropine (0.5–1.0 mg intravenously) as prophylaxis for bradycardia during balloon inflation in the carotid bulb; for restenoses following CEA, this may not be necessary. The monitoring nurse/CRNA should be alerted that balloon inflation may cause significant hemodynamic instability (bradycardia, hypotension).

8. The guidewire/embolic protection device (0.014-in.) is advanced across the lesion, with the aid of road-mapping. Care should be taken when inserting the device through the sheath valve, as the tip can be damaged at this juncture. If a protection device is utilized, it should be deployed into the distal extracranial ICA, just before its petrous (C3) segment. For balloon-occlusion devices, absence of flow in the ICA must be demonstrated; for filter devices, apposition of the device to the ICA must be documented, along with flow in the ICA through the device (and should be documented after each step during the intervention).

9. The lesion is predilated with a 4.0-mm coronary balloon. The balloon can be advanced into the distal CCA before crossing the lesion with the guidewire/ protection device to save time. I prefer rapid exchange/monorail balloons for this purpose. Typically, relatively low inflation pressures (4–6 mm Hg) are required to achieve balloon profile. After the predilation balloon is removed, another bifurcation angiogram is performed through the sheath (unless distal balloon occlusion is utilized, in which case the ICA will not be visualized; in these circumstances, the distal stent must be placed based on predetermined bony landmarks and the location of the CCA bifurcation).

10. The stent is then deployed after confirmation of accurate position. My preference is to utilize nitinol stents, most commonly extending a 10 mm (diameter) × 30 mm (length) stent from the ICA into the CCA, covering the ECA origin. Keep in mind that nitinol stents have a tendency to "jump" distally when rapidly deployed (despite manufacturers' claims to the contrary), which may cause one to miss the target lesion. As such, I typically expose/deploy two or three stent rings and wait for 5–7 sec, allowing the

distal stent to become well-opposed and attached to the ICA above the lesion. Subsequently, the remainder of the stent can be deployed more rapidly with little worry that it will migrate. Remember, the diameter of the stent must be sized to the largest portion of the vessel, typically the distal CCA (and not the ICA); it is important to avoid unopposed stent in the CCA, which may become a nidus for thrombus formation. Unconstrained stent diameter should be at least 10% (approximately 1–2 mm) larger than the maximum CCA diameter.

11.	If necessary, the lesion is postdilated with a 5-mm balloon; larger balloons are rarely necessary. A residual stenosis of 20% or so is completely acceptable; the goal is protection from embolic stroke, not necessarily a perfect angiographic result.

12.	A completion angiogram of the carotid bulb/bifurcation and distal extracranial ICA is performed *before* removing the guidewire/device wire to assure that a dissection has not occurred. Severe vasospasm can sometimes be encountered (and can mimic dissection). Watchful waiting and, on occasion, administration of vasodilators through the sheath (my preference is nitroglycerine in 100-μg aliquots) will usually resolve this problem. On occasion, the guidewire must be removed before spasm will completely resolve, but this should be undertaken only after dissection is excluded. After the guidewire is removed, a completion angiogram of the carotid and intracranial circulation is performed in two views.

13.	I typically do not reverse the heparin anticoagulation, and obtain access-site hemostasis with a percutaneous closure device, typically the Perclose device.

Following the procedure, the patient is monitored in the recovery area for approximately 30 min, and is then transferred to a monitored floor. Admission to an intensive care unit is typically not necessary. Patients are allowed to ambulate in 2–3 hr if a closure device is utilized, and allowed to resume a regular diet. An occasional patient will suffer prolonged hypotension from carotid sinus stimulation; this can be managed with judicious fluid administration, pharmacological treatment of bradycardia, and occasionally with intravenous pressors such as dopamine. A rare patient will experience prolonged hypotension that must be treated with oral agents; phenylephrine and midodrine are both acceptable for this purpose.

A duplex ultrasound is obtained before hospital discharge as a baseline study. Subsequent ultrasound examinations are performed at 6 mo, 1 year, and yearly thereafter. Neurological evaluation is performed at approximately 24 hr postprocedure, and then following the schedule of duplex studies. Patients are treated with ASA for life and clopidogrel for 6 weeks. For patients being treated for postendarterectomy restenosis, cilastozol (Pletal) may be utilized at a dose of 50 mg BID, barring medical contraindications. While not proven, there is some evidence in the coronary literature to suggest that it may inhibit restenosis secondary to intimal hyperplasia; I have anecdotal experience in several patients who developed in-stent restenosis following CAS whose lesions regressed following initiation of this treatment regimen.

Conclusion

Regardless of the exact technique utilized for CAS, proper patient selection, procedural standardization, and meticulous attention to detail are mandatory for success. The majority of patients with carotid occlusive disease are still best treated with endarterectomy; 60% of the author's carotid practice remains surgical. Carotid angioplasty, once felt to be an experimental in nature, is now considered a complementary procedure in the treatment of patients with carotid artery stenosis.

11

Technique of Carotid Bifurcation Angioplasty and Stent Placement: How I Do It

KARTHIKESHWAR KASIRAJAN

Emory University, School of Medicine, Atlanta, Georgia, U.S.A.

The purpose of this chapter is to describe one method for balloon angioplasty and stent placement in the treatment of carotid bifurcation occlusive disease. Carotid angioplasty and stenting (CAS) is an investigational procedure. There are no large prospective randomized trails comparing this to the "gold standard" endarterectomy. However, the recent announcement of the results of the SAPPHIRE trial and the publication of several other studies have suggested that carotid artery stenting can be performed with acceptable immediate and durable late outcomes (1–5). To date, no stent or emboli protection systems have been approved by the Food and Drug Administration (FDA) for use in carotid stenting. However, the approval of PercuSurge Guardwire (Medtronic AVE, Santa Rosa, CA) and the FilterWire (Boston Scientific) for coronary saphenous vein graft stenosis has allowed, for the first time, the "off-label" application of an emboli protection device. The field of distal emboli protection devices is rapidly developing and devices may be approved in the very near future. A comprehensive review of all available techniques for CAS is not the goal of this article. Instead, the author hopes that some of the lessons learned during the early stages in the development of CAS may assist the reader in entering the field of CAS.

The technique of CAS may be divided into the following steps:

1. Preprocedural evaluation
2. Patient preparation

3. Femoral access
4. Aortic arch angiogram
5. Selective common carotid cannulation and angiogram
6. Selective external carotid cannulation
7. Common carotid sheath access
8. Crossing ICA stenosis, predilatation, stenting, and postdilatation
9. Completion angiogram
10. Access site management
11. Postoperative care and follow-up

Preprocedural Evaluation

All patients are seen by an independent neurologist and an NIH stroke scale is completed, as we still consider CAS an investigational procedure. A CT or MRI of the brain is obtained in symptomatic patients to evaluate for preprocedural pathological changes. Initial duplex evaluation is performed of both carotids. Patients are started on antiplatelet therapy; aspirin 81 mg daily in addition to Clopidogrel (Plavix®) 75 mg bid for a minimum of 2 days before the procedure. In all cases, patients should have received clopidogrel (total dose 300 mg) before the intervention. In patients with an absent femoral pulse, we have performed a transbrachial approach. This approach is significantly more challenging compared to the transfemoral approach, with need for a larger selection of reversed angle catheters. Hence the technique of transbrachial CAS is not discussed any further. Currently, at our institution, certain patients are preferentially

Table 1 High-Risk Patient Subgroups for Carotid Endarterectomy

1. Restenosis following previous carotid endarterectomy
2. Patients >80 years of age (Recent CREST data suggests otherwise)
3. Radiation therapy to neck region
4. Radical neck dissection, or other major neck surgery
5. Tracheostomy or other risk factors for wound infection
6. Contralateral carotid artery occlusion
7. Carotid dissection
8. Contralateral recurrent laryngeal nerve palsy
9. High lesions (above C2)
10. Low common carotid lesions
11. Tandem lesions ≥70% stenosis
12. Inability to extend neck (cervical fusion, cervical osteoarthritis, unstable C-spine)
13. Chronic obstructive pulmonary disease (FEV1 <30% predicted)
14. Myocardial infarction within previous 6 weeks
15. Unstable angina (resting pain with EKG changes)
16. History of angina with two or more major diseased coronary arteries with >70% stenosis
17. Congestive heart failure (NYHA Class III or IV)
18. Liver failure with elevated prothrombin time

offered CAS based on the superior results of CAS compared to CEA in this patient subgroup (Table 1).

Patient Preparation

The procedure is performed under local anesthesia with minimal or no sedation to facilitate continuous neurological monitoring. An arterial line is placed for continuous pressure monitoring and EKG leads for cardiac monitoring. Temporary pacer pads should be readily available. Patients should have a detailed explanation of the need for continuous neurological monitoring. Techniques such as squeezing a rubber doll aids in simple and effective neurological monitoring during the procedure. Because of the minimal use of sedation, patients are often apprehensive and may develop reactive systemic hypertension. Hence it is important to document the patient's baseline blood pressure during the prior clinic visit. We avoid acutely reducing the blood pressure during the intervention with pharmacological agents, as poststent hypotension/bradycardia is not uncommon (6,7).

Access

The right common femoral approach is the most convenient for catheter manipulations by the right-handed surgeon. We routinely use a micropuncture set (21-guage needle) for the initial femoral access; this has significantly reduced the number of femoral access complications, especially in the event of adjunctive GIIb–IIIa agent use. Following guidewire access, a 5-Fr introducer sheath is placed in the common femoral artery. The author's inventory choices are listed in Table 2.

Table 2 Inventory Commonly Used During
Carotid Angioplasty and Stenting

Micropuncture set (Medi-Tech, Boston Scientific)
260-cm angled Glidewire (Medi-Tech, Boston Scientific)
5-Fr standard access sheath
Pigtail catheter
Vertebral catheter (Cook Inc.)
VTK catheter100 cm, (Cook Inc.)
0.038-in. Extra Stiff Amplatz® Wire-260 cm, short floppy tip (Cook Inc.)
Pinnacle Destination GFr, 90 cm (Boston Scientific)
0.014-in. Balance® Wire (BMW, Guidant Inc.) or available filter devices. (8)
Savvy® balloon 2 × 40 mm; 3 × 40 mm; 4 × 40 mm;
   5 × 40 mm; 6 × 40 mm; 5 × 20mm; and 6 × 20mm
   (Cordis Inc.)
Ranger® balloon (SciMed Inc., Maple Grove, MN)
Precise® Stent (Cordis Inc.), 5–10 mm diameter and
   lengths from 2 to 4 cm
Perclose® 6-Fr (Perclose Inc.)

Aortic Arch Angiogram

Arch manipulations with guidewires and catheters carry a small but significant risk of neurological events. Hence it is the authors practice to administer 5000 IU of heparin before any aortic arch manipulation. A 260-cm angled Glidewire (Medi-Tech, Boston Scientific, Natick, MA) is then placed into the ascending aorta followed by a pigtail catheter. An initial arch angiogram is performed with the image intensifier (I–I) in approximately a 45° LAO position. The origins of the arch vessels are better exposed in this oblique projection (Figs. 1 and 2). The pigtail catheter is subsequently withdrawn over a 260-cm-angled glide wire. Resist attempts to leave the Glidewire in place if inadvertent selective cannulation of the common carotid artery is achieved while withdrawing the pigtail catheter from the aortic arch. It is almost impossible to withdraw the pigtail catheter from the artic arch while maintaining glidewire access in the common carotid artery. The fewer the manipulations in the arch and neck vessels, the lower the risk of an embolic event. Vessels that originate below the apex of the aortic arch in a more proximal location, are often more difficult to selectively cannulate (Fig. 3). The author would caution against carotid stenting in this setting of a "difficult arch" until the operator has become quite comfortable with selective cannulation of the common carotid arteries in this situation. Experience with a minimum of 20 selective diagnostic carotid angiograms is suggested as a prerequisite before one proceeds with CAS procedures.

Selective Common Carotid Cannulation

Selective cannulation of the arch vessels are technically the most challenging and critical portion of CAS procedures. Most intent-to-treat failures are secondary to inability to

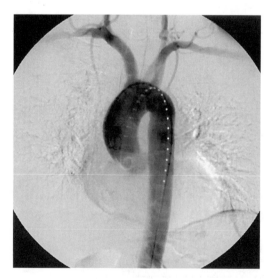

Fig. 1 Aortic arch angiogram in the straight A–P projection.

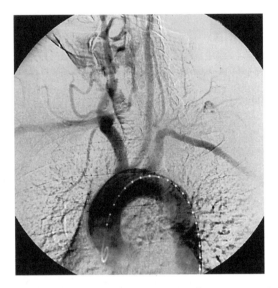

Fig. 2 Left-anterior-oblique ($\approx 45°$) projection demonstrates the origin of the arch vessels better.

selectively cannulate the common carotid arteries. The author has almost always been able to accomplish this with just two preshaped catheters; a vertebral catheter or a reversed angle Vitek catheter (VTK). The I–I is maintained in its fixed position (LAO) and the bony landmarks may be used to guide vessel cannulation. Road-mapping techniques and simple marks made with a dry-erase pen on the screen may also help guide selective common carotid cannulation. The catheter of first choice has almost

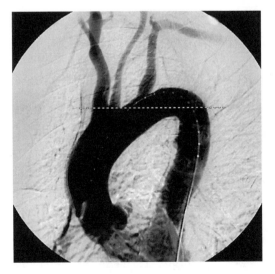

Fig. 3 A "difficult arch"—the takeoff of the innominate and left common carotid proximal to the apex of the aortic arch—makes their selective cannulation more cumbersome.

always been a vertebral catheter. The angle formed by the vertebral catheter along with the tip angle on an angled Glidewire is adequate to cannulate the common carotid artery in most patients. The right common carotid is often easier to cannulate than the left common carotid. Once the Glidewire has accessed the common carotid artery, the vertebral catheter is advanced over the Glidewire for selective angiograms of the common carotid artery.

Reversed-angle catheters such as the VTK (Fig. 4) are best reformed in the proximal descending aorta and then moved proximally, especially for cannulation of the left common carotid artery. The VTK is my catheter of choice for the "difficult arch" with branch vessels arising in the ascending aorta. Reversed-angle catheters such as VTK and Simmons cannot be easily advanced into the branch vessels; they are used only to access the origin of the branch vessels for a selective angiogram of the carotid arteries. Because of the reverse angle, forward motion on these catheters will only further advance the catheter proximally in the aortic arch. Catheter access to the common carotid artery following access with the reversed-angle catheter requires a subsequent catheter exchange. This requires the Glidewire be placed in the common carotid artery and the reversed-angle catheter is withdrawn over the guidewire and replaced with the vertebral catheter. If the Glidewire cannot be maintained in the common carotid while withdrawing the reversed-angle catheter, selective cannulation of the external carotid may be required using road-mapping techniques before catheter withdrawal. Reversed-angle catheters have a tendency to flip the guidewire as they exit the femoral sheath; hence the Glidewire needs to be immediately grasped after the tip of the reversed-angle catheter is seen exiting the femoral sheath. Once selective cannulation of the common carotid artery is performed, angiograms are performed with a

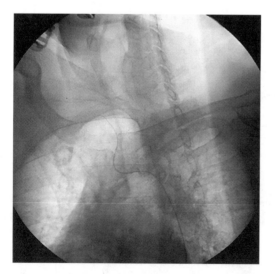

Fig. 4 A reversed-angle catheter with a Glidewire in place used to cannulate the origin of the innominate artery.

10- or 20-mL syringe filled with half strength contrast. The carotid bifurcation is best visualized in the ipsilateral oblique position (~60° ipsilateral oblique). Multiple views may be needed to best open the carotid bifurcation, as the next step would involve selective cannulation of the external carotid artery. Lateral and AP intracranial images are then obtained (20-mL syringe half strength contrast) to identify any intracranial pathology and to document the intracranial circulation before CAS. A certain amount of experience must be gained in interpretation of intracranial images. Identifying small embolic events may be quite difficult without experience in reading intracranial images. After images are obtained, failure to recognize an intracranial embolus may be detrimental to the patient and a medical-legal disaster.

Selective External Carotid Cannulation

This is always carried out using road-mapping techniques. Blind guidewire and catheter manipulation in the carotid artery must be avoided at all times. Selective external carotid cannulation is quite easily accomplished with a 260-cm angled Glidewire and the vertebral catheter. In case of a tight external stenosis, a Tracker-18 ([BS]3-Fr catheter with a 0.018 wire) may be used and the 0.018 wire is then exchanged for a stiffer 0.018 guide wire (Roadrunner-Cook, Inc., Bloomington, IN) and predilated with a 2-mm Savvy balloon. The balloon is then withdrawn and a vertebral catheter is passed into the external carotid artery over the Roadrunner guidewire. An attempt should be made to reach as distally on the external carotid artery as possible. This allows adequate guidewire length for the subsequent placement of the Pinnacle destination (PD) sheath. The Glidewire is then withdrawn from the vertebral catheter and a 260-cm Amplatz superstiff wire is taken into the external carotid artery. It is helpful to inject a little contrast into the vertebral catheter to confirm external carotid placement. Contrast injections into the carotids should not be performed unless free back flow of blood is noticed at the back end of the injection catheter. In the external carotid artery, blood back flow may at times be difficult because of the tight fit of the vertebral catheter in the external branches. In this event, the vertebral catheter is slowly withdrawn until good back flow is noted.

Common Carotid Sheath Access

The vertebral catheter is withdrawn leaving the Amplatz guidewire in the external carotid artery. The 5-Fr sheath in the groin is subsequently withdrawn. A 6-Fr, 90-cm-long PD sheath is then advanced over the Amplatz guidewire into the common carotid artery. It is helpful to image the tip of the Amplatz wire in the external carotid during this maneuver. If the tip of the guidewire is found to move back, it indicates that the sheath is not appropriately advancing over the guidewire. Stop at this point and image lower down to visualize the location of the tip of the PD sheath. If difficulty is encountered, it is often in the aortic arch. Techniques for advancing a sheath in a "difficult arch" are detailed in Table 3.

Table 3 Techniques to Advance the Shuttle Sheath Across a "Difficult Arch"

1. Make sure adequate length of the Amplatz guidewire is located in the external carotid artery. It may help to recannulate a more distal branch of the external carotid artery for a longer guidewire "purchase" in the artery. (Use a short floppy tip Amplatz wire)
2. It has helped in a few situations to soak the PD sheath in warm saline before insertion; this makes it more supple and easier to take the angle of a "difficult arch."
3. If the Amplatz guidewire can be palpated against to the skin, firm pressure against the neck may help fix the guidewire while advancing the sheath. Care must be taken not to squeeze the carotid bifurcation, as this may result in an embolic event.
4. Consider substitution of the Amplatz guidewire for stiffer guidewires such as the Meier or Lunderquist, before advancing the Shuttle sheath.
5. Always remember there is another option—carotid endarterectomy!

The dilator in the PD sheath is much longer than most other dilators. It is helpful to identify the optimal length that you would want the dilator to protrude from the sheath tip and to lock the Y-adaptor on the back end of the dilator in this position. Once in the common carotid artery, withdrawing the dilator as the sheath is advanced makes the sheath move more efficiently in the common carotid artery. The Amplatz guidewire along with the dilator is then withdrawn and the carotid angiogram is repeated through the PD sheath with a road map of the ICA stenosis.

Crossing the Internal Carotid Artery Stenosis, Angioplasty, and Stenting

This may be performed with any one of a variety of distal protection devices that are currently being used in trials. The author has had most success with the PercuSurge Guardwire (Medtronic) because of its low crossing profile, compared to many of the filters currently in clinical trial. The PercuSurge is commercially available for coronary saphenous vein grafts and is not approved for CAS. In the author's experience, the incidence of transient neurological events is lower with the use of embolic protection devices. Before the availability of the PercuSurge, a 0.014 BMW (Guidant Inc., Temecula, CA) was the guidewire of choice to cross the ICA stenosis. The tip of the 0.014-in. guidewire is shaped appropriately to aid access to the ICA. After crossing the stenosis, the tip of the guidewire is placed close to the skull base. If the internal carotid artery is kinked, coiled, or tortuous, the guidewire is passed distally to the level of skull base. It is important to not advance the tip of the guidewire any further. The intracranial portion of the carotid artery is highly prone to dissection with guidewire manipulations (Fig. 5). It is easy for the operator to miss the guidewire moving distally, because the primary focus is at the ICA stenosis. I have routinely asked one of my assistants/observers to keep an eye on the tip of the guidewire and inform me of significant distal or proximal migration. Once the lesion has been crossed, it is predilated with a 2- or 3-mm Savvy balloon. A 4-cm-long balloon is routinely used.

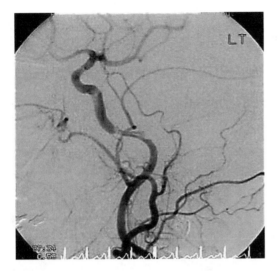

Fig. 5 Intracranial carotid artery dissection.

Shorter lengths have a tendency to "melon seed" and in the process may release embolic debris. The longer-length balloons have a tendency to expand at both ends (dog-boning) and thereby fix the balloon in place. I have routinely administered 0.5 mg of atropine before balloon dilatation, except in patients with a recurrent stenosis. The pressure used for predilatation is nominal for the balloon used. I use higher pressure (14–16 atm) only in heavily calcified stenoses. The duration of the predilatation depends on the appearance and behavior of the balloon. If the balloon immediately attains its full shape, the predilatation time is shorter. If the balloon attains its full shape slowly, the predilatation time is prolonged up to 120 sec, especially in calcified lesions, which have tendency for recoiling. The balloon is inflated only once and the inflation time varies depending on the lesion. I do not practice "primary stenting" without predilatation; it is my impression that postdilatation of the constricted stent is associated with more "scissoring" of the stent struts on the plaque with greater risk of embolization. If an occlusion balloon such as the PercuSurge is used for emboli protection, it is important to mark the site of ICA stenosis on the monitor, as the lesion cannot be angiographically visualized once the protection balloon has been inflated (Fig. 6a,b). The use of embolic protection filters have the advantage of allowing for continuous angiographic monitoring of the target lesion.

A variety of self-expanding stents are available for use. I have most commonly used the Precise stent (135-cm catheter length). A variety of diameters (6–10) and lengths of 2–4 cm should be available. The most common size I have used is the 8-mm × 3-cm stent. The self-expanding stent is deployed using the vertebral bodies as landmarks, or using dry-erase marks on the monitor. The self-expanding stent is postdilated with a 5 mm, or 6 × 20 mm balloon (Savvy®, Cordis Inc., Miami, FL) over the 0.014 wire, depending on the size of the internal carotid artery. A 5-mm balloon PTA is often adequate, rarely is a 6-mm PTA required post stent deployment. A residual

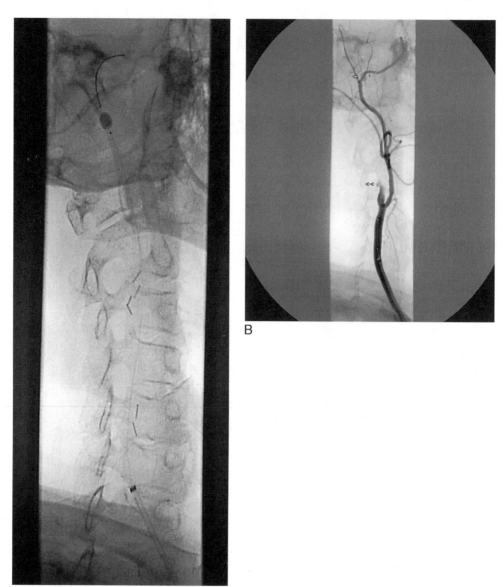

A

B

Fig. 6 (A) PercuSurge Guardwire with distal protection balloon inflated. (B) Note the inability of angiography to visualize the internal carotid artery following inflation of the distal protection balloon.

stenosis of <15% may be accepted, as the nitinol stents continue to expand with time. Following stent deployment, shorter (2 cm) balloons are used to dilate the narrow portion of the stent. Longer length may cause a dissection in the distal ICA, as these balloons may be larger than the unstented portion of the ICA. The balloon used for poststent PTA is always maintained within the stent. Nominal pressure is used to fully expand the balloon and the stent. The balloon is again slowly deflated. High pressures are not used. In heavily calcified stenoses, consider postdilating with Titan balloons (Cordis Inc.) that accept higher pressures. In most of the cases, the stent is placed across the bifurcation into the common carotid artery, crossing the origin of the external carotid artery (Fig. 7a,b). To cover the external carotid artery with the stent does not cause problems; our follow-up arteriograms and Duplex studies showed external carotid artery to be patent in all patients.

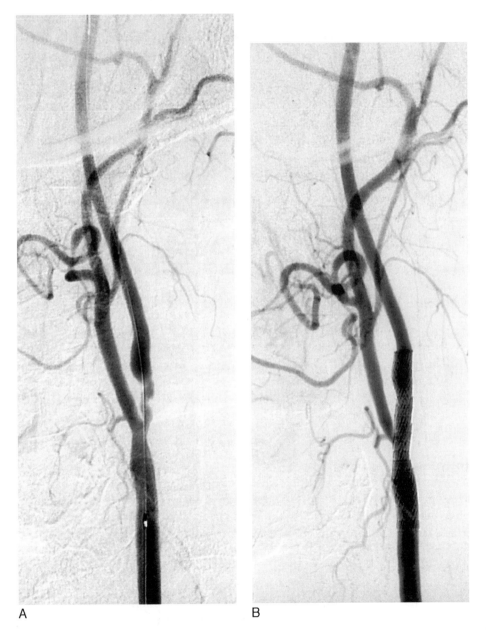

A   B

Fig. 7   (A) Internal carotid artery stenosis. (B) Stent is placed across the origin of the external carotid artery with no flow limitation.

If a Wallstent (Medi-Tech, Boston Scientific) of 8 × 20 mm is chosen and it expands to 8 mm, then the length would be 20 mm. However, there is a size differential between the internal and the common carotid arteries, the former being 5–6 mm and the latter 7–9 mm; hence the Wallstent does not expand to the full 8 mm and does not shorten to 20 mm. Instead, it ends up being 25–35 mm in length. Additionally, the continuous cell design of the Wallstent prevents it from adequate wall apposition at the shoulder region where the common carotid abruptly tapers to become the ICA. Hence, it has been my preference to use nitinol based stents.

In some cases, continued flow of contrast into an ulcer is seen (Fig. 8a,b). No attempt should be made to obliterate this communication by using larger balloons or higher pressures as this communication will seal off in the ensuing few weeks and is usually of no consequence. In a patient with a large ulcer (Fig. 9a,b), I have elected to offer the patient an endarterectomy as the end angiographic result of CAS is often unsatisfactory. These large ulcers may remain patent and in communication with the circulation, thereby acting as a source of embolic debris. Patients with >2-cm-long carotid lesions, dense calcification (seen on plain fluoroscopic images), and large ulcerated plaques are at a higher risk for embolization during CAS .

Kinks and bends in the ICA may pose a problem with stent implants. Deploy stents across kinks only if they are isolated (Fig. 10a,b). Avoid placing the distal end of the stent into kinks and tortuosities of the internal carotid artery if more than a single bend is noted. These cannot be eliminated and are only distally displaced and can become more exaggerated. A tortuous ICA should be considered a relative contraindication for CAS, as acute occlusions are more common following stent placement in these tortuous vessels.

If the external carotid artery becomes significantly stenosed with flow restriction or occluded after postdilatation of the stent, no attempt should be made to salvage the ECA. This is a very uncommon event and attempts to correct this may be quite difficult and result in further complications. The vasculature to the head and neck region supplied by the external carotid artery is abundant and occlusions of one or both external carotids are very well tolerated.

Completion Angiogram

Following CAS, final angiograms are acquired in the projection that had demonstrated the maximum stenosis. Extra attention is paid to the ICA immediately cephalad to the stent. Spasm in this segment may be encountered. With use of emboli protection devices, total ICA spasm may occasionally be seen, particularly if the embolic protection device is allowed to bob up and down during guidewire manipulation. A small dose of intra-arterial nitroglycerine (100–200 µg) is directly administered into the ICA (Fig. 11). A more proximal injection of nitroglycerine (common carotid artery) is often insufficient as this has a tendency to preferentially flow into the external carotid artery in the presence of an ICA spasm. Distal dissections are

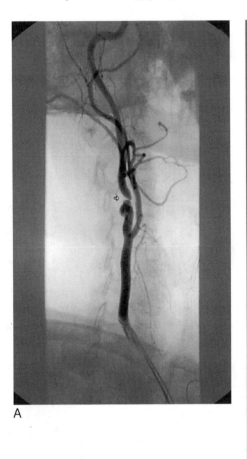

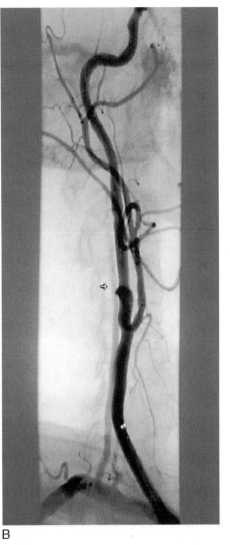

Fig. 8 (A) High-grade recurrent stenosis with ulcerated proximal plaque. (B) Postangioplasty and stenting; note flow of contrast into the plaque ulcer via the stent struts.

unusual and when present can be remedied with an additional stent of appropriate size. It is important not to lose guidewire access until the operator is satisfied of the final angiographic appearance.

We routinely acquire post-CAS intracranial angiograms. Most operators will do this as a routine, and all the current carotid stent investigational protocols call for repeat intracranial views. It also helps to learn to compare pre- and post intracranial images, as competent interpretation of these images takes practice.

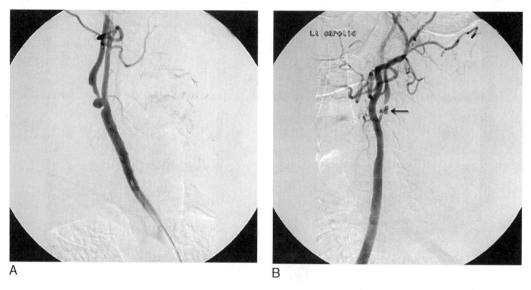

Fig. 9 (A) Large plaque ulcer seen on the diagnostic angiogram. (B) Complex ulcerated plaque—not an ideal case for carotid angioplasty and stenting.

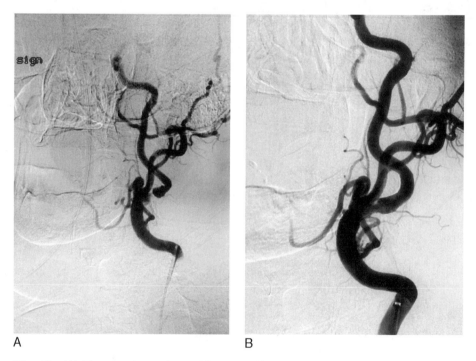

Fig. 10 (A) Tortuous internal carotid artery with proximal internal carotid artery stenosis. (B) Distal end of the stent is placed across the proximal kink, hence eliminating the acute angle.

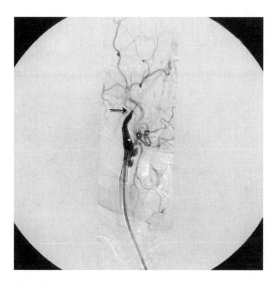

Fig. 11 Severe spasm of the internal carotid artery following use of a emboli protection device. Note that the vertebral catheter is selectively used to inject nitroglycerine into the internal carotid artery.

Access Site Management

At the present time, in suitable patients, access site hemostasis is achieved at the end of the procedure using a 6-Fr suture closure device (Perclose, Perclose Inc.; Redwood City, CA). If a calcified vessel is encountered during needle puncture, Perclose is not used. In this situation, the PD sheath is exchanged for a short 6-Fr sheath that would be removed once the ACT is less than 160 sec.

Postoperative Care and Follow-up

Patients are monitored in the intensive care unit overnight. It is not uncommon, especially in patients with a history of coronary artery disease to have a heightened response to carotid sinus distension. It may take 24–48 hr of ionotropic support before the carotid sinus adapts to the radial force of the self-expanding stents. Avoiding extreme oversizing of the stents helps to decrease the incidence of post-CAS bradycardia and hypotension. The presence of significant hypotension in the absence of bradycardia is unusual in the immediate postprocedure period; it is worth emphasizing that other causes, e.g., retroperitoneal bleed related to access site problems, should also be excluded as the cause.

If patients are doing fine, they are ambulated the next day. A neurologist is routinely involved in predischarge evaluation and a NIH stroke scale is completed before discharge. Routine carotid ultrasound exams are not obtained, with the exception of patients with neurological events or ICA spasm or dissection seen on the completion angiogram. Medications include ASA 81 mg PO qd indefinitely and Clopidogrel 75 mg PO qd × 1 mo. Follow-up includes 1 mo, 6 mo, and yearly clinical evaluation and duplex examination.

References

1. Al-Mubarak N, Iyer S, Roubin G, Vitek JJ. Is carotid stenting a viable treatment option for high-risk endarterectomy subsets? Stroke 2000; 31:289A.
2. Yadav JS, Roubin GS, Iyer S, Vitek JJ, King P, Jordan WD, Fisher WS. Elective stenting of the extracranial carotid arteries. Circulation 1997; 95:376–381.
3. Roubin GS, New G, Iyer SS, Vitek JJ, Al-Mubarak N, Kuntz RE. Immediate and late outcomes of carotid artery stenting in patients with symptomatic and asymptomatic carotid artery stenosis. Circulation 2001; 103:532–537.
4. Gaines PA. Carotid angioplasty and stenting. Br Med Bull 2000; 56:549–556.
5. Parodi JC, La Mura R, Ferreira LM, Mendez MV, Cersosimo H, Schonholz C, Garelli G. Initial evaluation of carotid angioplasty and stenting with three different cerebral protection devices. J Vasc Surg 2000; 32:1127–1136.
6. Kasirajan K, Matteson B, Marek J, et al. Comparison of non-neurological events in high-risk patients treated by carotid angioplasty versus endarterectomy. Am J Surg 2003; 185(4):301–304.
7. Qureshi AI, Luft AR, Lopes DK, Lanzino G, Fessler RD, Sharma M, Guterman LR, Hopkin LN. Postoperative hypotension after carotid angioplasty and stenting: report of three cases. Neurosurgery 1999; 44:1320–1323.
8. Kasirajan K, Schneider PA, Kent KC. Emboli Protection Filters for Cerebral Protection during carotid angioplasty and stenting. JEVT 2003; 10:21–27.

12

Cerebral Protection Devices for Carotid Stenting: Technique and Results

TIMOTHY M. SULLIVAN

Mayo Clinic, Rochester, Minnesota, U.S.A.

While enthusiasm continues to grow for carotid angioplasty and stenting (CAS) as an alternative to carotid endarterectomy (CEA), its "Achilles heel" remains the risk of distal (cerebral) embolization during the procedure, especially for de novo atherosclerotic lesions, where the potential for embolization of atheromatous material is substantial. These particles, by their nonthrombotic nature, are not likely amenable to cerebrovascular rescue techniques (i.e., catheter-directed lysis); therefore prevention of embolization is paramount. Jordan et al. (1) reviewed transcranial Doppler (TCD) data from a series of CEA ($n = 76$) and CAS ($n = 40$) procedures. The mean number of microemboli, detected by TCD in the CAS cohort (74.0 emboli per lesion), was significantly greater than in the CEA group (8.8 emboli per lesion, $p = 0.0001$). Four patients in the CAS group had neurological events compared with one in the CEA group. Ohki et al. (2), in an ex vivo model of CAS using human atherosclerotic plaque in a flow model, found that substantial numbers of particles were released from the lesions during angioplasty; the majority were captured by the experimental filter device. Of note, the filter device itself produced very few particles due to its low crossing profile. Figure 1 illustrates this point in a patient treated by the author in 1996 with CAS (and monitored with TCD) prior to the advent of embolic protection devices.

Table 1 reviews the current results of CAS, with and without embolic protection. Only publications that appeared in peer-reviewed journals during the last 5 years and

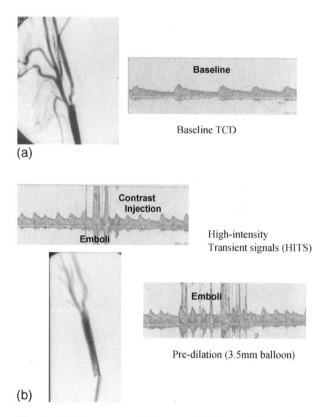

Fig. 1 (a) Symptomatic de novo left internal carotid stenosis. A 76-year-old male with previous radical neck dissection and radiation therapy. Baseline angiogram and TCD study, showing normal flow in the left middle cerebral artery. (b) High-intensity transient signals, denoting emboli, with contrast administration and predilation of the lesion, in the absence of an embolic protection device. The patient remained asymptomatic throughout the procedure.

included at least 50 patients are included. The self-reported multicenter registry reported by Wholey et al., because of the limitations of this type of data, was not included in the composite results. It seems remarkable that, although cerebral protection was only occasionally utilized, the risk of stroke and death is, overall, much lower than one might anticipate, given the high rate of embolization (documented by TCD) with CAS.

Preliminary (30-day) results from the SAPPHIRE trial of carotid angioplasty stenting with distal protection in high-risk patients has recently been reported (although not yet published). This trial, sponsored by Cordis Corporation, used a nitinol self-expanding stent and the Angioguard, a filter-type embolic protection device. The aim of the study was to prove *equivalency* of carotid intervention to carotid endarterectomy in a cohort of patients felt to be at high risk for surgery, based on a number of medical and anatomic criteria. Primary endpoints were stroke, death, and myocardial infarction (both Q-wave and non-Q). A total of 307 patients were randomized to angioplasty ($n = 156$) or surgery ($n = 151$), while 408 patients had angioplasty and were placed into a consecutive

Table 1 Current Results of Carotid Angioplasty/Stenting

Author, year	n (arteries)	% Asymptomatic	Cerebral protection	Stroke + death (%)
Yadav, 1997	126	41%	No	7.9
Jordan, 1997	107	36%	No	9.3
Henry, 1998	174	65%	Mixed	2.9
Bergeron, 1999	99	56%	No	2
Wholey, 2000	5210	Not stated	Mixed	5.07
Shawl, 2000	192	39%	No	2.9
Roubin, 2001	604	48%	Mixed	7.4
CAVATAS, 2001	251	4%	No	10
Brooks, 2001	53	0%	No	0
d'Audiffret, 2001	68	70%	Mixed	5.8
Reimers, 2001	88	64%	Yes	2.3
Paniagua, 2001	69	84%	No	5.6
Criado, 2002	135	60%	Mixed	2
Guimaraens, 2002	194	8%	Yes	2.6
Al-Mubarak, 2002	164	52%	Yes	2
Weighted average (excluding Wholey)	2324	42%	Mixed	5.3

registry. In the randomized group, the results were statistically equivalent with respect to stroke (3.8% stent vs. 5.3% CEA, $p = 0.59$), death (0.6% stent vs. 2.0%, $p = 0.36$), MI, the majority of which were non-Q (2.6% stent vs. 7.3% CEA, $p = 0.07$), and death + stroke (4.5% stent vs. 6.6% CEA, $p = 0.46$). The combined endpoint of death, stroke, and MI did reach significance in favor of stenting (5.8% stent vs. 12.6% CEA, $p = 0.047$). In the stent registry, the risk of death and stroke was 6.9%. These data will likely be used to support FDA approval, which is anticipated soon.

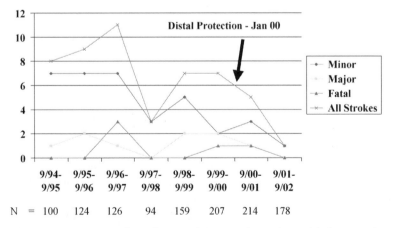

Fig. 2 Experience of Roubin et al., suggesting substantial decrease in stroke rate using routine embolic protection. (From Ref. 3.)

Roubin et al. (3) have reported on patients treated at the University of Alabama at Birmingham and at Lenox Hill Hospital in New York. Six hundred four arteries were treated in 528 consecutive patients over a 5-year period. This included patients treated with both balloon-expandable and self-expanding stents, with and without cerebral protection devices. The overall 30-day combined stroke/mortality was 8.1% (for 528 patients) and included a 5.5% rate of minor stroke, 1.6% major stroke rate, and 1% rate of nonneurologic death. When divided into yearly intervals, the risk of stroke and death reached a maximum of 12.5% in the period ending September 1997 and fell to a minimum of 3.2% the following year (Fig. 2). This rather dramatic change in results likely represents improvement in technology (filter devices, stents, and guidewires) as well as an improved ability of the investigators to select appropriate patients for intervention.

Types of Cerebral Protection Devices and Techniques for Use

This section will briefly review three types of embolic protection devices, as well as basic instructions for their use.

DISTAL OCCLUSION DEVICES

The most basic of devices, balloon-occlusion devices, simply cease flow in the internal carotid artery during the period of angioplasty and stenting. The PercuSurge Guard Wire (Medronic AVE) is a compliant balloon housed on a 0.014-in. guidewire, with a rather ingenious valve (microseal adapter) that allows the balloon to remain inflated when the inflation device is removed. Angioplasty balloons, catheters, and stents can then be loaded onto the wire and removed while the balloon occludes the internal carotid artery. At the completion of the interventional procedure, the static column of blood in the ICA is aspirated using a special catheter (Export catheter) to remove any embolic particles that may have accumulated. The balloon can be inflated from 3 to 6 mm in diameter, in 0.5-mm increments, depending on the size of the target artery. The device is approved for aortocoronary saphenous vein graft intervention and not for carotid or peripheral vascular use.

Suggestions for use:

1. As balloon-occlusion devices do not allow for antegrade flow in the internal carotid artery during the period of balloon inflation, a preprocedure contrast angiogram is suggested. In patients with an "isolated" ipsilateral cerebral hemisphere, balloon inflation may not be tolerated, even with induced hypertension and full heparin anticoagulation. In these patients, CAS with a filter device may be preferable.
2. Patients should be pretreated with ASA and clopidogrel and anticoagulated with heparin to an activated clotting time (ACT) of at least 300 sec.

3. The occlusion device should be prepped and tested on the back table (and all angioplasty balloons and stents opened and prepared) prior to crossing the carotid lesion. If a monorail system (both balloon *and* stent) is utilized, the 200-cm length PercuSurge may be utilized; for "over-the-wire" systems, the 300-cm wire is mandatory.

4. The Guard Wire is advanced across the target lesion and into the proximal petrous segment of the internal carotid artery (ICA). The predilation balloon is advanced into the distal common carotid artery (CCA) prior to balloon inflation.

5. The balloon is carefully inflated to a target diameter, based on preprocedure measurements of the ICA. As the balloon *approaches* the target diameter, contrast angiography of the ICA is performed. The *minimum* diameter necessary to achieve cessation of flow in the ICA is preferred; overinflation of the balloon can result in ICA dissection. On rare occasions, the distal ICA will be larger than 6 mm; in these cases, the balloon will not completely occlude the ICA. Patients with "isolated" hemispheres may become symptomatic during the period of balloon inflation, necessitating deflation. These patients typically become symptomatic within 60 sec of cessation of ICA flow. Should patients become symptomatic, the operator has several options: complete the procedure without balloon occlusion, complete the procedure with *intermittent* balloon occlusion, or switch to a filter-type device, if available.

6. The intervention on the internal carotid is performed "blind"; that is, one cannot angiographically visualize the ICA during balloon occlusion. The operator must rely on the fluoroscopic appearance of the stent, following postdilation, to assess the completed result. If, following balloon deflation and completion angiography, the lesion requires further angioplasty or stent placement, the occlusion balloon must be reinflated; this situation is even more pronounced when the ECA is occluded, as the static column of blood extends from the balloon proximally to the junction of the CCA and the aortic arch.

7. Following completion of the intervention, the static column of blood in the ICA is aspirated (three separate aspirations of 20 mL each). When the ECA is occluded (see above), one should consider more vigorous aspiration and perhaps flushing the sheath to expel debris from the common carotid artery. Flow is then restored as the balloon is deflated. A completion angiogram is mandatory before the wire is removed, making sure that an iatrogenic dissection has not occurred.

DISTAL FILTER DEVICES

Filter devices allow for continued flow into the intracranial ICA during intervention. They are typically 0.014-in. guidewire systems that have expandable and constrainable "baskets" or "umbrellas" near their distal ends; these baskets prevent particles of a

certain diameter from passing into the brain (Fig. 3). The filter is closed during placement and then opened when located in the appropriate position distal to the carotid
bifurcation lesion. Filter deployment mechanisms vary, but most are deployed by
withdrawing an outer catheter that covers and restrains the filter, thus permitting self-
expansion of the device. The Angioguard device (Cordis Corp.) was used in the
SAPPHIRE trial of high-risk patients; this device has 100-μm pores which allow smaller
particles (which presumably will not cause clinical events) to pass, trapping larger (and
presumably more dangerous) ones. At the time of this manuscript, the Filter Wire EX
(Boston Scientific) is the only filter device approved by the FDA. Like the PercuSurge, it
is approved for aortocoronary saphenous vein grafts and not for carotid or peripheral
applications. It is likely that the Angioguard will be the first filter device approved for
high-risk carotid applications.

Suggestions for use:

1. Unlike balloon-occlusion devices, filter devices are designed to maintain
   flow into the distal ICA during the course of intervention. Following
   placement of a sheath/guide into the CCA, the filter device is placed across
   the target lesion into a straight, normal segment of the extracranial ICA.
   Placing the device into a tortuous ICA may be quite difficult and perhaps
   relatively contraindicated. An ACT of 250 sec or greater is sufficient for
   filter-type devices.
2. As the crossing profile of filter-type devices are typically greater than standard guidewires or balloon-occlusion devices, on occasion, it may be difficult
   to cross extremely stenotic, tortuous, or calcified lesions. A "buddy wire" (a
   stiff guidewire placed into the external carotid artery) may be helpful in
   providing extra support to the filter device.
3. Confirmation that the edges of the device are well-opposed to the ICA, via
   several views of the device with different obliquity, is mandatory. If the
   device is not properly "aligned" with the ICA and it is not in contact with
   the vessel in 360°, embolic particles can "bypass" the filter.

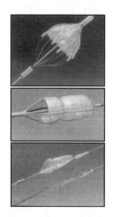

Angioguard

NeuroShield

FilterWire EX

Fig. 3 Examples of filter-type protection devices.

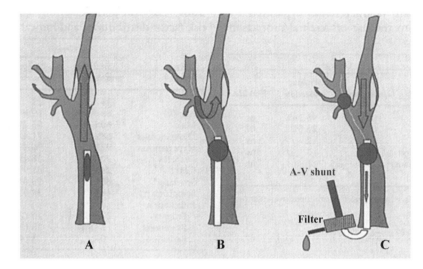

Fig. 4 Parodi flow-reversal system for cerebral protection during CAS.

4. Once deployed, and after *every* step of the intervention, flow of contrast through the device must be documented. If the device becomes filled with debris, it must be either aspirated (much like the PercuSurge device) or temporarily removed. When removing a full device, it is important not to recapture it completely, as debris may be extruded from it and embolize distally.

FLOW-REVERSAL DEVICES

Juan Parodi, MD, "inventor" of the aortic stent graft, has devised a rather ingenious device that reverses flow in the internal carotid artery (Fig. 4). This is accomplished by placing a large catheter into the CCA, occluding CCA flow with a balloon surrounding the catheter, and then placing an occlusion balloon in the ECA. The CCA catheter is connected to an external filter and then to the femoral vein, producing an arteriovenous fistula and reversal of flow in the ICA. Theoretically, intervention can be performed under complete protection, as antegrade flow in the ICA is never achieved until the procedure is terminated. Preliminary results with this device suggest that 25% of patients do not tolerate reversal of flow (i.e., become symptomatic with ICA flow reversal); in these cases, flow reversal can be performed intermittently until the procedure is completed. A combination of flow reversal with distal filter protection (during lesion crossing) is an intriguing possibility for near-complete protection during CAS.

Conclusions

While it may never be proven, it seems logical that most patients having CAS would benefit from embolic protection devices. With the availability of at least two devices, and with several more on the horizon, many operators have access to embolic protection devices even outside of industry- or FDA-sponsored trials. In my opinion, most patients with de novo carotid lesions should be treated with a protection device (although conclusive data are lacking). Patients with early restenosis following CEA, which is most frequently myointimal in nature and carries a lower risk of embolization, may safely be treated without a protection device. At the present time, however, most would agree that embolic protection is the standard of care for the majority of patients undergoing CAS.

References

1. Jordan WD Jr, Voellinger DC, Doblar DD, Plyushcheva NP, Fisher WS, McDowell HA. Microemboli detected by transcranial Doppler monitoring in patients during carotid angioplasty versus carotid endarterectomy. Cardiovasc Surg Jan 1999; 7(1):33–38.
2. Ohki T, Roubin GS, Veith FJ, Iyer SS, Brady E. Efficacy of a filter device in the prevention of embolic events during carotid angioplasty and stenting: an ex vivo analysis. J Vasc Surg Dec 1999; 30(6):1034–1044.
3. Roubin GS, New G, Iyer SS, et al. Immediate and late clinical outcomes of carotid artery stenting in patients with symptomatic and asymptomatic carotid artery stenosis. A 5-yr prospective analysis. Circulation 2001; 103:532–537.

13

Comparison of Cerebral Protection Devices for Carotid Artery Stenting

MARC BOSIERS and **KOEN DELOOSE**

AZ St. Blasius, Dendermonde, Belgium

PATRICK PEETERS and **JÜRGEN VERBIST**

Imelda Hospital, Bonheiden, Belgium

The importance of cerebral protection during carotid artery stenting (CAS) cannot be underestimated. Although the efficacy of these protection devices is not yet proven by any randomized trial, it is widely accepted that cerebral protection devices are essential for minimizing the neurological complication of CAS. Experimental and clinical evidence suggests that the embolization of potentially hazardous particles is reduced with the routine use of these devices during CAS (1). The immediate success of CAS cannot merely be attributed to the selected cerebral protection device; it also depends upon the experience of the interventionalists (2). All cerebral protection devices are designed to safely capture and remove possible debris during the different procedural steps in order to prevent any embolization to the cerebral circulation. Three conceptually different methods, each having its own advantages and disadvantages, have been developed thus far to prevent neurological complications during CAS. These methods include distal occlusion devices, distal filter devices, and proximal occlusion devices.

Distal Occlusion Devices

WORKING PRINCIPLE OF DISTAL OCCLUSION DEVICES

Distal occlusion devices were developed following the principle applied by Theron in 1996 during his first successful attempt to create cerebral protection during CAS (Fig. 1)

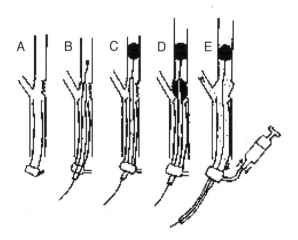

Fig. 1 Distal occlusion device. The working principle of the distal occlusion technique as described by Theron et al. (3). (A) A sheath is placed in the common carotid artery. (B) The lesion is crossed with a distal occlusion balloon. (C) Inflation of the distal occlusion balloon stops forward flow in the internal carotid artery. (D) Carotid angioplasty and stent placement is performed with cerebral protection. (E) The carotid bifurcation is aspirated and flushed before system removal.

(3). By occluding the internal carotid artery (ICA) with an inflated balloon at its segment in between the lesion and the cerebral circulation, debris could be prevented from entering the brain during the procedure. Aspiration and flushing of the carotid arteries after balloon angioplasty and stent placement remove the debris from the carotid bifurcation either by flushing into the external carotid artery (ECA) or aspirating through the sheath in the common carotid artery (CCA).

DIFFERENT DISTAL OCCLUSION DEVICES ON THE MARKET

PercuSurge Guardwire	(Medtronic)
Tri-Activ	(Kensy Nash Corp.)
Guardian	(Rubicon-Abbott)

PercuSurge Guardwire (Medtronic).   The best-known distal occlusion device is the PercuSurge Guardwire, which consists of a simple balloon mounted on a 0.014-in. guidewire (Fig. 2). The advantage of this device is its low crossing profile (0.036 in.) almost equaling the standard guidewire size (0.035 in.). The manual active aspiration needed after CAS to remove the debris makes the procedure more laborious in comparison to other devices.

Henry et al. (4) have shown a technical success rate of 99.5% using the PercuSurge Guardwire during CAS. The distal occlusion balloon was tolerated in 95.7% of the patient population. In the remaining 4.3% of the cases, the intracerebral collateralization

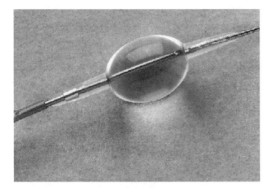

Fig. 2 PercuSurge Guardwire. The PercuSurge Guardwire consists of a simple balloon mounted on a 0.014-in. guidewire. The balloon is inflated to temporarily occlude the internal carotid artery distal to the lesion being treated.

was insufficient to provide adequate oxygen to the brain. In these patients, the distal occlusion balloon was deflated in between the different steps of CAS, increasing the risk of emboli migration during the procedure. Nevertheless, this is not reflected in the stroke/death rate at 30 days which was 2.7%.

Tri-Activ (Kensy Nash Corp.). The Tri-Activ distal protection device is composed of three components: a guidewire with distal protection balloon, a 4-Fr flush catheter, and an active peristaltic pump extraction device (Fig. 3). Active aspiration by means of

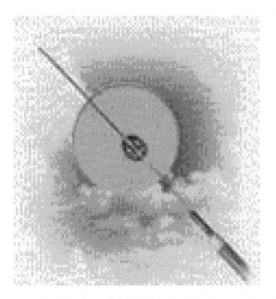

Fig. 3 Tri-Activ. The Tri-Activ distal protection device includes a guidewire with distal protection balloon, a 4-Fr flush catheter, and a peristaltic pump extraction device.

Table 1 Advantages and Disadvantages of Distal Occlusion Devices[a]

Advantages	Disadvantages
Complete protection of distal ICA	Interruption blood flow during protection
Low crossing profile	Potential dissection/spasm in distal ICA
High flexibility	Potential embolization via patent ECA
One size fits all—no sizing issue	No angiographic evaluation of the lesion possible during protection since flow is stopped

[a] These devices are available outside the United States for clinical use. These devices are not approved for use in association with CAS in the United States.

the peristaltic pump secures a continuous aspiration and removal of debris from the carotid circulation.

ADVANTAGES AND DISADVANTAGES OF DISTAL OCCLUSION DEVICES

The principle of occluding the ICA in between the lesion and the brain creates complete protection of the distal ICA and prevents emboli from migrating to the cerebral circulation. However, complete blockage of the distal ICA has disadvantages; this approach interrupts blood flow to the brain and adversely influences oxygen supply to the brain in patients with insufficient intracerebral collateralization. Although this problem can be solved by restoring cerebral oxygen delivery by deflating the distal protection balloon between the different stages of CAS, this decreases the quality of the cerebral protection. Another disadvantage of complete ICA occlusion is that angiographic control of the carotid lesion during protection is impossible. There is also a small chance of embolization via branches of the ECA, which is not occluded. Latex balloons to occlude the vessel make sizing of the devices simple since all vessel diameters are covered by only one balloon size. Nevertheless, balloon inflation should be done cautiously since the required pressure implies a potential risk of spasm and dissection at the distal ICA. A major advantage of the distal occlusion devices is their low crossing profile and high flexibility compared to distal filtration devices, facilitating device delivery (Table 1).

Distal Filter Devices

WORKING PRINCIPLE OF DISTAL FILTER DEVICES

The reasoning behind distal filters is the most intuitive of the cerebral protection devices. Debris is captured in an umbrella-like filter placed in the ICA between the lesion and the brain. After the CAS procedure, a specially designed retrieval device is advanced to a location immediately proximal to the filter for removal of the debris-filled device from the body (Fig. 4). There are two different systems to deliver the filter distal to the lesion. The filter can be directly affixed to a guidewire that is used to cross the lesion and stays in place for the rest of the procedure. Another possibility is to cross the lesion with a

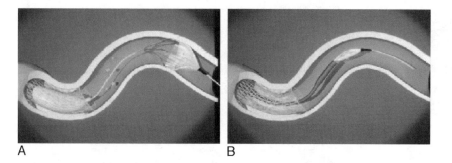

A   B

Fig. 4   Distal filter device. (A) The working principle of the distal filter technique: debris is captured in an umbrella-like filter placed in the ICA between the lesion and the brain. (B) After the CAS procedure, a retrieval device is advanced to a location immediately proximal to the filter for removal of the debris-filled device from the body.

guidewire without filter, after which the filter is brought into place by means of a special delivery device.

DIFFERENT DISTAL FILTER DEVICES ON THE MARKET

Angioguard XP	(Cordis)
Neuroshield	(MedNova)
FilterWire EX	(Boston Scientific)
FilterWire EZ	(Boston Scientific)
AccuNet	(Guidant)
SPIDER	(ev3)
Interceptor	(Medtronic)
Rubicon filter	(Rubicon Medical)

Angioguard XP (Cordis).   The Angioguard XP filter consists of a polyurethane filter affixed to a guidewire with a soft atraumatic tip (Fig. 5). The filter is kept open by 8 nitinol struts that give the filter the general configuration of an umbrella. Visibility of the device is secured by radiopaque markers on the proximal end on 4 of the 8 struts. The pore size of the filter is 100 μm, and the system has a crossing profile between 3.2F and 3.9F. The filter is available in five different sizes, including diameters of 4, 5, 6, 7, and 8 mm. The Sapphire Trial evaluated the use of Angioguard XP for CAS in high-risk patients and is the first randomized trial that suggested the superiority of CAS with cerebral protection over carotid endarterectomy (CEA) in any patient population (5). Combined stroke/ death/myocardial infarction (MI) rates were 5.8% for CAS versus 12.6% for CEA.

Neuroshield (Mednova).   The Neuroshield has a filter element with a pore size of 140 μm. Filter delivery differs from the other devices in that the lesion is first crossed with a special 0.014-in. guidewire having a 0.018-in. tip (Fig. 6). After lesion passage, the

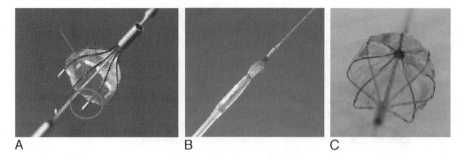

Fig. 5 Angioguard XP. The Angioguard XP filter consists of a polyurethane filter affixed to a guidewire with a soft atraumatic tip. (A) Fully deployed filter with nitinol struts and radiopaque markers. The filter is kept open by 8 nitinol struts that give the filter the general configuration of an umbrella. Visibility of the device is secured by radiopaque markers on the proximal end on 4 of the 8 struts. (B) The Angioguard filter is removed by closure within the Recapture Sleeve. (C) The Angioguard collects debris released from the treated lesion.

filter is brought up with a 3F delivery catheter and is affixed between a proximal stop and a distal olive at the proximal part of the 0.018-in. guidewire tip. Macdonald et al. (6) compared the results of CAS in 75 patients treated under Neuroshield protection to 75 cases without use of a cerebral protection device. This study showed that CAS using the Neuroshield device was safer than CAS without protection: combined rates of stroke and death at 30 days were 4.0% and 10.7%, respectively.

FilterWire EX (Boston Scientific).   The FilterWire EX consists of a wind-sock-type polyurethane filter with a proximal radiopaque nitinol loop affixed to a 0.014-in. guidewire (Fig. 7). The pore size of the filter is 80 μm and the delivery system has a crossing profile of 3.9F. The proximal nitinol loop secures the filter's wall adaptation and makes it a one-size-fits-all device that can accommodate arterial diameters between 3.5 and 5.5 mm. The eccentric design of the filter necessitates angiographic control for positioning of the filter. Complete wall apposition of the filter is only guaranteed if the radiopaque marker on the guidewire at the nitinol loop shows it to be at the arterial wall. Otherwise, the risk of incomplete protection remains (Fig. 8). We evaluated the Filter-Wire EX during CAS in 100 patients with severe ICA stenosis. The combined 30-day stroke and death rate was 2.0% in a population of mostly symptomatic patients (69%). In this study, visible debris was found in 56.9% of the filters used (7).

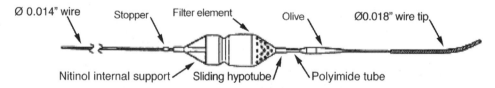

Fig. 6 Neuroshield. The Neuroshield Filter delivery method differs from the other devices; the lesion is first crossed with a special 0.014-in. guidewire with a 0.018-in. tip.

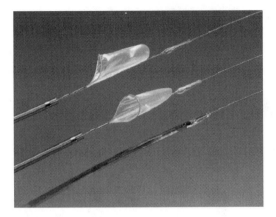

Fig. 7   FilterWire EX. The FilterWire EX consists of a wind-sock-type polyurethane filter with a proximal radiopaque nitinol loop on a 0.014-in. guidewire.

FilterWire EZ (Boston Scientific).   The FilterWire EZ is the newer generation of the FilterWire EX filter (Fig. 9). Just as its predecessor, the FilterWire EZ has a polyurethane filter with a proximal radiopaque nitinol loop. The pore size of the filter is 110 μm, and the crossing profile of the delivery system is downsized to 3.2F. A relocation of the wire more central in the lumen of the filter makes multiplanar control no longer necessary, as the proximal loop will secure good wall apposition in all arteries

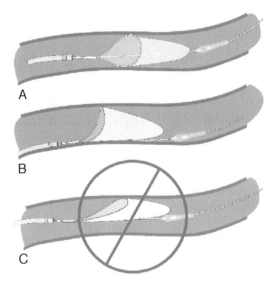

Fig. 8   Positioning the FilterWire EX. Complete wall apposition of the filter is only guaranteed if the radiopaque marker on the guidewire at the nitinol loop shows it to be at the arterial wall. (A) Control in single plane gives appearance of complete wall apposition. (B) Multiplanar evaluation may confirm good wall apposition. (C) Detailed evaluation could show that the guidewire is not against the wall and the filter is not in reasonable position to provide protection.

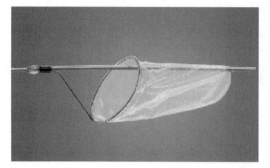

Fig. 9 FilterWire EZ. The FilterWire EZ is the newer generation of the FilterWire. The FilterWire EZ has a polyurethane filter with a proximal radiopaque nitinol loop.

between 3.5 and 5.5 mm in diameter. Improved features of this newer version of the FilterWire are its better visibility and its greater flexibility, permitting the filter to be effective in more tortuous arteries.

RX Accunet (Guidant). The RX Accunet is an umbrella-like polyurethane filter that remains open and is affixed to the vessel wall by a stent-like nitinol structure (Fig. 10). Blood flows in through large proximal openings and debris are captured at the filter's membrane which has a constant pore size of 125 μm. The filter is available in four sizes (4.5–5.5–6.5–7.5 mm). Corresponding crossing profiles are 3.5F for the two smaller filters and 3.7F for the two larger devices.

Spider (ev3). The Spider filter is characterized by its wind-sock-like nitinol mesh basket, making the pore size variable from the proximal end up to the distal tip (Fig. 11). The filter captures debris as small as 50 μm. The proximal radiopaque gold loop increases the visibility of the device and gives an optimal fitting of the nitinol basket to the wall. The Spider system differs from the other distal filter devices in that the lesion first can be crossed with a standard guidewire, enabling the operator to choose a 0.014-in. wire which makes crossing the lesion simpler and safer. After lesion passage, the 2.9F

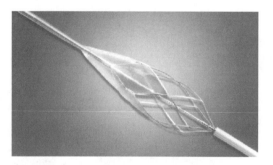

Fig. 10 Accunet. The RX Accunet is an umbrella-like polyurethane filter that is apposed to the vessel wall by a stent-like nitinol structure. Blood flows in through large proximal openings and debris are captured at the filter's membrane.

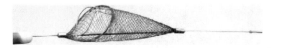

Fig. 11 Spider. The Spider filter has a wind-sock-like nitinol mesh, with a variable pore size. The proximal radiopaque gold loop increases the visibility of the device and enhances fitting of the nitinol basket to the wall.

delivery system is advanced distal to the lesion. The original guidewire is then removed and the wire with the Spider basket affixed on the top is brought into place. The crossing profile of the delivery system is 2.9F for all of the five available filter sizes (3, 4, 5, 6, and 7 mm). The nonrandomized Protect Trial on the use of the Spider during CAS in 50 patients showed a stroke/death rate of 4% at 30 days. Histological exam of the used filters revealed that material was captured in 85% of the examined filters.

Interceptor (Medtronic). Blood flows into the nitinol interceptor through four large proximal holes, and debris is captured by the nitinol maze which has a constant pore size of 100 μm (Fig. 12). The filter comes in two sizes (5.5 and 6.5 mm), and the crossing profile of the delivery system of both sizes is 2.9F.

Rubicon filter (Rubicon Medical). With its crossing profile of less than 2F, the Rubicon filter's crossing profile is the lowest of all distal cerebral protection devices (Fig. 13). To this date, the device is under development and still experimental. The filter membrane has a pore size of 100 μm, and the filter diameters are 4, 5, and 6 mm.

ADVANTAGES AND DISADVANTAGES OF DISTAL FILTER DEVICES

Many surgeons consider the principle of placing a basket between the carotid lesion and the brain to be an appealing concept. The most important feature of distal filtration

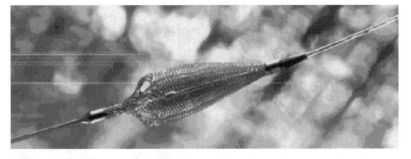

Fig. 12 Interceptor. Blood flows into the nitinol interceptor through four large proximal holes and debris is captured by the nitinol maze.

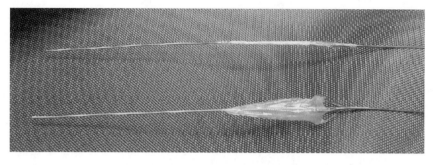

Fig. 13 Rubicon filter. The Rubicon filter's crossing profile is the lowest of all distal cerebral protection devices.

devices is the maintenance of blood flow to the brain. One advantage is that angiographic control of the carotid lesion is possible during all steps of the procedure. Yet far more important is that cerebral oxygen delivery is not impeded with the protection device in place. Should the filter occlude during the procedure due to debris collection or thrombosis, then a number of solutions exist. The debris may be removed by aspirating the filter with a 5-Fr vertebral diagnostic or multipurpose catheter, brought up through the introducer sheath. In those cases where flow blockage by an occluded filter causes acute neurological symptoms, instant removal of the filter is required. The procedure may be continued after inserting a new protection device or, if this is not possible, without any protection device. Filter thrombosis is prevented by full heparinization at the start of procedure and by selecting a filter device with sufficient pore size. Pore sizes between approximately 80 and 140 μm are recommended for they are large enough to prevent filter thrombosis and small enough to offer sufficient embolic protection. The filter design of most devices requires larger crossing profiles than those of the distal occlusion devices, potentially making passage of the filter in very tight or tortuous lesions more difficult. But the current process of further downsizing the crossing profiles and the improvement of the flexibility of the filter system components facilitates the use of the filtration devices in already very difficult anatomies. Most available filter devices

Table 2 Advantages and Disadvantages of Distal Filter Devices[a]

Advantage	Disadvantages
Preservation of flow	Larger crossing profile
Angiographic lesion control during protection is possible	Importance of exact diameter sizing (in some cases)
Less spasm in distal ICA compared to distal occlusion devices	Difficulties in crossing very tight/tortuous lesions
	Potential thrombosis or occlusion of filter with debris

[a] These devices are available outside the United States for clinical use. These devices are not approved for use in association with CAS in the United States.

are manufactured in different sizes. To guarantee optimal vessel fitting and full protection, exact preprocedural vessel diameter sizing is mandatory. With distal filtration devices, less force needs to be applied to the arterial wall than with occlusion balloons, and thus have a considerably lower risk on spasm or wall dissection (Table 2).

Proximal Occlusion Devices

WORKING PRINCIPLE OF PROXIMAL OCCLUSION DEVICES

Proximal occlusion systems are characterized by two compliant balloons, one to place in the common carotid artery and another placed in the external carotid artery. This way, a reversed-flow protection is created, allowing the surgeon to stent a lesion in the internal carotid artery without risking cerebral embolization of dislodged debris during the procedure.

DIFFERENT PROXIMAL OCCLUSION DEVICES ON THE MARKET

Parodi Anti-Emboli System	(ArteriA)
Mo.Ma	(Invatec)

Parodi Anti-Emboli System (Arteria). The Parodi Anti-Emboli System is a reversed-flow system, consisting of two parts (Fig. 14). First, there is the Parodi Anti-Emboli Catheter (PAEC), a flexible dual lumen sheath with a low-pressure balloon at the distal end. Second, there is the Parodi External Balloon (PEB), an over-the-wire, low-profile balloon mounted on a radiopaque guidewire. After arterial access with the 10-Fr introducer sheath, the PAEC is advanced up to the common carotid artery, where it will serve as an arterial suction device. The distal PAEC balloon is dilated in the CCA, and the PEB balloon is placed in the ECA. A vacuum is created resulting in reversed blood flow. After establishing retrograde flow, surgeons can choose between continuous or intermittent flow reversal as well as passive or active suction. The passive suction is created by an arteriovenous shunt, creating a physiological pressure gradient guiding emboli out of the arterial system through an external filter into the venous system. Whitlow et al. (8) reported a series of 75 procedures on symptomatic patients: 95% of patients tolerated proximal occlusion and reversed flow with this device and the stroke/death rate at 30 days was 0%. Similar results were published by Adami et al. (9) who performed 30 procedures on 15 symptomatic and 15 asymptomatic patients. Flow reversal was successful in 93% of the cases and there were no strokes or deaths.

Mo.Ma (Invatec). The Mo.Ma device is a no-flow protection device designed to prevent cerebral embolization during CAS by means of two compliant elastomeric rubber balloons mounted on a 5-Fr distal end of the guiding catheter (Fig. 15). For this system, an 11F introducer sheath is required. Inflating the distal balloon in the external

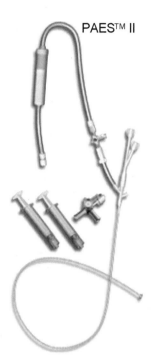

PAES™ II

Fig. 14 Parodi Anti-Emboli System. The Parodi Anti-Emboli System is a reversed-flow system. The Parodi Anti-Emboli Catheter (PAEC) is a flexible dual lumen sheath with a low-pressure balloon at the distal end. After arterial access, the PAEC is advanced into the common carotid artery, where it will serve as an arterial suction device. The distal PAEC balloon is dilated in the CCA to stop forward flow.

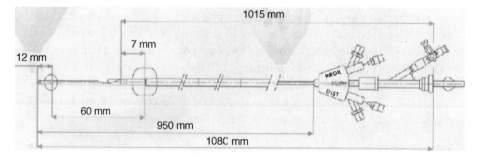

Fig. 15 Mo.Ma device. The Mo.Ma device is a no-flow protection device designed to prevent cerebral embolization during CAS by inflating two compliant elastomeric rubber balloons to isolate the carotid bifurcation.

Table 3 Advantages and Disadvantages of Proximal Occlusion Devices[a]

Advantage	Disadvantages
Complete protection prior to lesion manipulation	Large introducer size
Ability to treat tight/tortuous lesions	Potential dissection/spasm in CCA or ECA
Ability to use guidewire of choice	Interruption of blood flow during protection
	Device handling more laborious

[a] These devices are available outside the United States for clinical use. These devices are not approved for use in association with CAS in the United States.

carotid artery and the proximal one in the common carotid artery blocks blood flow in the carotid arteries. After stenting and/or dilatation, the blood is actively aspirated through the sheath, after which both balloons are deflated to restore normal flow.

ADVANTAGES AND DISADVANTAGES OF PROXIMAL OCCLUSION DEVICES

The major advantage of proximal occlusion is that they do not require lesion passage prior to establishing complete cerebral protection. Once the occlusion balloons are in place, the surgeon can use his guidewire of choice, making it possible to cross even tight or tortuous lesions (Table 3).

The bulkiness and rigidity of these devices make them less maneuverable. Therefore the steps to be undertaken to maneuver the protection device into the carotid circulation are more laborious than with the other types of cerebral protection devices. In addition, ICA and CCA blockage impedes blood supply to the brain in patients with insufficient intracerebral collateralization. Solving this by deflating the distal protection balloon between the different stages of CAS so that cerebral oxygen delivery is restored lowers the efficacy of the cerebral protection. Characteristic to the use of balloons in peripheral arteries is the potential danger of dissection or spasm in the common and external arteries.

Conclusion

Coincidental with the introduction of cerebral protection devices, the neurological complication rates during CAS appear to have decreased considerably over the past few years. Other simultaneous developments that may also be responsible for improved results include lower-profile devices and more operator experience with this procedure. Cerebral protection devices have been developed to decrease the risk of embolization during CAS. None of the devices can guarantee a complete emboli-free procedure since any supra-aortic endovascular manipulation, even a simple diagnostic carotid angiogram, includes a risk of cerebral embolization. The actual delivery of each type of cerebral protection device can itself be an emboligenic event. Patient selection for CAS and clinical and technical experience are of key importance in achieving low complication rates.

Since all the devices have their assets and downsides, it is virtually impossible to acclaim one specific device as being the best, only taking into account product characteristics. We advise the selection of one or two different devices and gaining the experience required to use them well.

References

1. Müller-Hülsbeck S, Jahnke T, Liess C, Glass C, Paulsen F, Grimm J, Heller M. In vitro comparison of four cerebral protection filters for preventing human plaque embolization during carotid interventions. J Endovasc Ther 2002; 9:793–802.

2. Ahmadi R, Willfort A, Lang W, Schillinger M, Alt E, Gschwandtner ME, Haumer M, Maca T, Ehringer H, Minar E. Carotid artery stenting; effect of learning curve and intermediate-term morphological outcome. J Endovasc Ther 2001; 8:539–546.

3. Theron JG, Payelle GG, Coskun O, Huet HF, Guimaraens L. Carotid artery stenosis: Treatment with protected balloon angioplasty and stent placement. Radiology 1996; 201:627–636.

4. Henry M, Henry I, Klonaris C, Masson I, Hugel M, Tzvetanov K, Ethevenot G, Le BE, Kownator S, Luizi F, Folliguet B. Benefits of cerebral protection during carotid stenting with the PercuSurge GuardWire system: Midterm results. J Endovasc Ther 2002; 9:1–13.

5. Yadav JSapphire investigators. Stenting and Angioplasty with Protection in Patients at High Risk for Endarterectomy. Chicago: American Heart Association, November 2002.

6. Macdonald S, McKevitt F, Venables GS, Cleveland TJ, Gaines PA. Neurological outcomes after carotid stenting protected with the Neuroshield filter compared to unprotected stenting. J Endovasc Ther 2002; 9:793–802.

7. Bosiers M, Peeters P, Verbist J, Schroë K, Deloose K, Lauwers G, Stockx L. Belgian experience with FilterWire EX in the prevention of embolic events during carotid stenting. J Endovasc Ther, 2003; 10:695–701.

8. Whitlow PL, Lylyk P, Londero H, Mendiz OA, Mathias K, Jaeger H, Parodi J, Schonolz C, Milei J. Carotid artery stenting protected with an emboli containment system. Stroke 2002; 33:1308–1314.

9. Adami CA, Scure A, Spinamano L, Galyagni E, Antoiucci D, Farello GA, Maglione F, Manfrini S, Mangialardi N, Mansueto GC, Mascoli F, Nardelli E, Tealdi D. Use of the Parodi Anti-Embolysm system in carotid stenting: Italian study results. J Endovasc Ther 2002; 9:147–154.

14

Neurorescue During Carotid Stenting: Catheter-Based Techniques and Patient Management

PETER A. SCHNEIDER

Hawaii Permanente Medical Group, Honolulu, Hawaii, U.S.A.

MICHAEL B. SILVA, JR.

Texas Tech University, Lubbock, Texas, U.S.A.

The purpose of this chapter is to provide an algorithm for recognizing and managing an acute neurological event during or immediately after carotid stent placement. A major concern about carotid stenting that has delayed its development is the possibility of cerebral emboli as a result of endoluminal manipulation of the carotid bifurcation. Although clinically significant neurological events are less common with carotid angioplasty and stenting (CAS) than many experts initially thought they would be, stroke occurs after 2% to 7% of cases (1–6). Surgeons performing CAS must be ready to manage these events. The rationale for neurorescue therapy is discussed, as well as the supporting evidence, tools, techniques, and protocol.

What Are the Mechanisms of Perioperative Stroke?

Acute stroke during a cerebrovascular procedure, such as carotid arteriography or carotid stent placement, may be due to ischemia or hemorrhage. This is an important distinction since the management of these entities varies significantly from each other. Ischemia is much more common and may be due to emboli (thrombus, atherosclerotic plaque, or both), thrombosis (associated with an intracranial occlusive lesion, iatrogenic injury, or a hypercoagulable state), or low flow (such as an ischemic watershed area). Hemorrhage during carotid stent placement is considered in a later section.

When an acute neurological deficit occurs during carotid arteriography or carotid stent placement, the likely cause is the embolization of dislodged atherosclerotic plaque or catheter-generated thrombus (Table 1). The tendency of the guidewire and catheter to attempt to lurch forward while advancing into the common carotid artery must be continuously monitored. Arch or branch vessel origins that are laden with friable plaque may also pose a risk of plaque dislodgment during catheter manipulation. Occasionally, catheter-induced spasm or arterial injury may cause thrombus formation (see Chapter 19). This can be minimized by using heparin, reducing catheter time in the artery, moving the catheter occasionally in the artery if multiple runs are required, and using vasodilators as needed. Other mechanisms that may cause ischemic stroke in this setting are poor perfusion, arterial injury, or the iatrogenic administration of air bubbles or other incompatible substances.

Stroke associated with carotid arteriography using modern techniques probably occurs in less than 1% of cases (see Chapter 4) (7,8). Carotid arteriography has been made safer by improvements in catheters, guidewires, contrast, and technique. Improved imaging equipment has also shortened procedure times and decreased the catheter indwelling time. Nevertheless, carotid arteriography does occasionally cause stroke. Some of the studies of intra-arterial thrombolysis for acute stroke have included patients who had stroke associated with carotid arteriography (9).

Transcranial Doppler studies performed during carotid stent procedures have shown evidence of cerebral emboli during guidewire placement, predilatation, stent placement, and post-stent dilatation (10,11). In addition, other events may occur in association with carotid access, stent placement, or use of a distal protection device. Events such as stent thrombosis, distal internal carotid artery (ICA) spasm, and arterial damage and thrombosis associated with distal protection devices are discussed in Chapter 19 (12). Air emboli may also occur and there is no method for reversing this when it occurs. Air may be introduced through a faulty valve mechanism, may be contained in administered solutions, or may result from rupture of an angioplasty balloon. When an air bubble disperses and moves more distally into the vasculature, it occludes the smaller branches and eventually the capillary bed, thus preventing any possible collateral back flow. Since air does not dissolve, it can cause profound ischemia and prevent recovery of brain tissue by occluding deep matter end arteries that have no collaterals.

Despite the multitude of possible mechanisms for an acute neurological event, there are a few specific issues to address when stroke occurs. (1) How severe is the neurological deficit? (2) Is the stent site patent and free of thrombus? (3) Can a distal cerebral embolus be identified?

Table 1 Mechanisms of Acute Ischemic Stroke During Carotid Stent Placement

Mechanism	Establish carotid access	Cross lesion and place cerebral protection	Stent placement, balloon angioplasty	Retrieve cerebral protection device and completion arteriogram
Dislodge plaque	Arch, proximal CCA, or bifurcation plaque dislodged by guidewire, catheter, or sheath.	Bifurcation plaque dislodged by crossing lesion with guidewire or cerebral protection device.	Dislodged bifurcation plaque may escape cerebral protection device.	Captured material may be spilled and escape into distal circulation.
Form thrombus	Catheter- or sheath-based thrombus may embolize.	Thrombus may form under low-flow conditions with cerebral protection device across critical ICA stenosis.	A full filter, a distal dissection, a new kink may cause thrombus formation.	Thrombus associated with cerebral protection device may embolize.
Cause low flow	Sheath may occlude inflow by creating kink or by prohibiting flow if there is a proximal CCA lesion.	Low flow may occur with device placed across critical lesion.	Distal occlusion balloon stops flow. Filter with small pore size or that is full of debris may cause low flow. Hypotension from carotid dilation.	Cerebral protection device may cause spasm in distal ICA.
Injure artery	Arch or proximal CCA injury due to catheter or sheath manipulation.	Bifurcation or ICA may be injured by passing cerebral protection device.	Overdilation may rupture artery. Stent placement may cause kink. Balloon dilation may cause dissection distal to stent.	Arterial injury may occur during removal of cerebral protection device.
Introduce bubbles or unwanted solutions	Could happen at any time with a break in technique or equipment failure.	Could happen at any time with a break in technique or equipment failure.	Could happen at any time with a break in technique or equipment failure.	Could happen at any time with a break in technique or equipment failure.

CCA = common carotid artery; ICA = internal carotid artery.

How Is a Perioperative Neurological Event Recognized?

A comprehensive and documented preoperative neurological examination is critical. This will serve as the patient's neurological baseline for comparison during and after carotid stenting. Many decisions may be made regarding the patients' care that are based on this exam. Is there a neurological change or is the patient just sedated? Is this a minor or major change from baseline? Should thrombolytic therapy be administered or should supportive care only be performed? These are some of the difficult questions that must be answered in a matter of minutes, and the appropriate actions must be prepared ahead of time.

When a neurological event occurs during the procedure, it may present as a focal motor deficit, seizure, hemineglect, or a decreased level of consciousness. Often the first signs are yawning or confusion, which can be fairly subtle. The sooner a neurological problem can be identified, the better it is for the safe conduct of the procedure. The development of a new deficit will significantly influence the conduct of the case in terms of the sequence of maneuvers, the initiation of supportive care and medications, and the search for a cause. Patients with a decreased level of consciousness or confusion can be very challenging to evaluate and manage. It may also be difficult to assess whether patients have developed a deficit after they become confused. Subtle neurological changes are exceedingly challenging to detect when the patient is under the drapes.

Most neurological events are self-limited and resolve without mechanical intervention. When a neurological event occurs, specific treatment modalities are initiated. The medical management of acute stroke is accompanied by a specific decision tree analysis to assess the cause. If a severe or worsening neurological deficit is present and a specific branch vessel occlusion is identified, catheter-based neurorescue is performed. The management of stroke is discussed in the next section.

How Is a Perioperative Neurological Event Managed?

When a neurological event is suspected during carotid stent placement, specific maneuvers are undertaken to manage the patient and to perform ongoing assessment to help determine the next management steps (Table 2). The part of the procedure during which the problem occurred will help to determine the sequence of events. In general, a bailout by backing away from stent placement is not a reasonable option. If the deficit occurs before the stent is placed, it is not usually an option to stop the procedure. The stent should be rapidly placed and the perfusion to the brain optimized. If a distal embolus has occurred, access to this area must be through the stented carotid artery. If a plaque has been destabilized by manipulation, the only way to stabilize it is to go ahead with stent placement. If an ischemic area in the brain has become clinically symptomatic, the best way to reverse it or to limit damage is to restore perfusion. When a deficit occurs early in the case, proceed rapidly to stent placement if at all possible while carrying out the decision tree that is outlined in this section (Fig. 1).

Table 2 Major Steps in Managing an Acute
Neurological Deficit During Carotid Stent
Placement

Assess the patient.
   Neurological
   Hemodynamic
   Coagulation
Optimize hemodynamics and anticoagulation.
Assess vasculature.
   Stent site
   Cerebral arteries
Treat significant defect at stent site.
Reassess the patient's neurological status.
Treat cerebral artery emboli with neurorescue techniques.

Initially, one should confirm that the patient has an adequate airway. This can be challenging in the confused patient or when a decreased level of consciousness has occurred. Check for hypoxia. Supplemental oxygen should be administered. If the patient requires intubation for inability to protect the airway or for hypoventilation, hyperventilation should be instituted to reduce pCO_2 and induce cerebral vasodilation. A hemodynamic assessment is also performed and hypotension should be corrected. Consider elevating systemic blood pressure to improve cerebral collateral perfusion. A systolic blood pressure of 160 mm Hg or more is desirable. Check the anticoagulation status by performing an activated clotting time. The ACT should be maintained at greater than 250 sec. Dexamethasone should be administered (20 mg) to help reduce cerebral swelling and injury. If hypertension and bradycardia are occurring spontaneously (Cushing's response), especially if there is a depressed level of consciousness, be suspicious of increased intracranial pressure, possibly due to hemorrhage.

After hemodynamic optimization, another neurological exam should be performed. Some patients will have developed neurological impairment on the basis of hypoperfusion and will improve. Others may have had a transient ischemic attack resulting from a passing embolus and the deficit may clear after a few minutes.

Adjust the anticoagulation status based on the results of the next few maneuvers. If a fleeting, subtle, or transient deficit has occurred or it resolves with hemodynamic improvement, additional heparin and/or IIb/IIIa receptor inhibitors should be considered. If the ACT is less than 250, additional heparin should be administered to prevent propagation of thrombus and/or generation of sheath thrombus.

When a neurological deficit is identified, the vasculature must be assessed as soon as the patient's vital signs have been evaluated and as they are being stabilized. An arteriogram of the stent site and the cerebral artery runoff is performed through the sheath. The angiographic assessment of the patient with a neurological deficit is described in a section below. Arteriographic assessment is required even if the neurological event is only transient. Those patients with persistent neurological impairment should

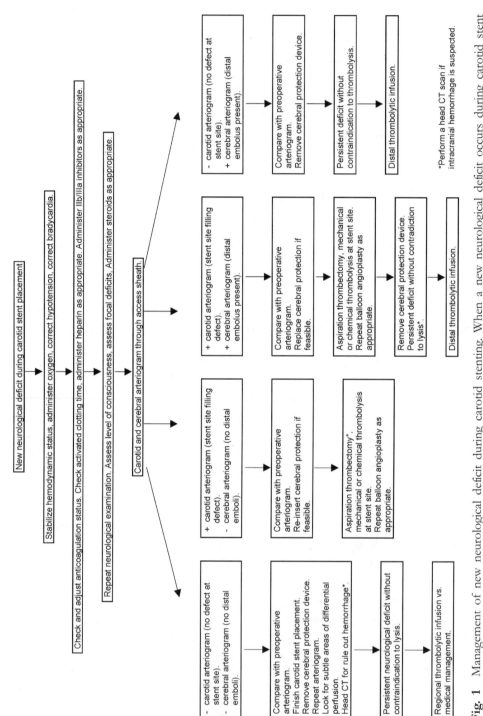

Fig. 1 Management of new neurological deficit during carotid stenting. When a new neurological deficit occurs during carotid stent placement, management is performed in a methodical manner so that as information is accumulated, the appropriate maneuvers can be performed in an attempt to reverse cerebral ischemia and preserve cerebral function.

be considered for adjunctive treatment. If there is evidence of a filling defect in the stent or in the distal cerebral artery, IIb/IIIa receptor inhibitors should be administered intravenously if they have not already been started.

If there is a filling defect at the stent site, it must be treated. Aspiration, thrombectomy, mechanical thrombolysis, or chemical thrombolysis with thrombolytic agents or intra-arterial IIb/IIIa inhibitors are options. The carotid access sheath maybe aspirated vigorously. A larger caliber straight or angled catheter, 5 or 6 Fr, or a long guiding catheter may be advanced through the sheath and into the thrombus. Aspiration is performed while withdrawing the catheter from distal to proximal. If a 90-cm length carotid access sheath is being used, a catheter length must be selected accordingly. The effluent is filtered to evaluate the content of the material. Platelet-rich thrombus may indicate that intra-arterial IIb/IIIa inhibitor is the appropriate next step. Aspiration should be performed until the effluent is clear of thrombus or particles.

After optimizing the hemodynamics and anticoagulation and ensuring that the stent site is patent and is a not a source for continuing embolization, the patient should be reassessed. Patients with major neurological deficits and with angiographic evidence of distal emboli may be acceptable candidates for neurorescue techniques, including catheter directed thrombolysis. The precise indications for the use of neurorescue techniques to treat a neurological event during carotid stenting are unclear at present. Because the combination of a persistent and severe neurological deficit in the setting of an identified cerebral embolus in a patient who is a candidate for thrombolysis is an uncommon situation, it will take some time for the indications to be clarified. Technical options for managing distal emboli are listed in Table 3.

Patients with a sudden major deficit and no angiographically identifiable embolus are a challenging group in which to decide upon a treatment course. The differential diagnostic possibilities of seizure or intracranial hemorrhage should be considered (see next section). A very small but well-placed embolus to a branch of the MCA or a shower of microemboli could also produce this clinical scenario. An aggressive approach would be to treat these patients with a regional thrombolytic infusion into the middle cerebral artery with the intention of dissipating the thrombus or platelet aggregates that may have showered into the smaller arterial branches of the brain. Minor deficits without angiographic evidence of emboli may be treated with supportive care alone or possibly IIb/IIIa inhibition.

Table 3　Neurorescue Techniques: Options for Treating Distal Cerebral Emboli

---

Catheter-directed chemical thrombolysis: TPA or UK
IIb/IIIa receptor inhibitors: intravenous or intra-arterial
Balloon angioplasty
Thrombus maceration
Aspiration thrombectomy
Snare removal of embolus

Time frame of new neurological deficit associated with carotid stent placement

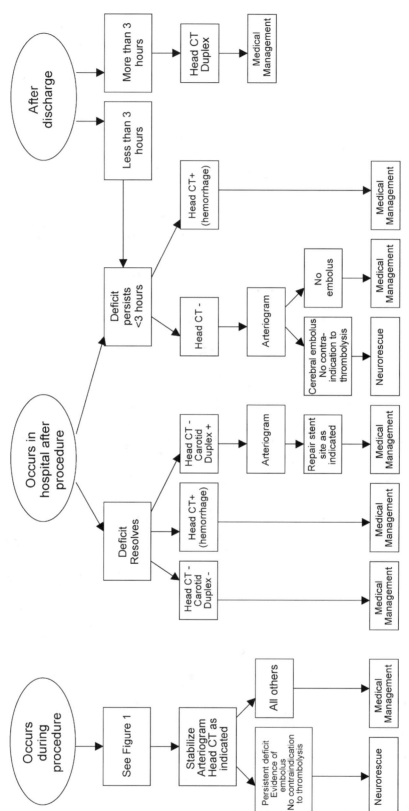

Fig. 2 Neurorescue versus medical management of new neurological deficits during the perioperative period for carotid stent placement. The timing of the occurrence of the neurological deficit affects its management in the perioperative period for carotid stent placement. Other important factors include the following: whether the deficit persists, whether an embolus is identified, whether the carotid stent site contains filling defects that could produce more emboli, whether the patient presents within 3 hr of developing the new neurological deficit, and whether the patient is a candidate for thrombolysis.

Stroke that occurs in association with carotid stent placement may occur during the procedure, but also may occur later in the perioperative period (Fig. 2). A substantial number of events occur hours to days after the carotid stent procedure (13–15). In one study, 26% of the strokes occurred more than 24 hr (and up to 14 days) after the carotid stent procedure (13). In another study, 71% of the perioperative neurological deficits (10 of 14) associated with carotid stent placement in 111 patients, occurred after the procedure was concluded (15). This presents logistical challenges to intracranial thrombolysis. Medical management is usually most appropriate in patients who have resolved or improving neurological deficits, intracranial hemorrhage, poor candidacy for thrombolysis, no identifiable cerebral embolus, or delayed presentation. Neurorescue should be considered when the neurological deficit is severe and persistent, there is a cerebral embolus, the patient is a good candidate for thrombolysis, and the patient presents within 3 hr of the event.

How Is Intracranial Hemorrhage Recognized?

When a patient develops an acute neurological deficit during a cerebrovascular procedure, the likelihood is that it is related to ischemia and not hemorrhage. Although hemorrhage occurs very uncommonly, it still occurs with a greater frequency after CAS than after carotid endarterectomy (3.8% vs. 0.6%) and should be considered in the differential when neurological symptoms develop in the perioperative period (16). In addition, the basic treatment options for ischemia and hemorrhage are quite different and may make things worse if incorrectly applied.

Patients who have had recent strokes prior to CAS are at high risk for intracranial hemorrhage during the stent placement procedure. Any patient who has had a stroke within 4 to 6 weeks of CAS should not undergo thrombolysis because of the possibility of making the patient worse by converting the previous ischemic stroke to an area of hemorrhage. Patients who are undergoing carotid stent placement because of recent transient ischemic attacks should undergo CT scanning of the brain prior to CAS to look for the possibility of a silent cerebral infarct. If this has not been done and the patient develops a neurological deficit during CAS, consideration should be given to placing the stent, securing cerebral inflow, and moving the patient for a head CT before administering any thrombolytic agents. If a patient develops a neurological deficit during CAS and there is no sign of distal cerebral embolus, intracranial hemorrhage should be considered as a possibility. If thrombolytic agents are administered to a patient with unrecognized cerebral hemorrhage, the chance of worsening the situation is increased significantly. Some neurorescue options are still available without the use of chemical thrombolysis, but catheter-based thrombolytic infusion has been a mainstay of this developing treatment (Table 3).

There are some signs that one may find in the setting of acute hemorrhage that may indicate the diagnosis (Table 4). Patients who have had a previous stroke are at increased risk, also patients with a long-term history of diabetes, hypertension or small-

Table 4   Evaluation of Cerebral Ischemia Versus Intracranial Hemorrhage

	Cerebral ischemia	Intracranial hemorrhage
Clinical	Neurological deficit	Headache
	No pain or pain not prominent	Decreased level of consciousness
		Cushing's response
History	Nonspecific	Previous stroke
		Previous hemorrhage
		Diabetes, hypertension
		Intracranial occlusive disease
Angiographic	Filling defect, vessel occlusion	Blush of extravascular contrast
	Distal embolus	Mass effect

vessel intracranial disease. A patient that complains of headache and develops a sudden loss of consciousness may have cerebral hemorrhage. Clinically, hemorrhage may cause signs of increased intracranial pressure, such as pain (headache) and hypertension with bradycardia (Cushing's response). Angiographically, one might not see anything that is apparently abnormal. However, any mass effect, extravascular blush, extravasation, or tissue shift is important.

What Is the Rationale for Catheter-Based Neurorescue Therapy?

The concept of catheter-based neurorescue makes intuitive sense. When brain damage occurs as a result of embolization, endovascular techniques may be used to remove or dissolve the embolic material and reverse ischemic damage. There is good motivation to improve over the medical management of acute stroke. The mortality for an untreated middle cerebral artery occlusion ranges from 12% to 28% and survivors have a high likelihood of significant disability (17–19).

Intravenous thrombolytic has been shown to improve outcome when administered within 3 hr of the onset of neurological deficit (20). There was no difference in mortality, but there was a 30% relative improvement in neurological function at 3 months after intravenous tissue plasminogen activator (TPA) administration was compared to placebo. The only FDA approved protocol for the use of thrombolytic agents to treat acute stroke is for systemic TPA to be administered intravenously within 3 hr of acute, de novo stroke (0.9 mg/kg, 10% as a bolus and the rest over an hour to a maximum of 90 mg). Several other studies have shown that intravenous TPA had no benefit if administered 3 to 6 hr after the onset of the stroke or could even make things worse (21–24). The cerebral artery recanalization rate for intravenous thrombolytic therapy ranges from 21% to 43% (25). Intravenous TPA was more efficacious at dissolving distal cerebral artery thrombus and less successful at recanalizing main cerebral artery occlusions. Patients with thrombus in the proximal middle cerebral artery tend to be helped the least by the intravenous TPA protocol (26).

The idea behind catheter-based intra-arterial thrombolysis of the cerebral arteries, as compared with the approved intravenous protocol, is to improve results by lowering the dose of thrombolytic required by direct administration, improving recanalization rates, and extending the treatment window for acute stroke. The idea that neurorescue could be used to treat stroke during carotid stent placement is extrapolated from studies suggesting that the acute treatment of newly presenting stroke with emergent intra-arterial thrombolytic therapy provides improved outcomes. The best evidence and only level 1 evidence for intra-arterial thrombolytic treatment of acute stroke comes from a single trial. Early Intra-arterial Prourokinase Trial (PROACT II) was a prospective, randomized comparison of catheter-directed intracranial prourokinase vs. systemic intravenous heparin (9). Prourokinase is not commercially available. The study did not include a comparison arm that was composed of patients treated with the only approved thrombolytic therapy for acute stroke, that is, intravenous TPA. Recanalization of cerebral arteries occurred in 67% of patients vs. 17% treated with heparin alone. There was no significant difference in mortality or in early outcome. There was a 15% absolute benefit in neurological status in the thrombolytic group at 90 days (40% had a Rankin score of 2 or less after intra-arterial prourokinase vs. 25% of those treated with heparin). The rate of identifiable intracranial hemorrhage was 28% after intra-arterial cerebral thrombolysis and 6% with heparin and the rate of clinically significant intracranial hemorrhage was 10.2% after intra-arterial thrombolysis and 1.8% in controls. Mortality in both groups was the same at 90 days. Intracranial hemorrhage that occurs in association with thrombolysis for acute stroke continues to be the major concern of this method of treatment.

There has been no prospective, randomized comparison of intravenous thrombolytic vs. catheter-directed, intra-arterial thrombolysis in acute stroke. The nationwide standard for the treatment of acute stroke is intravenous TPA administered within 3 hr of the event, not a catheter-directed intracranial approach. There is no agent approved by the FDA for catheter-directed intra-arterial cerebral thrombolysis. There is no standard protocol, standard of practice, or national credentialing standard for catheter-directed intracranial thrombolysis (27,28).

In addition to these areas of ambiguity, there are two major issues that remain unresolved with regard to catheter-based intra-arterial thrombolysis for acute stroke at the time of carotid stent placement. (1) De novo acute stroke is not the same as stroke that may occur during carotid stent placement, which is often due to plaque contents, rather than thrombus. The particles released during carotid stent placement are a combination of cholesterol crystals and lipoid masses from atherosclerotic carotid bifurcation plaque, neither of which dissolves or can be removed by thrombolytic therapy (29–31). The second major unresolved issue is a conglomeration of unknowns that are associated with brain function and cerebrovascular physiology that require study before catheter-based thrombolysis can be standardized. Some of these are listed here. (1) The brain is more tolerant of emboli than was previously thought, so not every embolus requires treatment. (2) The clinical effects of emboli are highly variable and do not necessarily correlate with size. (3) Manipulation of the carotid bifurcation produces atheroemboli that cannot be dissolved and usually cannot be removed. (4) The recovery from stroke is highly variable, with some patients recovering from initially profound deficits; therapy that makes the condition worse should be avoided. (5) Thrombolytic therapy and endovascular cerebral artery manipulation have a risk of complications, including intracranial hemorrhage. Despite these many issues requiring study, it is likely that the future of cerebral tissue preservation in these challenging situations will be largely catheter based.

There are many different procedures that are more commonly performed than CAS that have a risk of embolic stroke. These include coronary bypass, heart valve replacement, percutaneous coronary interventions, valvuloplasty, cardiac electrophysiology studies and treatments, cardioversion, carotid arteriography, arch vessel surgery, and carotid endarterectomy. The potential need for neurorescue techniques has not played a prominent role in the development of these procedures. Nevertheless, there has been an extensive discussion about the potential need for neurorescue techniques during CAS. There are several reasons for this. CAS is different from many procedures that have gone before it. There is an open surgical alternative that is proven and safe and has a low stroke rate (see Chapter 16). Carotid stent and cerebral protection systems and the techniques for placement are rapidly developing. There is a huge potential market for CAS. There is a large and able workforce across several medical disciplines that is planning to participate in carotid stenting. Each discipline is determined to point out its respective strengths and others' weaknesses in the endovascular management of carotid disease. There is significant political heat over who "owns" carotid stenting and who will be permitted to practice it. The actual need for neurorescue during carotid stenting is reported at a rate of about 1% (32) The benefits of neurorescue during carotid stenting appear to be more theoretical than real since the results have been so poor when reported. This is discussed in the next section.

In summary, current use of intracranial, catheter-directed thrombolysis and other rescue techniques makes sense and there is reason to be optimistic about future developments using these methods. However, intra-arterial thrombolysis for acute de novo stroke is supported by marginal evidence that demonstrates marginal benefit. Treatment in patients who sustain a neurological deficit during carotid stent placement has even less proof. This is an attractive concept, but it is not the standard of care and its validity is unproven.

What Are the Results of Neurorescue Therapy for Stroke During Carotid Stent Placement?

The published results of neurorescue during CAS have been poor. In the largest study to date, 27 of 450 patients undergoing carotid stent placement developed neurological deficits (6%) (32). Twenty-two neurological deficits resolved or nearly resolved on medical management alone and 5 patients were treated with intracranial thrombolysis. Three of these patients died of stroke (60% mortality) and 2 experienced some improvement, but neurological deficits persisted. These results cannot be the basis for a rational standard.

Intracranial thrombolytic therapy has its own high morbidity. In the PROACT II study, the intracranial hemorrhage rate was 28% (9). Hemorrhagic transformation of an acute stroke may occur in up to 39% when intra-arterial cerebral artery thrombolysis is performed (33). Patients in these studies underwent CT brain imaging prior to treatment to help avoid the potential disaster of administering thrombolytic treatment to a patient with an underlying intracranial hemorrhage. In the setting of an acute, intra-procedural, neurological event, it may not be logistically feasible to first perform axial brain imaging to rule out intracranial hemorrhage, making the risk of intracranial thrombolytic therapy in this setting even higher.

As carotid stenting develops, questions related to neurorescue that will hopefully be addressed include indications, timing, agent of choice, protocol for use, and results and risks of treatment. Most of the neurological deficits that have occurred as a result of carotid stent placement in published series have been minor and/or resolved or significantly improved spontaneously and would not be candidates for this treatment (14,34–36). Deciding who is a candidate for neurorescue remains a major challenge.

Angiographic Assessment of the Patient with Acute Neurological Deficit During Carotid Stenting

When a neurological deficit develops, the arterial anatomy must be reevaluated (Table 5). The evaluation of acute arterial occlusion in the brain is different than in other vascular beds since the exact location of the lesion is of profound importance and the signs of

Table 5 Potential Angiographic Findings During Evaluation of the Cerebral Arteries when a Patient Develops a Neurological Deficit Due to Distal Emboli During Carotid Stenting

Major cerebral arteries
  Absence of cerebral artery
  Abrupt cutoff of contrast column
  Occlusion
  Vessel stub
  Filling defect
  Retrograde flow, delayed flow during late images
Smaller branches of cerebral arteries
  Absence of parenchymal blush during initial phase of arteriogram
  Delayed or sluggish flow in a specific area
  Stagnant contrast in a specific area
  Collateral artery filling
  Luxury perfusion (from collaterals) during late images

vessel occlusion may be subtle. Contrast is administered through the side arm of the sheath. A major advantage of treating periprocedural stroke with directed thrombolysis is that there are comparison preoperative arteriograms in most cases. Careful analysis of the intraprocedural cerebral arteriogram is performed and it is compared with preoperative anterior–posterior and lateral arteriograms.

An abrupt cutoff, vessel stub, or notable absence of the distal internal carotid artery, the anterior cerebral artery, or the middle cerebral artery may be observed. An embolus to the origin or M1 segment of the middle cerebral artery may be visible. An M2 branch occlusion may be difficult to identify since it may be one of several branches. In general, the occlusion of smaller but essential branches that supply important regions of the brain, such as the lenticulostriate arteries, may be subtle and difficult to identify. Special attention should be given to the proximal MCA and the region where the lenticulostriate arteries originate. The status of these vessels and the collaterals in this area often determine the prognosis and the time available to treat the patient before ischemia becomes irreversible.

More often than the identification of a filling defect or an abrupt cutoff, subtle signs reveal the location of the occlusion. Angiographic clues to distal arterial emboli must be pursued. Look for signs of differential perfusion of the cerebral territories. Slow antegrade flow in a vessel while the rest of the vasculature shows a normal transit time to the arteriolar phase is a significant sign. An absence of the usual parenchymal blush in one area may indicate the area of emboli. Late images may show luxury perfusion as collateral flow feeds a specific area while all other regions have progressed to the venous phase. Retrograde flow or significant collateral artery filling may also indicate a proximal occlusion. Delayed or sluggish filling of a cerebral branch vessel, especially if it continues into the venous phase of contrast clearing the rest of the brain, is evidence of an arterial occlusion. This underscores the necessity of complete images of the arterial, parenchymal, and venous phases with cerebral angiography.

The thrombus may move, propagate, or disperse during the study, and this may also occur during attempts to perform neurorescue. The precise length of an occlusion may not be accurately reflected by the filling of contrast into the artery distal to the lesion. A patent arterial segment distal to the occlusion but with stagnant flow may not opacify with contrast if collateral perfusion is under low pressure. A comfortable familiarity with cerebral anatomy is essential to discover these subtle angiographic findings. An accurate assessment of the patient's current and previous neurological exams helps in determining the clinical severity of the event and assists in planning the necessary course of action.

How Can You Tell the Clinical Importance of an Intracranial Occlusion?

The worst outcome of episodes of cerebral embolization are associated with "T occlusions," that is, occlusion of the distal internal carotid artery that extends into the

M1 and A1 segments. The mortality in this setting is 50% to 90% (37–39). With more focal arterial occlusions, the specific location of the cerebral artery lesion is far more important than the tissue mass served by the occluded artery. A very small but well-placed infarction in the motor cortex may have much more severe sequelae than a much larger zone of infarction in the frontal or occipital lobes. When a significant neurological deficit occurs due to an embolus, the embolus is usually large enough to occlude a major cerebral artery (38,40,41). When an embolus lodges in a major cerebral artery, the vessel is usually patent distal to the embolus but with very slow or stagnant flow. If collateral perfusion is able to keep brain tissue alive long enough to perform thrombolysis, the results may be excellent (14). However, if end arteries are occluded, especially important ones like the lenticulostriate arteries, the likelihood of a good result is low. When a middle cerebral artery occlusion occurs, for example, the collateral blood supply is usually from the anterior cerebral artery through pial branches. The anterior cerebral artery usually receives collateral blood supply from the contralateral anterior cerebral artery through the anterior communicating artery. The posterior cerebral artery receives blood supply through the posterior communicating artery. A focal, proximal occlusion with good collaterals may be less threatening than a smaller, more distally placed embolus to an area with no collateral perfusion. If thrombus is instrumented aggressively enough to break it up without dissolving it, multiple distal branches may become occluded. In summary, when an occlusion occurs, the clinical significance may vary from none to profound, based on the location of the occlusion and underlying collateral pathways (both major cerebral arteries and pial collaterals).

The lenticulostriate arteries, as mentioned above, originate from the proximal middle cerebral artery (lateral group) and the anterior cerebral artery (medial group). This is the blood supply to the basal ganglia, deep white matter of the frontal and parietal lobes and the internal and external capsule. The lateral lenticulostriate arteries may arise from the M1 or M2 segments. An occlusion along the proximal MCA where these arteries originate causes severe ischemia and reduces the time available to perform any rescue maneuvers. Lenticulostriate arteries have little or no collateral pathways. If embolization during CAS results in an occlusion of the segment supplying the lenticulostriate arteries, an attempt should be made to recanalize it as soon as possible. Occlusion of the distal MCA or even the very proximal MCA in the setting of good collaterals to the MCA segment perfusing the lenticulostriates may not be as significant as occlusion of the segment that gives rise to the lateral lenticulostriate arteries (40). In general, higher cerebral artery recanalization rates after thrombolysis for stroke are associated with better outcomes (38,41,42). However, establishing major artery inflow may not always be helpful and could be harmful if it results in occlusion of the lenticulostriate arteries. A proximal major artery occlusion with good collaterals may be preferable to the potential of breaking up an embolus and passing numerous emboli into smaller distal branches. Therefore, in addition to the location of the lesion, the clinical condition of the patient is essential in determining the importance of an intracranial occlusion.

The status of the deep perforators (end arteries such as the lenticulostriate arteries) and the pial collaterals distal to an occlusion determines the time available until irreversible ischemia occurs and also the prognosis. Occlusion of the distal internal carotid artery at its bifurcation usually produces profound ischemia and carries a poor prognosis (T occlusion). If both the anterior cerebral artery (ACA) and middle cerebral artery (MCA) are occluded, there will be no collateral flow between the two territories. If the proximal MCA thrombus extends into the segment that originates the lenticulostriate arteries, the degree of ischemia is worse and the time to irreversibility is less. If the M1 segment that gives rise to the lenticulostriate arteries is patent, it is at the furthest possible location from any collateral flow. Thrombus located at the internal carotid artery (ICA) bifurcation may be dislodged mechanically by probing it with a guidewire or microcatheter, at least permitting the restoration of flow to the lenticulostriate arteries (43). Immediate chemical thrombolysis should be initiated. The clinical effects of an occlusion of the origin of the MCA depend on the pial collaterals from the anterior cerebral artery and the posterior cerebral arteries and their ability to backfill the distal MCA and the lenticulostriate arteries. If collateral perfusion is poor, the outcome will be similar to occlusion of the entire M1 segment and resultant infarct in the internal capsule. When the entire M1 segment fills with thrombus, the lenticulostriate arteries are deprived of perfusion. In this case, the time to perform rescue is shortened and the degree of pial collaterals is less important. Immediate intervention should be undertaken. The outcome of more distal MCA occlusions, such as at the distal M1 segment (distal to the lenticulostriates) or the M2 segments, depend on collateral flow. When these types of occlusions are accompanied by neurological deficits during the case, thrombolysis should be performed.

The risk of intracranial hemorrhage with thrombolysis seems to correlate somewhat with the location of the occlusion. Patients with occlusion of the distal internal carotid artery with patency of the circle of Willis and the lenticulostriate arteries have a lower risk of hemorrhage with thrombolysis (44). Patients with distal ICA and proximal MCA occlusion and occlusion of the lenticulostriate arteries usually have the densest neurological deficit and are at highest risk for hemorrhage with thrombolysis.

What Are the Indications for Rescue Therapy During Carotid Stenting?

The above discussion reveals that there are many factors that help to determine whether to proceed with neurorescue therapy, including the severity of the neurological deficit, the cerebral anatomy (whether an occlusion can be identified and is treatable), and the patient's risk of hemorrhage with thrombolytic therapy (Table 6). If patients have a severe and persistent or worsening neurological deficit despite aggressive medical management, anticoagulation, and intravenous IIb/IIIa inhibitors, they should be considered for neurorescue techniques including chemical thrombolysis. If a cerebral embolus can be identified (or an abnormality in cerebral flow localized to a specific area) in the clinical setting described, neurorescue is indicated. If no cerebral embolus or flow

Table 6 Indications for Neurorescue Techniques

Severe neurological deficit that is not responding to medical management
Identification of embolus or occlusion on cerebral arteriogram
   Regional thrombolysis may be appropriate in some patients without identification of an
     embolus
Low risk of intracranial hemorrhage with thrombolysis
Presentation within 3 hr of the event

---

abnormality or vessel absence can be identified on arteriography, other causes of neurological deficit should be sought before resorting to rescue techniques. The possibility of unrecognized cerebral hemorrhage should be considered in this setting. Patients at high risk for intracranial hemorrhage due to recent stroke, even if it is a silent infarct, should not be treated with chemical thrombolysis. A clinically significant hemorrhage as a result of thrombolysis may convert a disabling event into a life-threatening situation. If no thrombus is identified and there is no contraindication to thrombolysis, consideration should be given to going ahead with treatment in a patient with an acute neurological change during CAS.

Technique of Catheter-Based Neurorescue in the Cerebral Arteries

Catheter-based neurorescue is composed of several techniques (Table 3). The equipment required is listed in Table 7. Intra-arterial cerebral thrombolysis has been performed with TPA or urokinase (UK), neither of which has proven superiority. Reported doses for UK administration in this setting are 250,000 to 1.5 million units (17,45,46). TPA doses have ranged from 5 to 20 mg, well below the intravenous dose for acute stroke (17,47).

When an embolus is identified, an arteriographic road map of the arteries leading to it is made. The carotid access sheath is left in place with its tip in the common carotid artery. Placement of the sheath tip through the stented carotid segment may generate more thrombus and emboli and may decrease inflow to the area intended for neurorescue. A 3 Fr microcatheter is advanced through the carotid guide sheath and into the artery just proximal to the clot. The catheter generally tends to advance into the middle cerebral artery. An end-hole microcatheter permits the most accurate delivery of thrombolytic agent. The microcatheter usually advances to the area with forward

Table 7 Equipment Required for Neurorescue

Microguidewires, 0.014 in. with varying levels of stiffness
Microcatheters, 3 Fr
Angioplasty balloons, 1 to 2.5 mm in diameter, rapid exchange
Small caliber snares

---

pressure alone. TPA is reconstituted in sterile water then diluted in normal saline at a concentration of 2 mg per 5 mL. Mixing TPA in a solution that is more dilute than 1 mg per 5 mL may cause precipitation. To be prepared for the whole case, it may be best to mix 20 mg in 50 mL since the usual dose required is somewhere between 5 and 10 mg of TPA. At this juncture, there are varying levels of aggressiveness with which one may proceed with catheter-directed thrombolysis. One option is to infuse thrombolytic just proximal to the clot for 20 min and recheck to evaluate the progress. There is no set protocol for infusion, but a rate of infusion of 0.2 mg/min is reasonable. This results in the administration of 4.0 mg of TPA in 10 mL of solution over 20 min.

Another approach is to advance the microcatheter beyond the occluding thrombus. Initially, the microcatheter is advanced to the artery segment just proximal to the thrombus. The length of the occluded segment is usually 5 mm or less. Probe the clot with a neuroguidewire and gently attempt to cross the occluded vessel with the neuroguidewire. Probing the thrombus often reestablishes some antegrade flow. The guidewire itself may disrupt or disperse the thrombus. This is then followed by the microcatheter. Because the thrombus and the microcatheter occupy the small vessel lumen, the artery may not be possible to road-map at this point. The catheter advancement must be done cautiously since it may be without much guidance. After advancing the microcatheter across the occluded segment, the neuroguidewire is removed slowly and steadily while holding the hub of the microcatheter vertically and dripping heparinized saline into the hub to prevent air bubbles from being introduced. The tiny microcatheter lumen and the potentially very slow rate of backbleeding distal to the clot are a setup for suction to develop in the catheter. Dilute contrast in a 3-mL syringe is used to perform an arteriogram of the distal cerebral artery to confirm location and intra-arterial position. Very gentle pressure is applied by hand and contrast flow is observed on the fluoroscopic monitor for it is easy to cause arterial injury and leakage of the blood–brain barrier in this setting. Contrast extravasation or a Cushing's response may be signs of vessel perforation. Usually, the arteriogram reveals stagnant flow since inflow is limited to whichever collaterals are functioning.

TPA is administered distal to the clot with a very slow infusion. The microcatheter is slowly withdrawn while infusing thrombolytic into the clot. The thrombolytic is infused with a 10-mL syringe. Approximately 1.0 mg of TPA is administered distal to the clot (2.5 mL). TPA is then administered into the clot (1.0 mg) as the catheter is slowly withdrawn. The catheter tip has a radiopaque marker and this is carefully observed as it moves since the infusion is not interrupted for repeat arteriography. A fair amount of pressure is applied by hand to inject through a microcatheter using a 10-mL syringe. After infusing 2.0 mg (5 mL of solution), the catheter tip is placed just proximal to the clot and a constant infusion of TPA is performed. TPA infusion is performed at the rate of 0.2 mg/min (or 0.5 mL of solution per minute) for 20 min, for a total of 4.0 mg. This requires that 10 mL of solution be infused over the 20-min period.

Total TPA dose at this point is 6.0 mg, a fairly high dose of TPA considering the small amount of thrombus involved. If the patient improves before a 20-min infusion has been completed, a repeat arteriogram is performed. The whole dose of TPA may not be required. During this time, the patient is supported in any way necessary. After the infusion, a repeat arteriogram is performed through the microcatheter to evaluate the result. If thrombus persists, the infusion is repeated. If the infusion alone had been performed initially, without lacing of the clot with TPA, an attempt to cross the occluded vessel is made at this point. Careful attention should be given to the lenticulostriate arteries and clearance of the M1 segment. The maximal dose of TPA is considered to be approximately 20 mg but doses as high as 40 mg have been reported.

If the occlusion does not resolve, there may be an atherosclerotic stenosis at this location that has thrombosed or formed a landing zone for an embolus. Comparison with preprocedure cerebral arteriograms is useful. If the lesion can be crossed with the guidewire, balloon angioplasty of the lesion may be performed to open the artery. Residual stenosis is common after intracranial balloon angioplasty since induced spasm or perforation is to be avoided. Balloons in the range of 1.0 to 2.5 mm are used. The reestablishment of antegrade flow is the goal rather than a perfect cosmetic result. A disadvantage of this approach is that thrombus may disperse and occlude many smaller arteries downstream. Balloon angioplasty of cerebral vessels may also cause dissection, spasm, or perforation. Intracranial stents are not well developed and bailout maneuvers for complications of PTA are limited. A microsnare may also be used to retrieve a well-organized clot that is resistant to chemical thrombolysis.

Conclusion

Much remains to be resolved regarding the use of neurorescue for patients with neurological complications during carotid stent placement. Catheter-based techniques will probably play a major role in cerebral tissue preservation in patients who sustain strokes as a result of carotid stenting. It is likely that experience, technique, and technology will continue to improve. However, because these techniques are only required rarely after carotid stenting, it is unlikely that level 1 evidence will be achieved for neurorescue. Since most events resolve with medical management alone and thrombolysis has an associated risk, only the patients with the worst prognosis will be treated and this will continue to skew the results to be less favorable. Although neurorescue techniques have potential benefits in patients with new neurological deficits during carotid stenting, it is not the standard of care and may turn out to have worse results than other options in some patients. The risk of intracranial hemorrhage as a result of thrombolysis remains a significant concern.

References

1. Diethrich EB, Ndiaye M, Reid DB. Stenting in the carotid artery: initial experience in 110 patients. J Endovasc Surg 1996; 3(1):42–62.
2. Wholey MH, Wholey MH, Jarmolowski CR, Eles G, Levy D, Buecthel J. Endovascular stents for carotid artery occlusive disease. J Endovasc Surg 1997; 4(4):326–338.

3. Yadav JS, Roubin GS, Iyer S, Vitek J, King P, Jordan WD, Fisher WS. Elective stenting of the extracranial carotid arteries. Circulation 1997; 95(2):376–381.

4. Cremonesi A, Manetti R, Setacci F, Setacci C, Castriota F. Protected carotid stenting. Clinical advantages and complications of embolic protection devices in 442 consecutive patients. Stroke, 2003; 34:1936–1941.

5. Reimers B, Corvaja N, Moshiri S, Sacca S, Albiero R, Di Mario C, Pascotto P, Colombo A. Cerebral protection with filter devices during carotid artery stenting. Circulation 2001; 104(1):12–15.

6. Roubin GS, New G, Iyer SS, Vitek JJ, Al Mubarak N, Liu MW, Yadav J, Gomez C, Kuntz RE. Immediate and late clinical outcomes of carotid artery stenting in patients with symptomatic and asymptomatic carotid artery stenosis: a 5-year prospective analysis. Circulation 2001; 103(4):532–537.

7. Warnock NG, Ganghi MR, Bergvall U. Complications of intraarterial digital subtraction angiography in patients investigated for cerebral vascular disease. Br J Radiol 1993; 66:855–858.

8. Fayed AM, White CJ, Ramee SR, Jenkins JS, Collins TJ. Carotid and cerebral angiography performed by cardiologists: cerebrovascular complications. Catheter Cardiovasc Interv 2002; 55:277–280.

9. Furlan A, Higashida R, Weschler L, Gent M, Rowley H, Kase C, Pessin M, Ahuja A, Callohan F, Clark WM, Silver F, Rivera F. Intra-arterial prourokinase for acute ischemic stroke: the PROACT II Study: a randomized controlled trial. JAMA 1999; 282:2003–2011.

10. Orlandi G, Fanucchi S, Fioretti C, Acerbi G, Puglioli M, Padoleccia R, Sartucci F, Murri L. Characteristics of cerebral microembolism during carotid stenting and angioplasty alone. Arch Neurol 2001; 58:1410–1413.

11. Coggia M, Goeau-Brissonniere O, Duval JL, Leschi JP, Letort M, Nagel MD. Embolic risk of the different stages of carotid bifurcation balloon angioplasty: an experimental study. J Vasc Surg 2000; 31:550–557.

12. Cremonesi A, Manetti R, Setacci F, Setacci C, Castriota F. Protected carotid stenting: clinical advantages and complications of embolic protection devices in 442 consecutive patients. Stroke 2003; 34:1936–1941.

13. Wholey MH, Wholey MH, Tan WA, Toursarkissian B, Bailey S, Eles G, Jarmolowski C. Management of neurological complications of carotid artery stenting. J Endovasc Ther 2001; 8:341–353.

14. Criado FJ, Lingelbach JM, Ledesma DF, Lucas PR. Carotid artery stenting in a vascular surgery practice. J Vasc Surg 2002; 35:430–434.

15. Qureshi AI, Luft AR, Janardhan V, Suri MF, Sharma M, Lanzino G, Wakhloo AK, Guterman LR, Hopkins LN. Identification of patients at risk for periprocedural neurological deficits associated with carotid angioplasty and stenting. Stroke 2000; 31:376–382.

16. Morrish W, Grahovac S, Douen A, Cheung G, Hu W, Frab R, Kalapos P, Wee R, Hudon M, Agbi C, Richard M. Intracranial hemorrhage after stenting and angioplasty of extracranial carotid stenosis. Am J Neuroradiol 2002; 21:1911–1916.

17. Zeumer H, Freitag HJ, Zanella F. Local intra-arterial fibrinolytic therapy in patients with stroke: urokinase versus recombinant tissue plasminogen activator (r-TPA). Neuroradiology 1993; 35:159–162.

18. Chambers BR, Norris JW, Shurvell BL, Hachinski VC. Prognosis of acute stroke. Neurology 1987; 37:159–162.

19. Brott T, Boguslavsky J. Treatment of acute stroke. N Engl J Med 2000; 343:710–722.

20. The National Institute of Neurological Disorders and Stroke rt-PA Stroke Study Group. Tissue plasminogen activator for acute ischemic stroke. N Engl J Med 1995; 333:1581–1587.

21. Clark WM, Wissman S, Albers GW, Jhamandas JH, Madden KP, Hamilton S. Recombinant tissue plasminogen activator (alteplase) for ischemic stroke 3 to 5 hours after symptom onset. The ATLANTIS Study: a randomized controlled trial. JAMA 1999; 282:2019–2026.

22. ECASS II Investigators. Randomized double blind placebo controlled trial of thrombolytic therapy with intravenous alteplase in acute ischemic stroke (ECASS II). Lancet 1998; 352:1245–1251.

23. The Multicenter Acute Stroke Europe Study Group. Thrombolytic therapy with streptokinase in acute ischemic stroke. N Engl J Med 1996; 335:145–150.

24. Hacke W, Kaste M, Fieschi C. Intravenous thrombolysis with recombinant tissue plasminogen activator for acute ischemic stroke. N Engl J Med 1995; 333:1581–1587.

25. Sasaki O, Shigekazu T, Koike T. Fibrinolytic therapy for acute embolic stroke: intravenous, intracarotid and intra-arterial local approaches. Neurosurgery 1995; 36:246–252.

26. Tomsick T, Brott T, Barsan W, Broderick J, Haley EC, Spilker J, Khoury J. Prognostic value of the hyperdense middle cerebral artery sign and stroke scale score before ultraearly thrombolytic therapy. Am J Neuroradiol 1996; 17:79–85.

27. Executive Committee of the ASITN. Intra-arterial thrombolysis: ready for prime time? Am J Neuroradiol 2001; 22:55–58.

28. ASITN. Standards of Practice. Intra-arterial thrombolysis. http://www.asitn.org. pp. 1–10

29. Tubler T, Schluter M, Dirsch O, Sievert H, Bosenberg I, Grube E, Waigand J, Schofer J. Balloon-protected carotid artery stenting: relationship of periprocedural neurologic complications with the size of the particulate debris. Circulation 2001; 104:2791–2796.

30. Whitlow PL, Lylyk P, Londero H, Mendiz OA, Mathias K, Jaeger H, Parodi J, Schonholz C, Milei J. Carotid artery stenting protected with an emboli containment system. Stroke 2002; 33:1308–1314.

31. Martin JB, Pache JC, Treggiari-Venzi M, Murphy KJ, Gailloud P, Puget E, Pinzolato G, Sugiu K, Guimaraens L, Theron J, Rufenacht DA. Role of distal balloon protection technique in the prevention of cerebral embolic events during carotid stent placement. Stroke 2001; 32:479–484.

32. Wholey MH, Wholey MH, Tan WA, Toursarkissian B, Bailey S, Eles G, Jarmolowski C. Management of neurological complications of carotid artery stenting. J Endovasc Ther 2001; 8:341–353.

33. Kidwell CS, Saver JL, Carneado J, Bayre J, Starkman S, Duckwiler G, Gobin YP, Janan R, Vespa P, Villablanca JP, Liebeskind DS, Vinuela F. Predictors of hemorrhagic transformation in patients receiving intra-arterial thrombolysis. Stroke 2002; 33:717–724.

34. Vitek JJ, Roubin GS, Al-Mubarek N. Carotid artery stenting: technical considerations. Am J Neuroradiol 2000; 21:1736–1743.

35. Tan KT, Cleveland TJ, Berczi V, McKevitt FM, Venables GS, Gaines PA. Timing and frequency of complications after carotid artery stenting: what is the optimal period of observation? J Vasc Surg 2003; 38:236–243.

36. Kastrup A, Groschel K, Krapf H, Brehm BR, Diegans J, Schulz JB. Early outcome of carotid angioplasty and stenting with and without cerebral protection devices: a systematic review of the literature. Stroke 2003; 34:813–819.

37. Molina CA, Alvarez-Sabin J, Montaner J, Abilleira S, Arenillas JF, Coscojuella P, Romero

F, Codina A. Thrombolysis-related hemorrhagic infarction: a marker of early reperfusion, reduced infarct size, and improved outcome in patients with proximal middle cerebral artery occlusion. Stroke 2002; 33:1551–1556.

38. Zaidat OO, Suarez JI, Santillan C, Sunshine JL, Tarr RW, Paras VH, Selman WR, Landis DM. Response to intra-arterial and combined intravenous and intra-arterial thrombolytic therapy in patients with distal internal carotid artery occlusion. Stroke 2002; 33:1821–1826.

39. Rabinstein AA, Wijdicks EF, Nichols DA. Complete recovery after early intraarterial recombinant tissue plasminogen activator thrombolysis of carotid T occlusion. Am J Neuroradiol 2002; 23:1596–1599.

40. Arnold M, Schroth G, Nedeltchev K, Loher T, Remonda L, Stepper F, Sturzenegger M, Mattle HP. Intra-arterial thrombolysis in 100 patients with acute stroke due to middle cerebral artery occlusion. Stroke 2002; 33:1828–1833.

41. Kucinski T, Koch C, Eckert B, Rother J, Zeumer H. Collateral circulation is an independent radiological predictor of outcome after thrombolysis in acute ischemic stroke. Neuroradiology 2003; 45:11–18.

42. Labiche LA, Al-Senani F, Wojner AW, Grotta JC, Malkoff M, Alexandrov AV. Is the benefit of early recanalization sustained at 3 months? A prospective cohort study. Stroke 2003; 34:695–698.

43. Quershi AI, Siddiqui AM, Suri MF, Kim SH, Ali Z, Yahia AM, Lopes DK, Boulos AS, Ringer AJ, Saad M, Guterman LR, Hopkins LN. Aggressive mechanical clot disruption and low-dose intra-arterial third generation thrombolytic agent for ischemic stroke: a prospective study. Neurosurgery 2002; 51:1319–1327.

44. Theron J, Courtheoux P, Casasco A, et al. Local intraarterial fibrinolysis of the carotid territory. Am J Neuroradiol 1989; 10:753–765.

45. Mori E, Tabuchi M, Yoshida T, Yamadori A. Intracarotid urokinase with thromboembolic occlusion of the middle cerebral artery. Stroke 1988; 19:802–812.

46. Casto L, Caverni L, Camerlingo M, Censori B. Moschini L, Servalli MC, Partziguian T, Belloni G, Mamoli A. Intra-arterial thrombolysis in acute ischemic stroke. J Neurol Neurosurg Psychiatry 1996; 60:667–670.

47. Quershi AI, Suri MF, Shatla AA. Intraarterial recombinant tissue plasminogen activator for ischemic stroke: an accelerating dosing regimen. Neurosurgery 2000; 54:100–108.

15

Technical Tips for Carotid Angioplasty and Stenting

PETER A. SCHNEIDER

Hawaii Permanente Medical Group, Honolulu, Hawaii, U.S.A.

The purpose of this chapter is to summarize the technical tips one might consider in carotid bifurcation angioplasty and stenting.

Patient Selection

- Factors that most influence patient selection for carotid stenting are medical comorbidities, arterial access issues, and aortic arch and carotid artery anatomy and pathology.
- Patients considered for carotid intervention should be neurologically stable.
- The patient must be able to follow commands in order to permit safe carotid stenting.
- Patients with severely compromised cardiac or pulmonary status, who cannot lie flat on the fluoroscopy table due to shortness of breath, will not tolerate carotid intervention.
- Severe renal insufficiency precludes a patient from undergoing carotid intervention because contrast administration is required.
- Patients who are allergic to antiplatelet agents or at high risk of hemorrhagic complications from prolonged antiplatelet therapy should not undergo endovascular carotid intervention.
- Patients who are morbidly obese or have a large abdominal pannus present a formidable femoral access challenge. Arterial access may be difficult to achieve,

catheter torque response is diminished, and control of the puncture site after the procedure is often poor.

- Access via the brachial artery for carotid intervention depends on whether arterial branch angles of the aortic arch and its branches can be negotiated.
- Significant aortoiliac tortuosity or occlusive disease compromises the movement of guidewires and catheters and the precise placement of angioplasty balloons and stents in the carotid artery.
- Aortic aneurysm along the femoral to carotid route presents a significant risk of distal embolization during carotid sheath placement.
- A carotid and cerebral arteriogram should be performed as a separate procedure prior to the carotid stent. Baseline AP and lateral images of the extracranial and intracranial cerebral circulation are required before intervention.
- Variations in the anatomic configuration of the arch and great vessels are common and the operator must be able to manage these and achieve stable carotid access.
- Pathological factors involving the aortic arch that may limit patient selection for carotid intervention include the presence of severe aortic calcification or evidence of diffuse aortic wall irregularity.
- Patients with atherosclerotic ostial stenosis of the innominate, right common carotid and left common carotid arteries require angioplasty and stenting during carotid bifurcation intervention. Occasionally, the extent of proximal disease may preclude a safe carotid intervention. Examples may include stenotic lesions with atherosclerotic disease that appears soft or pedunculated, severely calcified stenotic lesions not responsive to angioplasty and stenting, and long diffuse stenoses involving the entire length of the common carotid artery.
- Severe tortuosity of the internal carotid artery may prevent carotid stenting. Marked acute angulation, kinks, and coils, particularly within a few centimeters distal to the bifurcation, leaves inadequate working room for protection and stenting. If a stent straightens an artery in one segment, the curvature is usually displaced to another segment where a new kink may form. Some of the cerebral protection devices, especially the filters, will be too stiff to pass through a kinked or coiled segment. Cerebral protection devices may not have complete arterial wall apposition when opened in tortuous segments.
- Other conditions that may preclude a patient from being selected for carotid intervention are related to their inherently high risk for embolism or thrombosis. These include the presence of a preocclusive internal carotid artery stenosis, a carotid artery luminal filling defect indicating the possibility of acute thrombus, a soft pedunculated-appearing stenotic lesion, and severe carotid artery bifurcation calcification.
- Possible indications for carotid stent placement include patients at "high risk" for carotid endarterectomy. These factors may include the following: severe cardiac disease requiring coronary PTA or CABG; history of congestive heart failure. Severe chronic obstructive pulmonary disease requiring home oxygen; FEV-1 <20% predicted. Chronic renal failure currently on dialysis. Prior carotid endarterectomy (restenosis). Contralateral vocal cord paralysis. Surgically inaccessible

lesions at or above the second cervical vertebra; inferior to the clavicle. Radiation-induced carotid stenosis. Prior ipsilateral radical neck dissection. Contralateral internal carotid occlusion.

Arch Assessment

- The initial arch aortogram should be obtained in the optimum left anterior oblique projection to give the widest arc possible.
- Access of an arch branch for intervention becomes more challenging in the progression from aortic arch segment I to segment III (Fig. 1, Chapter 2).
- When planning the initial branch vessel catheterization, the relative complexity of the access can be estimated from the location of the vessel's origin as it relates to the fulcrum point of the arch (Chapter 2, Fig. 3, and Chapter 6, Fig. 4).
- Segment I arteries are the most straightforward to catheterize and access with a high likelihood of success.
- Segment II catheterizations are more challenging. This segment of the arch is bisected into IIa and IIb categories, with the degree of catheterization difficulty increasing from IIa to IIb subdivisions.
- Segment III arteries are the most challenging to catheterize, with the origin of the target artery caudal to the horizontal line of the arch fulcrum.
- Disease or anatomic variations of the arch and its branches must be considered in a patient's potential candidacy for carotid stent placement.

Carotid Arteriography

- Informed consent includes an understanding of the risk of stroke.
- Perform a carotid duplex examination prior to angiogram.
- Make a plan for arterial access based upon physical exam.
- Access choices for arteriography in order or preference are either femoral artery, left brachial artery, or right brachial artery.
- Use a protocol for the procedure.
- After placing the flush catheter in the arch, rotate the image intensifier into the LAO position until the arch reaches its widest possible arc.
- Clear bubbles from catheters, stopcocks, and tubing.
- Label syringes.
- Use a sheath to diminish friction at the access site.
- Administer heparin.
- Wipe all guidewires and catheters liberally with heparin–saline.
- Do not withdraw guidewire too rapidly. This helps to avoid microbubbles.
- Constant guidewire control is required. Watch guidewire tip. Prevent it form jumping forward as the selective catheter is advanced. Do not allow the guidewire to cross the bifurcation while advancing selective catheter.

- Backbleed the catheter before flushing.
- Do not administer flush or contrast if the catheter is not backbleeding because this is may introduce air.
- Puff contrast to confirm catheter position before performing any pressure injections.
- Adjust the pressure and volume of contrast injection to the situation.
- Start low if uncertain about how much pressure and volume are required to fill out the carotid bifurcation.
- Flush the catheters every few minutes with heparin–saline.
- Don't flush cerebral catheters with too much volume. A few milliliters of heparin–saline will clear the catheter and help prevent thrombus formation.
- Be specific about the information you need.
- Keep it as simple as possible and be methodical in the sequence of events.

Selective Catheterization of the Carotid Arteries

- Maintain the image intensifier in the LAO position after performing the arch aortogram.
- Assess the arch for disease to be certain it is safe to perform selective catheterization.
- Use bony landmarks from the arch aortogram to assist in catheterizing the carotid arteries (Chapter 4, Fig. 10).
- Choose a couple of simple curve catheters and a couple of complex curve catheters and become very familiar with them.
- Use the "surf and turf" classification to help choose a selective cerebral catheter (Chapter 4, Table 6). The carotid stent procedure is facilitated by the use of simple curve catheters whenever possible.
- After placing the selective cerebral catheter into the arch, withdraw the guidewire into the catheter shaft to permit the catheter head to take its appropriate shape.
- Maneuvering selective cerebral catheters is detailed in Chapter 4.
- If the chosen selective catheter doesn't go, try another choice.
- After the catheter has engaged the orifice of the arch branch, adjust the catheter with slight turns and/or advancement to permit the catheter to be better seeded in the artery before advancing the guidewire.
- Advance the guidewire slowly out of the catheter tip since it may occasionally push the catheter out of the carotid artery.
- If the catheter does not advance easily into the artery, consider having the patient take a deep breath, turn the head, or cough.

Carotid Artery Sheath Access

- Pull everything ahead of time and make sure everything fits through the sheath you plan to use.
- Make sure the guidewire, balloon catheters, and stent deployment catheters are long enough to accommodate the length of the sheath selected.

- Assess the arch by analyzing the anatomy during the planning phase of the case. Access of an arch branch for intervention becomes more challenging in the progression from segment I to segment III (Chapter 2, Fig. 1).

- Anticipate the likely level of challenge posed by the anatomy (especially the arch) in each case. Some assessment of this may be made during selective catheterization at the time of the initial arteriogram.

- The peak of the inner curve of the aortic arch acts as a fulcrum over which the sheath must be placed to enter all arteries in segment III and some arteries in segment II, such as arteries originating in segment IIb (Chapter 6, Fig. 4).

- Each additional turn or angle that is added to the femoral–carotid route adds to the level of challenge. Distal to the origin of each branch, angulation or tortuosity of the innominate or common carotid artery may also work against smooth sheath placement.

- Plaque in the arch or occlusive disease at the branch origin or in the proximal artery is a relative contraindication to sheath placement.

- An external carotid artery that is occluded or lacks adequate branches cannot be used for anchoring the stiff guidewire over which the sheath is passed. Consider an alternative method in this situation.

- Whether to use a guiding sheath or a guiding catheter is an important consideration and the two are compared in Chapter 6, Table 3.

- Use the lowest profile guiding sheath (6 Fr in most cases).

- Put the sheath in warm saline bath to improve its flexibility. (Be sure that your assistant does not put the nitinol stent in the same warm saline bath.)

- Use dilators at the femoral access site to prepare the arteriotomy and reduce friction at the groin level.

- Administer heparin anticoagulation (typically 100mg/kg body mass) after arterial access is gained and prior to manipulation of catheters in the aortic arch and brachiocephalic vessels.

- After selective catheterization of the common carotid artery, road-map the carotid bifurcation, paying careful attention to choose a view that provides minimal overlap of the internal and external carotid arteries and provides maximum visualization of the target lesion. Advance the Glidewire into the external carotid artery.

- After advancing the selective catheter into the origin of the external carotid artery, road-map the artery and pick a branch in which to anchor the exchange guidewire. Advance the selective catheter into a distal external carotid artery branch, as far distally as is possible. Contrast injections into the carotids should not be done unless free back flow of blood is noticed at the back end of the injection catheter. External carotid artery backbleeding may be decreased due to the tight fit of the catheter in the external branches. In this event, the selective catheter is slowly withdrawn until back flow is present.

- Remove the Glidewire and place the Amplatz superstiff guidewire. Place the Amplatz guidewire as far into the external carotid artery as possible, but don't perforate the distal branch.

- Take the slack out of the stiff guidewire before passing the carotid sheath. Use fluroroscopy to observe the course of the guidewire from the access site to the bifurcation. If there is slack in the guidewire, focus on the guidewire tip and slowly withdraw the guidewire until the tip begins to move.
- Use special maneuvers to help with sheath delivery when they are needed. These include having the patient take a deep breath, turning the patient's head, compressing the guidewire tip along the face or scalp, using a very short floppy tip on the superstiff guidewire, and using the push–pull technique.
- Do not perform mechanical dilation of the carotid lesion with the tip of the dilator as the sheath is advanced. Withdraw the dilator slightly if needed, as the sheath is advanced. In patients with short common carotid arteries, the sheath can be advanced over the dilator once the sheath edge (radiopaque marker) is past the origin of the common carotid artery.
- Do not force the sheath.
- Watch the guidewire tip as the sheath is advanced so the sheath is not permitted to pull the guidewire out of the external carotid artery. As the sheath enters the arch, position the image intensifier so that the following landmarks are visible: the tip of the sheath as it passes the fulcrum and approaches the intended arch branch, and the tip of the guidewire in the external carotid artery.
- Advance the sheath until it is well inside the common carotid artery. The tip of the sheath should be far enough so that it is visible in the inferior aspect of a 9-in. field of view and the cerebral protection device when placed in the internal carotid artery distal to the bifurcation is visible in the superior aspect of the same field.
- An alternative method of carotid access begins by placing the long carotid access sheath into the transverse arch over a guidewire. The dilator is removed, and an appropriate selective diagnostic catheter is advanced into the common carotid artery. If a 90-cm sheath is placed, a 125-cm selective catheter should be used. A stiff guidewire is advanced into the external carotid artery. Using the guidewire and catheter for support, the sheath (without dilator) is advanced into the common carotid artery. This technique risks "snowplowing" the edge of the sheath at the junction of the aortic arch and the innominate or left common carotid artery without the protection of the dilator. This disadvantage can be diminished by using a 6 Fr cerebral catheter over which to pass a 6 Fr sheath.
- Maintaining sheath access to the distal common carotid artery is crucial: once the superstiff exchange guidewire is removed, support for the stent placement procedure is provided almost entirely by the sheath. If the sheath backs up into the aortic arch during the case, it is usually not possible to advance it into the common carotid artery over a 0.014-in. guidewire or protection device.
- For patients with an occluded external carotid artery, sheath access to the common carotid may be difficult. A stiff guidewire can be placed into the distal common carotid artery, but maintained proximal to the lesion. Alternatively, a guidewire with variable diameter, such as a TAD wire (0.018-in. tip, enlarging to 0.035-in. more proximally, Mallinkrodt) can to used to cross the internal carotid lesion,

giving additional guidewire length to facilitate sheath advancement. This approach requires crossing the lesion twice.

Perioperative Management

- A CT or MRI of the brain is obtained in symptomatic patients to evaluate for preprocedural pathological changes. Initial duplex evaluation is performed of both carotids.
- Clopidogrel has a slower onset of action compared to aspirin, and patients should take clopidogrel for an appropriate period before angioplasty and stenting, usually 3 to 4 days pre and 4 to 6 weeks poststent. A high-dose load should be considered in patients preprocedure who have not been taking their clopidogrel. Aspirin should be taken lifelong.
- The activated coagulation time (ACT) is used to guide heparin administration. A goal ACT of 250 to 300 sec is achieved prior to intervention. The dosage of heparin should be reduced when glycoprotein IIb/IIIa receptor inhibitors are used.
- Some reports support the routine use of glycoprotein IIb/IIAa inhibitors to reduce ischemic complications associated with carotid stenting, whereas others have found either no benefit or higher complication rates. Glycoprotein IIb/IIIa inhibitors are likely indicated in certain patients at high risk for thrombotic complications. Preoperative administration of glycoprotein IIb/IIIa inhibitors may be indicated in patients who are actively having carotid territory symptoms or those patients who did not have an appropriate preoperative loading of clopidogrel. Intraoperative administration of glycoprotein IIb/IIIa inhibitors should be considered when the development of thrombus is suspected within the stent.
- Atropine should be given prior to angioplasty of native carotid stenoses (0.5–1.0 mg intravenously) as prophylaxis for bradycardia during balloon inflation in the carotid bulb. For recurrent stenosis following endarterectomy, this may not be necessary.
- The procedure is performed under local anesthesia with minimal or no sedation to facilitate continuous neurological monitoring. An arterial line is placed for continuous pressure monitoring and EKG leads for cardiac monitoring. Temporary pacer pads should be readily available. Patients should have a detailed explanation of the need for continuous neurological monitoring. Techniques, such as squeezing a rubber doll, aid in simple and effective neurological monitoring during the procedure. Due to the minimal use of sedation, patients are often apprehensive and may develop reactive systemic hypertension. Avoid acutely reducing the blood pressure during the procedure with pharmacological agents since poststent hypotension/bradycardia is not uncommon.
- A closure device may be considered in CAS patients, particularly when IIb/IIIa inhibitors are used.
- Patients are monitored in the intensive care unit overnight. It is not uncommon to have a heightened response to carotid sinus distension. It may take 24 hr or more

of ionotropic support before the carotid sinus adapts to the radial force of the self-expanding stents. Avoiding extreme over sizing of the stents helps to decrease the incidence of post-CAS bradycardia and hypotension.

- The presence of significant hypotension in the absence of bradycardia is unusual in the immediate post procedure period. Other causes, such as retroperitoneal bleeding related to access site problems, should also be excluded.

Carotid Bifurcation Angioplasty and Stenting

- Always perform a thorough baseline neurologic exam and cerebral runoff images prior to carotid intervention. Both will be important for comparison following angioplasty and stenting if any neurological issues arise.
- Following successful femoral sheath insertion, the patient is systemically anti-coagulated with intravenous heparin. Additionally, in patients at higher risk for emboli, a IIb/IIIa inhibitor, such as eptifibatide (Integrilin) or tirofiban (Aggrastat) is administered at relatively lower doses than typically used in the coronary system.
- The tip of the shuttle sheath should be securely placed within the common carotid artery above the patient's clavicle.
- A 0.014-in. guidewire, appropriate to the cerebral protection device to be deployed, is advanced across the internal carotid stenosis. If the Amplatz guidewire is left in the external carotid artery, the 0.014-in. guidewire will often preferentially cross the internal carotid stenosis (buddy wire technique).
- Since it is not uncommon for patients to have bradycardia and hypotension with carotid angioplasty, hemodynamic assessments are made continuously throughout the procedure.
- A carotid angiogram is performed through the guiding sheath to further delineate the carotid bifurcation and the stenosis. The image intensifier is placed in an optimal position to separate the origins of the internal and external carotid arteries.
- Rapid exchange or monorail balloons, stent delivery systems, and cerebral pro-tection devices save time by decreasing the required guidewire length.
- Carotid stenting may be performed with any one of a variety of distal protection devices that are currently being used in trials. These are covered in the next section. They are all based on a 0.014-in. platform. The tip of the 0.014-in. guidewire is shaped appropriately to aid access to the internal carotid artery. After crossing the stenosis, the tip of the guidewire is placed close to the skull base but not any further. The location for deployment of the cerebral protection device should be selected before placement. The intracranial portion of the carotid artery and its branches are prone to dissection with guidewire manipulations.
- The predilatation balloon can be advanced into the distal common carotid artery prior to crossing the lesion with the guidewire for the cerebral protection device to save time.
- After the lesion has been crossed and the cerebral protection device deployed, the stenosis is predilated with a 2- to 4-mm balloon. A 4-cm-long balloon is

used to avoid "melon seeding" and the potential release of embolic debris. The longer length balloons have a tendency to expand at both ends and fix the balloon in place. The pressure used for predilatation is nominal for the balloon used. Higher pressure is used only in heavily calcified stenoses. The duration of the predilatation depends on the appearance and behavior of the balloon. If the balloon immediately attains its full shape, the predilatation time is shorter. If the balloon attains its full shape slowly, the predilatation time is prolonged up to 120 sec. The balloon is inflated only once and the inflation time varies depending on the lesion.

- During balloon deflation, a 30-cc syringe may be used to aspirate blood from the sheath to reduce the particulate debris that may have entered the bloodstream with the PTA.

- After the predilation balloon is removed, another bifurcation angiogram is performed through the sheath when a distal protection filter is being used. Stent placement is based upon this road map. The use of cerebral protection filters has the advantage of allowing for continuous angiographic monitoring of the target lesion. When a distal balloon occlusion, such as the PercuSurge, is utilized, the internal carotid artery will not be completely visualized and the stent is placed based on predetermined bony landmarks and the location of the bifurcation. It is important to mark the site of internal carotid artery stenosis since the lesion cannot be angiographically visualized once the distal occlusion balloon has been inflated.

- The size of the predilatation angioplasty balloon in relation to the native artery is taken into account when deciding what size of stent to use. Both the internal carotid artery and the common carotid artery diameters are important considerations when selecting the stent.

- A self-expanding stent is used following angioplasty of the carotid stenosis. The stent is deployed after confirmation of accurate position. Usually, a 10-mm-diameter stent is extended from the internal carotid artery into the common carotid artery, covering the external carotid artery origin. Nitinol stents conform well to contour changes but have a tendency to "jump" distally when deployed rapidly. Deploy two or three stent rings, adjust location (usually by pulling back slightly), and wait a few seconds, allowing the distal stent to become well opposed and attached to the artery above the lesion. The remainder of the stent can be deployed more rapidly with little worry that it will migrate. Coaxial stent delivery catheters have significant internal friction that must be overcome during deployment. The diameter of the stent must be sized to the largest portion of the vessel, typically the distal common carotid artery. Unconstrained stent diameter should be at least 10% (approximately 1–2 mm) larger than the maximum common carotid artery diameter.

- If a Wallstent (Medi-Tech, Boston Scientific) of 10 × 20 mm is chosen and it expands to 10 mm, then the length of the stent would be 20 mm. However, there is a size differential between the internal and the common carotid arteries, the former being 4 to 6 mm and the latter being larger. Since the Wallstent does not expand to the full 10 mm, it does not shorten to 20 mm. Instead, it ends up being

30 mm or more in length. Additionally, the continuous cell design of the Wallstent prevents it from complete wall apposition at the bifurcation where the common carotid abruptly tapers to become the internal carotid artery.

- The self-expanding stent is postdilated with a 5 or 6 × 20-mm balloon over the 0.014-in. wire. A 5-mm balloon PTA is usually adequate and a 6-mm balloon may be required for a common carotid artery lesion. Following stent deployment, shorter (2 cm) balloons are used to dilate the narrow portion of the stent. Longer length may cause a dissection in the distal internal carotid artery. The balloon used for poststent PTA is maintained within the stent. Nominal pressure is used to fully expand the balloon and the stent.

- A residual stenosis is accepted, as the stents continue to expand with time. This avoids the potential complications of emboli or rupture with repeated angioplasty or overdilatation. A residual stenosis of 20% or so is completely acceptable; the goal is protection from embolic stroke, not necessarily a perfect angiographic result.

- In some cases, continued flow of contrast into an ulcer is seen. No attempt should be made to obliterate this communication by using larger balloons or higher pressures.

- Deploy stents across kinks only if they are isolated. Avoid placing the distal end of the stent into kinks of the internal carotid artery if more than a single bend is noted. These cannot be eliminated and are only displaced distally and can become more exaggerated.

- If the external carotid artery becomes significantly stenosed with flow restriction or occluded after post dilatation of the stent, no attempt should be made to salvage the artery. This is an uncommon event and attempts to correct this may be quite difficult and result in further complications.

- A completion angiogram of the carotid bifurcation and distal extracranial internal carotid artery is performed *before* removing the device guidewire. Extra attention is paid to the internal carotid artery just distal to the stent. Severe vasospasm can sometimes be encountered (and can mimic dissection), particularly if the embolic protection device is allowed to bob up and down during guidewire manipulation. Watchful waiting and administration of vasodilators (nitroglycerine in 100-μg aliquots) will usually resolve this problem. On occasion, the guidewire must be removed before spasm is resolved completely, but this should be undertaken only after dissection is excluded. Administration of nitroglycerine directly into the internal carotid artery appears to be effective. A more proximal injection of nitroglycerine through the sheath, into the common carotid artery, has a tendency to flow preferentially into the external carotid artery in the presence of an internal carotid artery spasm. Distal dissections are unusual and when present can be remedied with an additional stent of appropriate size. Some distal protection filters, such as the FilterWire, require removal of the guidewire to remove the filter itself. If there is concern about the integrity of the distal internal carotid artery and the filter must be removed, as a potential cause of spasm, consider capturing the filter and placing a 0.014-in. buddy guidewire through the stent before removing the filter and its guidewire. It is important not to lose guidewire access until the operator is satisfied of the final angiographic appearance.

- After the guidewire is removed, a completion angiogram of the carotid and intracranial circulation is performed in two views. This should include an AP and lateral view of the cervical region, as well as AP and lateral views of the intracranial anatomy.

Cerebral Protection Devices

- The guidewire for the cerebral protection device (0.014-in.) is advanced across the lesion, with the aid of road-mapping. Care should be taken when inserting the device through the sheath valve, as the tip can be damaged. The protection device should be deployed into the distal extracranial internal carotid artery, just proximal to its petrous segment. For distal occlusion balloon devices, absence of flow in the internal carotid artery must be demonstrated; for filter devices, apposition of the device to the artery wall must be documented, along with flow in the internal carotid artery through the device (and should be documented after each step during the intervention).

- The PercuSurge Guardwire distal occlusion balloon is commercially available for coronary saphenous vein grafts and is not approved for CAS. A major advantage of the distal occlusion devices is their low crossing profile and high flexibility compared to distal filtration devices, facilitating device delivery. Because balloon-occlusion devices do not allow for antegrade flow in the internal carotid artery during the period of balloon inflation, a preprocedure MRA or contrast angiogram is suggested. In patients with an "isolated" ipsilateral cerebral hemisphere, balloon inflation may not be tolerated, even with induced hypertension and full heparin anticoagulation. Patients with isolated hemispheres may become symptomatic during the period of inflation of the distal occlusion balloon, necessitating deflation. These patients typically become symptomatic within 60 sec of cessation of internal carotid artery flow. Should patients become symptomatic, the operator has several options: complete the procedure without balloon occlusion, complete the procedure with intermittent balloon occlusion, or switch to a filter-type device, if available.

- The PercuSurge should be prepped and tested on the back table (and all angioplasty balloons and stents opened and prepared) prior to crossing the carotid lesion. If a monorail system, both balloon and stent, is utilized, the 200-cm length PercuSurge may be used; for "over-the-wire" (coaxial) systems, the 300-cm wire is required. The PercuSurge is advanced across the target lesion and placed proximal to the petrous segment of the internal carotid artery. The predilation balloon is advanced into the distal common carotid artery prior to balloon inflation. The PercuSurge balloon is carefully inflated to a target diameter, based on preprocedure measurements of the internal carotid artery. The inner lumen of the wire is 0.009 in. and may take 30 sec to permit the contrast-saline mixture to expand the distal occlusion balloon. As the balloon approaches the intended diameter, angiography is performed to assess for the presence of flow past the occlusion balloon. The minimum diameter necessary to achieve cessation of flow in the internal carotid artery is preferred because overinflation of the balloon can cause spasm or dissection.

- The intervention on the internal carotid is performed "blind" when the Percu-Surge Guardwire is deployed because the internal carotid artery cannot be angiographically visualized during distal balloon occlusion. The operator must rely on the fluoroscopic appearance of the stent, following postdilation, to assess the completed result. If, following balloon deflation and completion angiography, the lesion requires further angioplasty or stent placement, the occlusion balloon must be reinflated; this situation is even more pronounced when the external carotid artery is occluded, because the static column of blood extends from the origin of the common carotid artery to the occlusion balloon in the distal internal carotid artery.

- Following completion of the intervention, the static column of blood in the internal carotid artery is aspirated (three separate aspirations of 20 cc each). When the external carotid artery is occluded, consider more vigorous aspiration of the sheath to remove debris from the common carotid artery. Flow is then restored as the balloon is deflated. A completion angiogram is mandatory before the guidewire is removed, making sure that an iatrogenic dissection has not occurred.

- Unlike distal occlusion devices, filter devices are designed to maintain flow in the distal internal carotid artery during the intervention. There are two different systems to deliver the filter distal to the lesion. The filter can be directly affixed to a guidewire that is used to cross the lesion and stays in place with the filter during the procedure. Another method is to cross the lesion with a guidewire without a filter, then advance the filter over the guidewire using a special delivery device.

- The filter device is placed across the lesion into a straight, normal segment of the extracranial internal carotid artery. Most filters are deployed by withdrawing a covering membrane that permits the self-expanding filter to take its shape. Debris is captured in the filter. After the CAS procedure, a retrieval device is advanced immediately proximal to the filter for recapture of the filter.

- As the crossing profile of filter devices is greater than standard guidewires or balloon-occlusion devices, it may be difficult to cross extremely stenotic, tortuous, or calcified lesions. A "buddy wire" (a stiff guidewire placed into the external carotid artery) may be helpful in providing extra support to the filter device.

- Should the filter occlude during the procedure due to debris collection or thrombosis then a number of solutions exist. The debris may be removed by aspirating the filter with a 5 Fr vertebral catheter brought up through the sheath. In those cases, where occlusion by debris causes acute neurological symptoms, rapid removal of the filter is required. The procedure may be continued after inserting a new cerebral protection device or, if this is not possible, without any kind of protection. Filter thrombosis is prevented by full heparinization at the start of procedure and by selecting a filter device with sufficient pore size. Pore sizes between approx. 80 and 140-μm are recommended for they are large enough to prevent filter thrombosis and small enough to offer sufficient embolic protection.

- Confirmation that the edges of the device are in contact with the wall of the internal carotid artery, via several views of the filter device with different obliquity, is mandatory. If the device is not properly "aligned" with the ICA and it is not in contact with the vessel in 360°, embolic particles can flow past the filter.
- Once deployed, and after each step in the intervention, flow of contrast through the device must be checked. If the device becomes filled with debris, it must be either aspirated (much like the PercuSurge device) or temporarily removed. When removing a full device, it is important not to recapture it completely, as debris may be extruded from it and embolize distally.
- The Angioguard XP filter consists of a polyurethane filter affixed to a guidewire with a soft atraumatic tip. The filter is kept open by eight nitinol struts. Visibility of the device is secured by radiopaque markers on the proximal end on four of the eight struts. The pore size of the filter is 100 μm and the system has a crossing profile between 3.2 and 3.9 Fr. The filter is available in five different sizes ranging from 4 to 8 mm in diameter.
- The Neuroshield has a filter element with a pore size of 140 μm. Filter delivery differs from the other devices in that the lesion is first crossed with a special 0.014-in. guidewire having a 0.018-in tip. After lesion passage, the filter is brought up with a 3 Fr delivery catheter and is affixed between a proximal stop and a distal olive at the proximal part of the 0.018-in guidewire tip.
- The FilterWire EX consists of a wind-sock-type polyurethane filter with a proximal radiopaque nitinol loop affixed on the 0.014-in guidewire. The pore size of the filter is 80 μm and the delivery system has a crossing profile of 3.9 Fr. The nitinol loop makes it a one-size-fits-all device that can accommodate arterial diameters between 3.5 and 5.5 mm. The eccentric design of the filter necessitates the angiographic control of the positioning of the filter.
- The FilterWire EZ is the newer generation of the FilterWire EX filter. The FilterWire EZ has a polyurethane filter with a proximal radiopaque nitinol loop. The pore size of the filter is 110 μm and the crossing profile of the delivery system is downsized to 3.2 Fr. A relocation of the wire more central in the lumen of the filter makes multiplanar control no longer necessary, as the proximal loop will secure good wall apposition in all arteries between 3.5 and 5.5 mm in diameter. Improved features of this newer version of the FilterWire are its better visibility and its greater flexibility, allowing the filter to tackle virtually every curvature.
- The RX Accunet is an umbrella-like polyurethane filter that is affixed to the vessel wall by a stentlike nitinol structure. Blood flows in through the big proximal openings and potential debris is captured at the filter's membrane which has a constant pore size of 125 μm. The filter is available in four sizes (4.5, 5.5, 6.5, and 7.5 mm). Corresponding crossing profiles are 3.5 Fr for the two smallest filters and 3.7 Fr for the biggest devices.
- The Parodi Anti-Emboli System is a reversed-flow system consisting of two parts. First, there is the Parodi Anti-Emboli Catheter (PAEC), a flexible dual-lumen

guidewire with a low-pressure balloon at the distal end. Second, there is the Parodi External Balloon (PEB), an over-the-wire, low-profile balloon mounted on a radiopaque guidewire.

- After arterial access with the 10 Fr introducer sheath, the PAEC is advanced to the common carotid artery, where it serves as an arterial suction device. The distal PAEC balloon is dilated in the common carotid artery and the PEB balloon is placed in the external carotid artery. This way, a vacuum is created, reversing the blood flow. After establishing retrograde flow, interventionalists can choose between continuous or intermittent flow reversal as well as passive or active suction. The passive suction is created by an arteriovenous shunt, creating a physiological pressure gradient guiding emboli out of the arterial system through an external filter into the venous system.

- The major advantage of proximal occlusion is that they do not require that the lesion be crossed to achieve cerebral protection. Once the occlusion balloons are in place, the surgeon can use the guidewire of choice, making it possible to cross even tight and tortuous lesions.

16

Summary of Results of Carotid Bifurcation Angioplasty and Stenting

MICHAEL T. CAPS

Hawaii Permanente Medical Group, Honolulu, Hawaii, U.S.A.

The purpose of this chapter is to review the existing safety and efficacy data on carotid artery stenting (CAS). During the late 1980s and early 1990s, a series of multicenter randomized controlled clinical trials (RCTs) conducted in Europe and North America demonstrated the superiority of carotid endarterectomy (CEA) plus medical management vs. medical management alone for the prevention of stroke among patients with atherosclerotic carotid bifurcation stenosis. Coincident with the development of catheter-based technologies including stents, stent delivery systems, and cerebral protection devices, CAS has emerged as a potentially viable alternative, especially among patients who are at higher risk for perioperative complications following CEA.

To evaluate this data in its proper perspective, the RCTs comparing CEA plus medical management vs. medical management alone, including NASCET (North American Symptomatic Carotid Endarterectomy Trial) (1,2), ECST (European Carotid Surgery Trial) (3,4), ACAS (Asymptomatic Carotid Atherosclerosis Study) (5), and the VA (Veterans Affairs) trials (6,7) will first be briefly reviewed. Because these trials have established the superiority of CEA plus medical management over medical management alone, ethical concerns prohibit the performance of trials comparing CAS vs. medical management—thus CEA has been established as a "gold standard" with which to compare CAS. To date, there have been three published randomized trials comparing CEA and CAS and there is at least one additional trial nearing publication. In addition, there are at least 10 ongoing RCTs and registries in Europe and North America. Clearly, this is a rapidly evolving field.

The majority of the published data on CAS consists of noncontrolled single-center case series, most without independent verification of outcome events. Given these shortcomings, an attempt has been made to review and condense these studies into crude estimates of safety and efficacy. In addition to the randomized trials, all published consecutive case series involving at least 50 carotid bifurcation angioplasty procedures were included in this analysis. Whenever possible, these studies were stratified according to the degree of arteriographic stenosis, whether the carotid lesion was associated with recent neurological symptoms, whether a stent was used, whether the stent was balloon-expandable or self-expanding, and whether a cerebral protection device was used.

Outcome measures in studies of carotid artery intervention have been inconsistently reported. Depending on availability, the following periprocedural outcome rates were extracted: death (stroke-related and non-stroke-related), disabling stroke (defined as requiring assistance with activities of daily living for > 30 days following the procedure), nondisabling stroke, transient ischemic attack (TIA), cranial nerve injuries (permanent and transient), access site complications such as hematoma, pseudoaneurysm, and infection, and periprocedural myocardial infarction. In addition, the following long-term outcomes were evaluated during follow-up: death, stroke (including all and ipsilateral strokes, disabling and nondisabling), TIA, and hemodynamically significant carotid artery restenosis. Finally, there are several relevant outcome measures that could not be evaluated because of the lack of or sparse availability including quality of life, hospital length of stay, intensive care unit length of stay, and hospital- and procedure-related costs.

Carotid Endarterectomy

The first successful carotid endarterectomy (CEA) was performed in 1953 by Michael DeBakey (8). Over the ensuing half century, this surgical procedure has been extensively studied and modified. It is beyond the scope of this chapter to discuss all of the technical controversies that still exist today regarding CEA, so I will simply list some of the more important ones here: general vs. local-regional anesthesia, selective vs. obligatory shunting, whether to patch and if so, the optimum patch material, eversion vs. standard open endarterectomy, and type (if any) of intraoperative cerebral monitoring. Suffice it to say that excellent results have been achieved using a variety of techniques in the major CEA trials and in clinical practice.

The frequency of CEA dramatically increased in the late 1970s and early 1980s, resulting in the expression of serious concern and outright challenges to the safety and efficacy of this procedure. In response, several multicenter RCTs were conducted in Europe and North America over the ensuing decade. These trials demonstrated a sizable reduction in the risk of stroke for patients with recent hemispheric symptoms randomized to receive CEA and a more modest reduction in stroke risk for asymptomatic patients. Tables 1 and 2 summarize the results of these trials. Because there is a paucity of RCT data for carotid artery stenting (CAS) and because the vast majority of

Table 1 Perioperative (30-day) Morbidity and Mortality Rates Following Carotid Endarterectomy in Randomized Clinical Trials Comparing Medical Therapy Alone vs. Medical Therapy Plus Carotid Endarterectomy

Trial	N	Any death (%)	Stroke death (%)	Nonstroke death (%)	Any nonfatal stroke (%)	Disabling stroke (%)	Nondisabling stroke (%)	Any stroke or death (%)	Disabling stroke or death	CN injury (%)	MI (%)
Symptomatic											
VA (7)	90	3.3	1.1	2.2	2.2	1.1	1.1	5.5	4.4	5.5	2.2
NASCET (76)	1415	1.1	0.6	0.5	5.4	1.8	3.7	6.5	2.9	8.6	1.0
ECST (77)	1745	1.0	0.6	0.4	6.1	2.6	3.5	7.0	3.6	NG	NG
Pooled	3250	1.1	0.6	0.5	5.7	2.2	3.5	6.8	3.3		
Asymptomatic											
VA (6)	211	1.9	0.5	1.4	2.4	NG	NG	4.3	NG	3.8	3.3
ACAS (9)	721	0.1	0.1	0.0	1.4	0.7	0.7	1.5	0.8	5.0	0.4
Pooled	932	0.5	0.2	0.3	1.6			2.1		4.7	1.1

Not an intent-to-treat analysis: Results include only patients who actually underwent CEA.

CN = cranial nerve. MI = myocardial infarction. NG = not given.

"Pooled" statistics not calculated in categories with incomplete data.

Table 2　Long-Term Reduction in Risk of Trial Endpoints Associated with Carotid Endarterectomy in Randomized Clinical Trials Comparing Medical Therapy Alone vs. Medical Therapy Plus Carotid Endarterectomy

Trial	N medical/ N surgical	End point	Length of follow-up	Incidence— medical (%)	Incidence— surgical (%)	Relative risk reduction (%)	Absolute risk reduction (%)	NNT
Symptomatic								
VA, ≥50% (7)	98/91	Ipsi CVA/TIA	11.9 mo	19.4	7.7	60.3	11.7	8.5
NASCET, ≥70% (1)	331/328	Ipsi CVA/Surg. death	2 years	26	9	65.4	17	5.9
NASCET, 50–69% (2)	428/430	Ipsi CVA/Surg. death	5 years	22.2	15.7	29.3	6.5	15.4
ECST, ≥80% (77)	172/257	Major stroke/death	3 years	26.5	14.9	43.8	11.6	8.6
Asymptomatic								
VA (6)	233/211	Ipsi CVA	4 years	9.4	4.7	50.0	4.7	21.3
VA (6)	233/211	Ipsi CVA/death	4 years	44.2	41.2	NS	NS	NS
ACAS (5)	834/828	Ipsi CVA/death	5 years	11.0	5.1	53.6	5.9	16.9

Data presented according to the intent-to-treat principle.

NNT = number needed to treat. NS = not significant. CVA = cerebrovascular attack. TIA = transient ischemic attack.

the CAS data comes from nonrandomized and noncontrolled case series and registries with major potential biases, these trials establish the benchmark results for CEA against which CAS must be compared. Therefore it is critical to have a firm understanding of the results that can be expected following CEA when performed by experienced surgeons.

Table 1 shows the perioperative (30-day) morbidity and mortality rates reported in NASCET, ECST, ACAS, and the VA Cooperative Trials. The data are stratified according to whether the trial was conducted in symptomatic vs. asymptomatic patients. Table 1 shows that stroke and death rates were considerably higher in the symptomatic than in the asymptomatic trials. Taking the weighted average of the "stroke or death" rates yields a value of 6.8% for the symptomatic trials and 2.1% for the asymptomatic trials. In NASCET, the rates of death and any nonfatal stroke were 1.1% and 5.4%, respectively. The corresponding statistics from ACAS were 0.1% and 1.4%. Overall, approximately one half of perioperative deaths in these trials were stroke-related. The rate of cranial nerve injury ranged from 3.8% to 8.6%. In most cases, these injuries were transient with either complete or nearly complete recovery. The rate of myocardial infarction in these studies was low.

It is important to note that the data presented in Table 1 pertain to patients who actually *received* surgery, not to those *randomized* to surgery. The goal of this exercise was to use the data from the large CEA trials to estimate the complication rates associated with CEA. Among patients randomized to surgery, there was a significant proportion who suffered strokes after randomization but before the planned date of surgery, often as a direct result of diagnostic arteriography. For example, in the ACAS Trial, 4 of 415 (1.0%) patients who underwent diagnostic carotid arteriography suffered strokes (9), and in the VA Asymptomatic Trial, the stroke rate was 3/714 (0.4%) (6). Because it is now widely held that CEA can safely be performed without preoperative arteriography (10–14) and because no comparison is being made with the medically treated patients, it is rational to consider perioperative morbidity/mortality rates outside the aegis of the intent-to-treat principle.

In contrast, the long-term outcomes of the medically vs. surgically treated patients in these same trials *was* analyzed according to the intent-to-treat principle. The term "medical" treatment refers to antiplatelet therapy, typically with aspirin, in addition to cardiovascular risk factor reduction. The table demonstrates considerable variation in size, end points evaluated, and length of follow-up among the different trials. The VA Symptomatic Trial, for example, although underpowered, demonstrated a significant reduction in the risk of ipsilateral stroke or transient ischemic attack at 11.9 mo (7). The NASCET Trial demonstrated a 17% reduction in the absolute risk of ipsilateral stroke or any surgical stroke or death at 2 years for patients with ≥70% carotid stenosis, corresponding to a number needed to treat (NNT) of 5.9 patients to prevent one stroke (1). The benefit was considerably more modest for patients with 50–69% narrowing (2). The final publication of the ECST demonstrated benefit only for patients with ≥80% carotid stenosis (15). It should be noted, however, that the method used for measurement of arteriographic stenosis in ECST, in which the carotid bulb and not the more distal internal carotid artery was employed as the reference diameter, was different from that used in the North American trials. In a recently published study in which ECST arteriograms were reread by blinded reviewers using NASCET measurement criteria, the ECST results were strikingly similar to NASCET (Table 2) (16).

Based on the previously mentioned clinical trials, the risk of stroke among medically treated patients with asymptomatic carotid stenosis is estimated at 2–4% per year, a risk that is considerably less than that observed among symptomatic patients (10–20% per year for the first 2 years following initial symptoms). As a result, the reduction in stroke risk afforded by CEA is a great deal more modest among asymptomatic than among symptomatic patients, despite the fact that perioperative risks are clearly lower in the asymptomatic group. In the ACAS trial, for example, which had exceedingly low perioperative morbidity and mortality rates, the absolute reduction in the risk of ipsilateral stroke or death was 5.9% over 5 years for an NNT of 16.9. Critics of the ACAS Trial assert that the surgical results were, in fact, *too* good and are not replicated in "real-world" practice by less-experienced surgeons. Medicare claims studies have shown that while perioperative morbidity and mortality rates are generally higher in community settings than in clinical trials, results approaching those seen in ACAS and NASCET are achievable in high-volume hospitals (17–20). Ideally, carotid artery interventions should only be performed by those who have documented low periprocedural stroke or death rates (<7% for symptomatic patients and <3% for asymptomatic patients), a principle that should apply to both CEA and CAS.

In addition to hospital volume and perhaps surgeon training and volume (21), there are several patient characteristics that have been associated with increased perioperative risk following CEA. These issues warrant careful consideration because CAS is currently being advocated for these higher-risk patients. Factors that may be important in CEA risk-stratification include systemic illness (especially cardiac, pulmonary, and renal), cervical scarring because of prior surgery or irradiation, carotid lesions that are difficult or impossible to access surgically, and contralateral internal carotid artery (ICA) occlusion. For example, in a review of 3061 consecutive CEAs performed over a 10-year period at the Cleveland Clinic, Oriel et al. (22) identified a high-risk subset of patients defined by the presence of severe coronary artery disease, chronic obstructive pulmonary disease, or renal insufficiency. The composite end point of perioperative death, stroke, or myocardial infarction occurred in 7.4% of the high-risk group vs. only 2.9% of the low-risk subset. While the operative management of postendarterectomy restenosis is technically more challenging than primary CEA, it is not clear whether the risk of perioperative death, stroke, or even permanent cranial nerve injury are elevated following reoperative surgery: The published reports are case series with (necessarily) small sample sizes and variable perioperative complication rates (23–27). The effect of contralateral carotid artery occlusion on perioperative morbidity and mortality following CEA is equally unclear. In the ACAS Trial, for example, there was no difference in perioperative stroke or death rates among patients with vs. without contralateral ICA occlusion (28), whereas adverse perioperative outcomes were significantly more common among those with contralateral ICA occlusion in the NASCET trial (29).

The risk of carotid artery restenosis following CEA has been incompletely reported in the aforementioned clinical trials that were primarily conducted to evaluate the risk of stroke and death in patients treated medically vs. surgically. The best data on postendarterectomy restenosis comes from clinical trials evaluating patching and eversion in which restenosis was evaluated as a primary end point. The results from these trials indicate that rates of hemodynamically significant ($\geq$50% to $\geq$60%) restenosis are lowest in patients treated with conventional CEA with patch closure or eversion endarterectomy, with rates ranging from 3% to 12% (30–32). In the ACAS Trial, 677 of 720 patients who underwent CEA completed sufficient duplex follow-up to be evaluated for restenosis. The $\geq$60% restenosis rate was 4.6% among patched patients and 16.7% following primary closure (33). In all studies, the proportion of patients requiring reintervention for restenosis following CEA has been considerably lower, ranging from 1% to 4%.

In summary, CEA is an operation that has been exceedingly well studied. When performed by competent surgeons, the operation is safe and effective, providing durable protection against stroke with low rates of recurrent carotid stenosis.

Carotid Angioplasty and Stenting

Because of its less-invasive nature, percutaneous treatment of carotid bifurcation stenosis has several potential advantages over CEA including the elimination of local surgical complications such as neck hematoma, infection, cranial nerve injury, and postoperative pain and scarring, in addition to reduced blood loss, cardiopulmonary complications, and hospital length of stay. Percutaneous balloon angioplasty of the carotid arteries was first reported in the late 1970s and early 1980s (34 35 36 37). Over the ensuing decade, several additional small and highly selected case series of carotid angioplasty without detailed outcome assessment were reported, but enthusiasm for the procedure was limited because of the fear of cerebral embolism. In 1994, Marks et al. (38) reported the first use of stents in the cervical carotid arteries. Shortly thereafter, balloon angioplasty of the carotid bifurcation was almost completely replaced by "stent-supported" angioplasty (CAS), coincident with rapid proliferation and interest in this procedure. The past several years have witnessed impressive technological advancements in endoluminal stents, stent delivery systems, and cerebral protection devices. Initial interest in rigid balloon-expandable stents has given way to highly flexible self-expanding stents delivered via small, atraumatic, and flexible guide sheaths and catheters. Despite these important advancements, the continued risk of dislodgment of atherosclerotic plaque has lead to the development of several devices designed to prevent debris from embolizing into the cerebral circulation. Together with these technological improvements, growing familiarity and expertise with the technique of CAS have resulted in improved periprocedural complication rates that, in many institutions, appear to be nearly equivalent to CEA.

The safety/efficacy data on CAS consists of several single-center case series and multicenter registries and three published RCTs comparing CAS with CEA, two of which were stopped early because of superior results in the CEA group. The results of the observational studies will be presented first, with an emphasis on the larger consecutive series, followed by a review of the ongoing and completed clinical trials evaluating CAS.

A summary of the largest observational studies of CAS, including single-center case series and multicenter registries, is shown in Table 3. The results of stent-supported angioplasty of the carotid arteries are superior to balloon angioplasty without stenting, presumably because of lower risks of distal embolization and recurrent stenosis with primary stent placement. The earlier studies of PTA without stenting are thus omitted from this analysis.

The largest early series of CAS performed without cerebral protection devices were reported by Dietrich et al. (39), Wholey et al. (40), and Yadav et al. (41). All studies included significant proportions of patients considered "high risk" for CEA based on the presence of cardiac, pulmonary, or renal disease, or a history of prior neck surgery or irradiation. All but the Dietrich series included both symptomatic and asymptomatic patients (the Dietrich series included only symptomatic individuals). Periprocedural

Table 3 Summary of Published Results of Observational Studies of CAS

Study	Publication year	Lesions (N)	Cerebral protection (%)	30-Day outcome Death (%)	Stroke (%)
Dietrich et al. (39)	1996	117	0	1.7	6.0
Wholey et al. (40)	1997	114	0	1.8	3.5
Yadav et al. (41)	1997	126	0	0.8	7.1
Henry et al. (47)	1998	174	18	0	2.9
Mathias et al. (52)	1999	799	NG		2.1
Shawl et al. (55)	2000	192	0	0	2.6
Wholey et al. (Global Experience) (57)	2000	5210	Very low	1.9	3.9
d'Audiffret et al. (45)	2001	83	18		4.4
Reimers et al. (53)	2001	88	100		1.1
Roubin et al. (54)	2001	604	0	1.6	5.8
Al Mubarak et al. (42)	2002	164	100	1.2	1.2
Criado et al. (44)	2002	135	0	0	2.2
Guimaraens et al. (46)	2002	194	100	1.9	1.0
Henry et al. (48)	2002	184	100	0.5	2.2
Koch et al. (78)	2002	167	0		7.5
MacDonald et al. (51)	2002	150	50	1.3	6.0
Whitlow et al. (56)	2002	75	100	0	0
Cremonesi et al. (43)	2003	442	100		2.0
Hobson et al. (49)	2003	114	0	1.8	0.9
ARCHeR	NP	513	100	2.3	5.3

NP = Not Published.

death rates ranged from 0.7% to 1.8%, stroke rates ranged from 3.6% to 7.1%, and stroke/death rates ranged from 5.3% to 7.9%. Following the publication of these initial reports, there has been a proliferation of similar reports characterized by a temporal trend demonstrating improvement in periprocedural stroke and death rates (42–57). Using data from Table 3, the weighted average of stroke rates from studies published 1996–1998, 1999–2001, and 2002–2003 was 4.7%, 3.8%, and 2.6%, respectively. The explanation for this trend is almost certainly multifactorial. Technical success, defined as less than 20% or 30% residual arteriographic stenosis at the completion of the procedure, was reported in excess of 95% of cases in all studies. The majority of these reports are notable for their poor documentation of the proportion of patients treated with prior neurological symptoms and very limited long-term follow-up data. Restenosis rates, when documented, have ranged from 1% to 9%, typically with mean follow-up times of less than 1 year.

In 1998 and again in 2000, Wholey et al. (57,58) published reviews of the "global" experience with carotid artery stent placement. In the 2000 report, which was obtained via surveys sent to 36 major interventional centers in Europe, Asia, North and South America, results were reported on 5210 CAS procedures performed in 4749 patients (57). Forty-six percent of the patients in this series were asymptomatic. The procedures were performed by cardiologists in 57%, radiologists in 30%, and by surgeons in 13%. Stent deformations occurred in 45 cases and were exclusively seen with the Palmaz balloon-expandable stent. Technical success, defined as less than 30% residual stenosis, was achieved in 98.8% of cases. Despite the fact that cerebral protection devices were used only in a small minority of cases, the morbidity/mortality rates reported were quite good. The rates of procedure-related death, nonprocedure-related death, disabling stroke, and nondisabling stroke were 0.8%, 1.1%, 1.4%, and 2.5%, respectively, for a combined stroke or death rate of 5.7%. The rate of recurrent carotid stenosis observed at 12 mo was exceedingly low at 3.5%. A "learning curve" with respect to periprocedural complications was observed, which was highest during the first 50 cases, and then stabilized. The combined stroke and death rate was 5.8% among symptomatic patients, a figure that favorably compares with NASCET results. The corresponding rate in asymptomatic patients was 3.4%; this is more than double the combined stroke and death rate reported in the ACAS Trial. Using data from the NASCET and ACAS Trials (Table 1), the expected stroke or death rate following CEA in a population of patients with a similar proportion of asymptomatic individuals is 4.2%. It must be acknowledged that the majority of patients in Wholey's series would not have been candidates for inclusion in ACAS or NASCET owing to the presence of medical comorbidities or previous neck surgery. The potential biases inherent in such a study, including its retrospective nature, the lack of independent assessment of outcome events, incomplete reporting of cases, lack of peer review for the majority of cases, and lack of a control group must also be acknowledged.

The rationale for the use of cerebral protection devices for CAS is compelling. Surgeons experienced with CEA have long recognized the potential to dislodge the friable material present in carotid bifurcation plaques (59). Studies of carotid stenting with transcranial Doppler monitoring have demonstrated frequent embolic signals prevalent during several stages of the carotid stenting procedure including lesion crossing, predilation, stent placement, and postdilation (60,61). Diffusion-weighted MRI scans performed before and after CAS in one study demonstrated embolic brain lesions in 37% of patients, of which 85% were clinically silent (62). There are three classes of embolic protection devices currently available: (1) balloon occlusion/aspiration devices; (2) filter devices; and (3) flow reversal devices. Pathological analysis of particles retrieved with the use of these devices demonstrates the presence of atherosclerotic debris in a large fraction of cases (48,53,56).

The clinical use of cerebral protection devices was first described by Theron et al. (63). Although case series in which such devices were used have generally demonstrated lower stroke rates than those in which embolic protection was not used (Table 3), all cerebral protection devices have the potential to cause arterial damage and adverse clinical sequellae. In a systematic review of the medical literature of CAS, Kastrup et al. (64) identified 2537 patients treated without vs. 896 treated with cerebral protection devices. The stroke or death rate was 5.5% following unprotected vs. 1.8% following protected procedures (P < 0.001). As was previously mentioned, the history of CAS has witnessed a temporal trend showing impressive improvements in complication rates. Since this trend is evident even in series limited to unprotected CAS procedures, it is likely related to several factors in addition to the increased usage of cerebral protection devices, including improved stent and stent delivery system technology and importantly, increased operator experience.

There are several other factors that appear to effect the periprocedural risks associated with CAS. For example, CAS has particularly low complication rates when performed for postendarterectomy restenosis (65–68). Because post-CEA restenotic lesions are because of myointimal hyperplasia, they tend to be smooth and less friable with a lower embolic potential than de novo atherosclerotic lesions. New et al. (68) published a multicenter registry of CAS for post-CEA restenosis in 358 carotid arteries (338 patients), the largest published series of interventions for this problem. The stroke or death rate was 3.6% including a disabling stroke rate of 0.8%, values that are quite comparable to morbidity/mortality rates for surgical treatment of post-CEA restenosis. Because of these encouraging results, obtained in the vast majority of cases without the use of cerebral protection devices, many centers have begun their CAS programs by focusing on these lower-risk patients.

As experience has been gained with CAS, several factors have emerged that may increase the difficulty of and/or risks associated with CAS. The ability to access the common carotid artery with a guide sheath or guide catheter is largely determined by the shape of the aortic arch and the location of the great vessel orifices. Other factors that may be associated with increased difficulty or risk include external carotid artery occlusion, excessive internal carotid artery tortuosity, and the presence of visible thrombus on preprocedural imaging studies. These factors will be discussed in more detail in other chapters of this text.

Another factor that may have an important impact on the safety of CAS is the periprocedural use of platelet glycoprotein IIb/IIIa inhibitors, such as abciximab. The use of these drugs, which is a common practice during CAS, is based on extrapolation from the coronary literature. While there are theoretical reasons to believe the risk of embolic ischemic stroke may be lower with the use of these drugs, preliminary data suggest high bleeding risks, including hemorrhagic strokes, with the use of these agents (69). In a retrospective review of 550 patients undergoing CAS, Wholey et al. (70) found neurological complication rates of 6.0% among the 216 patients treated with IIb/IIIa inhibitors compared with only 2.4% for the 334 patients treated with heparin only.

While there is currently a paucity of published RCT data comparing CAS with CEA, there are several ongoing clinical trials being conducted in Europe and North America (Table 4). The Carotid Revascularization Endarterectomy vs. Stent Trial (CREST) is a randomized trial designed to compare CAS and CEA among 2500 symptomatic patients with $\geq 50\%$ carotid stenosis and low perioperative risk profiles. The trial is sponsored by the National Institutes of Health and Guidant Corporation and employs the use of the Acculink™ stent and AccuNet™ filter. The CARESS study (Carotid Revascularization with Endarterectomy vs. Stenting Systems) is a multicenter registry designed to study CAS in both symptomatic and asymptomatic patients who are not candidates for CREST and includes a concurrent nonrandomized CEA cohort. Many of the ongoing clinical trials listed in Table 4 are industry-sponsored non-randomized registries of CAS in high-risk patients organized in an attempt to gain FDA approval for stents and cerebral protection devices. The ARCHeR Study (Acculink™ for Revascularization of Carotids in High-Risk Patients) is a recently completed but not yet published Guidant-sponsored registry of 513 patients treated with the Acculink™ stent and AccuNet™ filter. This study included both symptomatic and asymptomatic high-risk patients, including patients with postendarterectomy restenosis. The periprocedural death and stroke rates were 2.3% and 5.3%, respectively, values that are higher than previously published single-center series employing cerebral protection devices (Table 3).

There are currently three published RCTs comparing CAS and CEA, two of which were stopped early because of superior results in the CEA group (71–73) The results of these three trials are shown in Table 5. In 1998, Naylor et al. (71) reported their results with a single-center RCT conducted in the United Kingdom, which was stopped after only 17 patients were randomized. There were no complications in the surgical group, but five of the seven patients who underwent CAS suffered strokes, three of which were disabling at 30 days (Table 5). The second stopped trial was a multicenter RCT sponsored by the Schneider Corporation (72). Published in abstract form only, the trial randomized 219 symptomatic patients (107 CAS, 112 CEA) with $\geq 60\%$ stenosis to receive CAS with the Wallstent vs. CEA. The perioperative stroke or death rate was 12.1% for the CAS patients vs. 4.5% for the CEA group ($P = 0.049$, Table 4). The 1-year cumulative incidence of any ipsilateral stroke or procedure-related or vascular

Caps

Table 4 Summary of Completed and Ongoing Clinical Trials of CAS

Full name	Acronym	Trial type	Patients	N	Sponsor	Stent	Cerebral protection device	Status	Published
CAS vs. CEA (71)		RCT	Symptomatic	17	Single center	NS	NS	Stopped	Yes
Wallstent Trial (72)		RCT	Symptomatic	219	Schneider	Wallstent	None	Stopped	Abstract
Carotid and Vertebral Artery Transluminal Angioplasty Study (74)	CAVATAS	RCT	Symptomatic Asymptomatic	504	British Heart Foundation	Variable	None	Complete	Yes
Stenting and Angioplasty with Protection in Patients at High Risk for Endarterectomy	SAPPHIRE	RCT	Symptomatic Asymptomatic High Risk	307	Cordis	Precise	AngioGuard	Complete	No
Carotid Revascularization: Endarterectomy vs. Stent Trial	CREST	RCT	Symptomatic	2500	NIH	Acculink	Accunet	Ongoing	No
Endarterectomy vs. Angioplasty in patients with Severe Symptomatic carotid Stenosis	EVA-3S	RCT	Symptomatic	1000	French Government	NS	NS	Ongoing	No
International Carotid Stenting Study	ICSS (CAVATAS 2)	RCT	Symptomatic	2000	U.K. Stroke Association	NS	NS	Ongoing	No
Stent-Protected Percutaneous Angioplasty of the Carotid vs. Endarterectomy	SPACE	RCT	Symptomatic	1900	German Government, Boston Scientific, Guidant	NS	NS	Ongoing	No

Trial	Acronym	Type	Patients	N	Sponsor	Stent	EPD	Status	RCT
Medtronic AVE Carotid Stent with Distal Protection In the Treatment of Carotid Stenosis	MAVErIC II	Registry	Symptomatic Asymptomatic High Risk	300	Medtronic	Exponent	GuardWire	Ongoing	No
Acculink for Revascularization of Carotids in High-Risk Patients	ARCHeR	Registry	Symptomatic Asymptomatic High Risk	513	Guidant	Acculink	Accunet	Complete	No
Carotid Revascularization with Endarterectomy or Stenting Systems	CARESS	Registry	Symptomatic Asymptomatic	NS	ISIS	NS	NS	Ongoing	No
Boston Scientific/EPI: A Carotid Stenting Trial for High-Risk Surgical Patients	BEACH	Registry	High Risk	775	Boston Scientific	Wallstent Monorail	FilterWire EX	Ongoing	No
Carotid Artery Revascularization Using the Boston Scientific EPI FilterWire EX* and the EndoTex NexStent	CABERNET	Registry	High Risk	NS	Boston Scientific, EndoTex	NexStent	Epi Filter	Ongoing	No
Stenting of High-Risk Patients Extracranial Lesions Trial with Embolic Removal	SHELTER	Registry	High Risk	NS	Boston Scientific	Wallstent Monorail	PercuSurge	Ongoing	No

N = actual N for completed trials, projected N for ongoing trials. NS = not specified. RCT = randomized clinical trial.

Table 5 Summary of Results of Randomized Controlled Trials Comparing CAS with CEA

| Trial | Group | N | 30-Day outcomes | | | | Long-term outcomes | | | |
			Any death (%)	Any nonfatal stroke (%)	Any stroke or death (%)	MI (%)	Length of follow-up (years)	Endpoint	Incidence (%)	Restenosis (%)
CAS VS CEA (71)	CAS	7	0	71.4	71.4					
	CEA	10	0	0.0	0.0					
Wallstent (72)	CAS	107			12.1		1	Ipsi CVA/Surg	12.1	
	CEA	112			4.5		1	Vascular death	3.6	
CAVATAS (74)	CAS	251	2.8	7.2	10.0	0.0	3	Disabling	14.3	14.5
	CEA	253	1.6	8.3	9.9	1.2	3	CVA/death	14.2	4.0
SAPPHIRE (75)	CAS	156	0.6	3.8	4.4	2.6				
	CEA	151	2.0	5.3	7.3	7.3				

MI = myocardial infarction. CVA = cerebrovascular accident.

death was 12.1% and 3.6% for the CAS and CEA groups, respectively ($P = 0.02$, Table 5). A subgroup analysis of this trial demonstrated particularly poor CAS results in centers with limited carotid stenting experience.

The CAVATAS (Carotid And Vertebral Artery Transluminal Angioplasty Study) Trial (74) was a multicenter European RCT in which 504 (251 CAS, 253 CEA) symptomatic or asymptomatic patients with carotid stenosis were randomized to receive balloon angioplasty +/− stenting vs. CEA (Table 5). Only 26% of the CAS patients received stents. The periprocedural stroke or death rates (10.0% CAS, 9.9% CEA) and the 3-year disabling stroke or death rates (14.3% CAS, 14.2% CEA) were equivalent, and restenosis rates at 1 year were considerably higher ($P < 0.001$) in the CAS patients (14.5%) than in the CEA group (4.0%). The generalizability of this trial has been criticized because of the inordinately high perioperative complication rates in the surgical group (9.9% stroke or death, 8.3% stroke), rates that are considerably higher than in previously published RCTs (see Table 1). Furthermore, the trial that was published in 2001 is already outdated because of the low proportion of CAS patients who received stents.

The SAPPHIRE Trial (Stenting and Angioplasty with Protection in Patients at High Risk for Endarterectomy) is a recently completed but not yet published RCT sponsored by Cordis Corporation in which 307 (156 CAS, 151 CEA) patients were randomized to receive CAS using the Precise™ stent together with the AngioGuard™ embolic protection device vs. standard CEA (75). Randomized patients were considered "high risk" for CEA based on medical or anatomic factors. Symptomatic patients with ≥50% stenosis and asymptomatic patients with ≥80% carotid stenosis were included. The perioperative stroke or death rates were 7/156 (4.5%) and 11/151 (7.3%) for the CAS and CEA groups, respectively ($P = 0.3$). When perioperative myocardial infarction is included in this composite end point (2.6% CAS, 7.3% CEA), the difference becomes statistically significant in favor of the CAS group, but the clinical significance of these myocardial infarctions is not clear.* While this is an underpowered trial with unexpectedly high periprocedural stroke rates in the CEA group (5.3%), especially when one considers that the majority of patients were asymptomatic, the results indicate that among high-risk patients, CAS appears to compare favorably to CEA. Given the low stroke risk for asymptomatic patients with carotid stenosis, the question of whether asymptomatic patients who are considered "high risk" should be considered for any type of carotid artery intervention should be addressed.

Conclusion

Optimum management of patients with carotid bifurcation stenosis requires thorough familiarity with the natural history of the disease process as well as with *all* modes of

---

*Results at one year of follow-up show similar trends of note, the rate of carotid restenosis at one year in the stent group was similar to that for endarterectomy (<5%).

therapy including medical management, CEA, and CAS. Randomized controlled clinical trials comparing CEA with medical management have established CEA as the standard of care for the majority of patients with symptomatic and for highly selected patients with asymptomatic carotid bifurcation stenosis. These trials have established benchmark perioperative morbidity/mortality rates that can be achieved in standard-risk patients. The data on CAS consists of a limited number of flawed RCTs in addition to a large number of case series and registries with inherent biases. These studies indicate that periprocedural complication rates following CAS have markedly improved over the past decade, probably owing to many factors including improved technical skill and enhanced technology. Until additional RCTs comparing CAS with CEA are completed, CEA should be considered the treatment of choice for standard-risk patients with carotid stenosis requiring intervention. For patients considered at high risk for CEA, however, CAS is a viable alternative when performed in centers with established expertise and excellence.

References

1. Beneficial effect of carotid endarterectomy in symptomatic patients with high-grade carotid stenosis. North American Symptomatic Carotid Endarterectomy Trial Collaborators. N Engl J Med 1991; 325(7):445–453.
2. Barnett HJ, Taylor DW, Eliasziw M, Fox AJ, Ferguson GG, Haynes RB, Rankin RN, Clagett GP, Hachinski VC, Sackett DL, Thorpe KE, Meldrum HE. Benefit of carotid endarterectomy in patients with symptomatic moderate or severe stenosis. North American Symptomatic Carotid Endarterectomy Trial Collaborators. N Engl J Med 1998; 339(20):1415–1425.
3. MRC European Carotid Surgery Trial: interim results for symptomatic patients with severe (70–99%) or with mild (0–29%) carotid stenosis. European Carotid Surgery Trialists' Collaborative Group. Lancet 1991; 337(8752):1235–1243.
4. Randomised trial of endarterectomy for recently symptomatic carotid stenosis: final results of the MRC European Carotid Surgery Trial (ECST) [comment]. Lancet 1998; 351(9113):1379–1387.
5. Endarterectomy for asymptomatic carotid artery stenosis. Executive Committee for the Asymptomatic Carotid Atherosclerosis Study. JAMA 1995; 273(18):1421–1428.
6. Hobson RW, Weiss DG, Fields WS, Goldstone J, Moore WS, Towne JB, Wright CB. Efficacy of carotid endarterectomy for asymptomatic carotid stenosis. The Veterans Affairs Cooperative Study Group. N Engl J Med 1993; 328(4):221–227.
7. Mayberg MR, Wilson SE, Yatsu F, Weiss DG, Messina L, Hershey LA, Colling C, Eskridge J, Deykin D, Winn HR. Carotid endarterectomy and prevention of cerebral ischemia in symptomatic carotid stenosis. Veterans Affairs Cooperative Studies Program 309 Trialist Group. JAMA 1991; 266(23):3289–3294.
8. Strandness DE. Historical perspectives in cerebrovascular disease. In: Zierler RE, ed. Surgical Management of Cerebrovascular Disease. New York: McGraw-Hill, 1995:1–6.
9. Young B, Moore WS, Robertson JT, Toole JF, Ernst CB, Cohen SN, Broderick JP, Dempsey RJ, Hosking JD. An analysis of perioperative surgical mortality and morbidity in the asymptomatic carotid atherosclerosis study. ACAS Investigators. Asymptomatic Carotid Arteriosclerosis Study. Stroke 1996; 27(12):2216–2224.

10. Chervu A, Moore WS. Carotid endarterectomy without arteriography. Ann Vasc Surg 1994; 8(3):296–302.

11. Dawson DL, Zierler RE, Strandness DE Jr, Clowes AW, Kohler TR. The role of duplex scanning and arteriography before carotid endarterectomy: A prospective study. J Vasc Surg 1993; 18(4):673–680.

12. Dawson DL, Roseberry CA, Fujitani RM. Preoperative testing before carotid endarterectomy: A survey of vascular surgeons' attitudes. Ann Vasc Surg 1997; 11(3):264–272.

13. Loftus IM, McCarthy MJ, Pau H, Hartshorne T, Bell PR, London NJ, Naylor AR. Carotid endarterectomy without angiography does not compromise operative outcome. Eur J Vasc Endovasc Surg 1998; 16(6):489–493.

14. Shifrin EG, Bornstein NM, Kantarovsky A, Morag B, Zelmanovich L, Portnoi I, Aronovich B. Carotid endarterectomy without angiography. Br J Surg 1996; 83(8):1107–1109.

15. Randomised trial of endarterectomy for recently symptomatic carotid stenosis: final results of the MRC European Carotid Surgery Trial (ECST) [comment]. Lancet 1998; 351(9113):1379–1387.

16. Rothwell PM, Gutnikov SA, Warlow CP. Reanalysis of the final results of the European Carotid Surgery Trial. Stroke 2003; 34(2):514–523.

17. Birkmeyer JD, Siewers AE, Finlayson EV, Stukel TA, Lucas FL, Batista I, Welch HG, Wennberg DE. Hospital volume and surgical mortality in the United States. N Engl J Med 2002; 346(15):1128–1137.

18. Cebul RD, Snow RJ, Pine R, Hertzer NR, Norris DG. Indications, outcomes, and provider volumes for carotid endarterectomy. JAMA 1998; 279(16):1282–1287.

19. Kresowik TF, Bratzler D, Karp HR, Hemann RA, Hendel ME, Grund SL, Brenton M, Ellerbeck EF, Nilasena DS. Multistate utilization, processes, and outcomes of carotid endarterectomy. J Vasc Surg 2001; 33(2):227–234.

20. Kresowik TF, Hemann RA, Grund SL, Hendel ME, Brenton M, Wiblin RT, Adams HP, Ellerbeck EF. Improving the outcomes of carotid endarterectomy: results of a statewide quality improvement project. J Vasc Surg 2000; 31(5):918–926.

21. Pearce WH, Parker MA, Feinglass J, Ujiki M, Manheim LM. The importance of surgeon volume and training in outcomes for vascular surgical procedures. J Vasc Surg 1999; 29(5):768–776.

22. Ouriel K, Hertzer NR, Beven EG, O'hara PJ, Krajewski LP, Clair DG, Greenberg RK, Sarac TP, Olin JW, Yadav JS. Preprocedural risk stratification: identifying an appropriate population for carotid stenting. J Vasc Surg 2001; 33(4):728–732.

23. AbuRahma AF, Snodgrass KR, Robinson PA, Wood DJ, Meek RB, Patton DJ. Safety and durability of redo carotid endarterectomy for recurrent carotid artery stenosis. Am J Surg 1994; 168(2):175–178.

24. Gagne PJ, Riles TS, Jacobowitz GR, Lamparello PJ, Giangola G, Adelman MA, Imparato AM, Mintzer R. Long-term follow-up of patients undergoing reoperation for recurrent carotid artery disease. J Vasc Surg 1993; 18(6):991–998.

25. Hill BB, Olcott C, Dalman RL, Harris EJ Jr, Zarins CK. Reoperation for carotid stenosis is as safe as primary carotid endarterectomy. J Vasc Surg 1999; 30(1):26–35.

26. Mansour MA, Kang SS, Baker WH, Watson WC, Littooy FN, Labropoulos N, Greisler HP. Carotid endarterectomy for recurrent stenosis. J Vasc Surg 1997; 25(5):877–883.

27. Rockman CB, Riles TS, Landis R, Lamparello PJ, Giangola G, Adelman MA, Jacobowitz GR. Redo carotid surgery: An analysis of materials and configurations used in carotid

reoperations and their influence on perioperative stroke and subsequent recurrent stenosis. J Vasc Surg 1999; 29(1):72–80.

28. Baker WH, Howard VJ, Howard G, Toole JF. Effect of contralateral occlusion on long-term efficacy of endarterectomy in the asymptomatic carotid atherosclerosis study (ACAS). ACAS Investigators. Stroke 2000; 31(10):2330–2334.

29. Gasecki AP, Eliasziw M, Ferguson GG, Hachinski V, Barnett HJ. Long-term prognosis and effect of endarterectomy in patients with symptomatic severe carotid stenosis and contralateral carotid stenosis or occlusion: results from NASCET. North American Symptomatic Carotid Endarterectomy Trial (NASCET) Group. J Neurosurg 1995; 83(5):778–782.

30. AbuRahma AF, Hannay RS, Khan JH, Robinson PA, Hudson JK, Davis EA. Prospective randomized study of carotid endarterectomy with polytetrafluoroethylene versus collagen-impregnated Dacron (Hemashield) patching: Perioperative (30-day) results. J Vasc Surg 2002; 35(1):125–130.

31. Cao P, Giordano G, De Rango P, Zannetti S, Chiesa R, Coppi G, Palombo D, Peinetti F, Spartera C, Stancanelli V, Vecchiati E. Eversion versus conventional carotid endarterectomy: Late results of a prospective multicenter randomized trial. J Vasc Surg 2000; 31(1):19–30.

32. O'hara PJ, Hertzer NR, Mascha EJ, Krajewski LP, Clair DG, Ouriel K. A prospective, randomized study of saphenous vein patching versus synthetic patching during carotid endarterectomy. J Vasc Surg 2002; 35(2):324–332.

33. Moore WS, Kempczinski RF, Nelson JJ, Toole JF. Recurrent carotid stenosis: Results of the asymptomatic carotid atherosclerosis study. Stroke 1998; 29(10):2018–2025.

34. Bockenheimer SA, Mathias K. Percutaneous transluminal angioplasty in arteriosclerotic internal carotid artery stenosis. AJNR Am J Neuroradiol 1983; 4(3):791–792.

35. Kerber CW, Cromwell LD, Loehden OL. Catheter dilatation of proximal carotid stenosis during distal bifurcation endarterectomy. AJNR Am J Neuroradiol 1980; 1(4):348–349.

36. Mathias K. A new catheter system for percutaneous transluminal angioplasty (PTA) of carotid artery stenoses. Fortschr Med 1977; 95(15):1007–1011.

37. Wiggli U, Gratzl O. Transluminal angioplasty of stenotic carotid arteries: Case reports and protocol. AJNR Am J Neuroradiol 1983; 4(3):793–795.

38. Marks MP, Dake MD, Steinberg GK, Norbash AM, Lane B. Stent placement for arterial and venous cerebrovascular disease: Preliminary experience. Radiology 1994; 191(2):441–446.

39. Diethrich EB, Ndiaye M, Reid DB. Stenting in the carotid artery: Initial experience in 110 patients. J Endovasc Surg 1996; 3(1):42–62.

40. Wholey MH, Wholey MH, Jarmolowski CR, Eles G, Levy D, Buecthel J. Endovascular stents for carotid artery occlusive disease. J Endovasc Surg 1997; 4(4):326–338.

41. Yadav JS, Roubin GS, Iyer S, Vitek J, King P, Jordan WD, Fisher WS. Elective stenting of the extracranial carotid arteries. Circulation 1997; 95(2):376–381.

42. Al Mubarak N, Colombo A, Gaines PA, Iyer SS, Corvaja N, Cleveland TJ, Macdonald S, Brennan C, Vitek JJ. Multicenter evaluation of carotid artery stenting with a filter protection system. J Am Coll Cardiol 2002; 39(5):841–846.

43. Cremonesi A, Manetti R, Setacci F, Setacci C, Castriota F. Protected carotid stenting. Clinical advantages and complications of embolic protection devices in 442 consecutive patients. Stroke, 2003; 34:1936–1941.

44. Criado FJ, Lingelbach JM, Ledesma DF, Lucas PR. Carotid artery stenting in a vascular surgery practice. J Vasc Surg 2002; 35(3):430–434.

45. d'Audiffret A, Desgranges P, Kobeiter H, Becquemin JP. Technical aspects and current results of carotid stenting. J Vasc Surg 2001; 33(5):1001–1007.

46. Guimaraens L, Sola MT, Matali A, Arbelaez A, Delgado M, Soler L, Balaguer E, Castellanos C, Ibanez J, Miquel L, Theron J. Carotid angioplasty with cerebral protection and stenting: Report of 164 patients (194 carotid percutaneous transluminal angioplasties). Cerebrovasc Dis 2002; 13(2):114–119.

47. Henry M, Amor M, Masson I, Henry I, Tzvetanov K, Chati Z, Khanna N. Angioplasty and stenting of the extracranial carotid arteries. J Endovasc Surg 1998; 5(4):293–304.

48. Henry M, Henry I, Klonaris C, Masson I, Hugel M, Tzvetanov K, Ethevenot G, Le BE, Kownator S, Luizi F, Folliguet B. Benefits of cerebral protection during carotid stenting with the PercuSurge GuardWire system: Midterm results. J Endovasc Ther 2002; 9(1):1–13.

49. Hobson RW, Lal BK, Chaktoura E, Goldstein J, Haser PB, Kubicka R, Cerveira J, Pappas PJ, Padberg FT, Jamil Z. Carotid artery stenting: Analysis of data for 105 patients at high risk. J Vasc Surg 2003; 37(6):1234–1239.

50. Koch C, Kucinski T, Eckert B, Wittkugel O, Rother J, Zeumer H. Endovascular therapy of high-degree stenoses of the neck vessels—stent-supported percutaneous angioplasty of the carotid artery without cerebral protection. RoFo Fortschr Geb Rontgenstrahlen Neuen Bildgeb Verfahr 2002; 174(12):1506–1510.

51. Macdonald S, McKevitt F, Venables GS, Cleveland TJ, Gaines PA. Neurological outcomes after carotid stenting protected with the NeuroShield filter compared to unprotected stenting. J Endovasc Ther 2002; 9(6):777–785.

52. Mathias K, Jager H, Sahl H, Hennigs S, Gissler HM. Interventional treatment of arteriosclerotic carotid stenosis. Radiologe 1999; 39(2):125–134.

53. Reimers B, Corvaja N, Moshiri S, Sacca S, Albiero R, Di Mario C, Pascotto P, Colombo A. Cerebral protection with filter devices during carotid artery stenting. Circulation 2001; 104(1):12–15.

54. Roubin GS, New G, Iyer SS, Vitek JJ, Al Mubarak N, Liu MW, Yadav J, Gomez C, Kuntz RE. Immediate and late clinical outcomes of carotid artery stenting in patients with symptomatic and asymptomatic carotid artery stenosis: A 5-year prospective analysis. Circulation 2001; 103(4):532–537.

55. Shawl F, Kadro W, Domanski MJ, Lapetina FL, Iqbal AA, Dougherty KG, Weisher DD, Marquez JF, Shahab ST. Safety and efficacy of elective carotid artery stenting in high-risk patients. J Am Coll Cardiol 2000; 35(7):1721–1728.

56. Whitlow PL, Lylyk P, Londero H, Mendiz OA, Mathias K, Jaeger H, Parodi J, Schonholz C, Milei J. Carotid artery stenting protected with an emboli containment system. Stroke 2002; 33(5):1308–1314.

57. Wholey MH, Wholey M, Mathias K, Roubin GS, Diethrich EB, Henry M, Bailey S, Bergeron P, Dorros G, Eles G, Gaines P, Gomez CR, Gray B, Guimaraens J, Higashida R, Ho DS, Katzen B, Kambara A, Kumar V, Laborde JC, Leon M, Lim M, Londero H, Mesa J, Musacchio A, Myla S, Ramee S, Rodriquez A, Rosenfield K, Sakai N, Shawl F, Sievert H, Teitelbaum G, Theron JG, Vaclav P, Vozzi C, Yadav JS, Yoshimura SI. Global experience in cervical carotid artery stent placement. Catheter Cardiovasc Interv 2000; 50(2):160–167.

58. Wholey MH, Wholey M, Bergeron P, Diethrich EB, Henry M, Laborde JC, Mathias K, Myla S, Roubin GS, Shawl F, Theron JG, Yadav JS, Dorros G, Guimaraens J, Higashida R, Kumar V, Leon M, Lim M, Londero H, Mesa J, Ramee S, Rodriguez A, Rosenfield K,

Teitelbaum G, Vozzi C. Current global status of carotid artery stent placement. Catheter Cardiovasc Diagn 1998; 44(1):1–6.

59. Beebe HG, Archie JP, Baker WH, Barnes RW, Becker GJ, Bernstein EF, Brener B, Clagett GP, Clowes AW, Cooke JP. Concern about safety of carotid angioplasty. Stroke 1996; 27(2):197–198.

60. Coggia M, Goeau-Brissonniere O, Duval JL, Leschi JP, Letort M, Nagel MD. Embolic risk of the different stages of carotid bifurcation balloon angioplasty: An experimental study. J Vasc Surg 2000; 31(3):550–557.

61. McCleary AJ, Nelson M, Dearden NM, Calvey TA, Gough MJ. Cerebral haemodynamics and embolization during carotid angioplasty in high-risk patients. Br J Surg 1998; 85(6):771–774.

62. Theron JG, Payelle GG, Coskun O, Huet HF, Guimaraens L. Carotid artery stenosis: treatment with protected balloon angioplasty and stent placement. Radiology 1996; 201(3):627–636.

63. Kastrup A, Groschel K, Krapf H, Brehm BR, Dichgans J, Schulz JB. Early outcome of carotid angioplasty and stenting with and without cerebral protection devices: A systematic review of the literature. Stroke 2003; 34(3):813–819.

64. Hobson RW, Goldstein JE, Jamil Z, Lee BC, Padberg FT Jr, Hanna AK, Gwertzman GA, Pappas PJ, Silva MB Jr. Carotid restenosis: operative and endovascular management. J Vasc Surg 1999; 29(2):228–235.

65. Vitek JJ, Roubin GS, New G, Al Mubarek N, Iyer SS. Carotid angioplasty with stenting in post-carotid endarterectomy restenosis. J Invasive Cardiol 2001; 13(2):123–125.

66. Yadav JS, Roubin GS, King P, Iyer S, Vitek J. Angioplasty and stenting for restenosis after carotid endarterectomy. Initial experience. Stroke 1996; 27(11):2075–2079.

67. New G, Roubin GS, Iyer SS, Vitek JJ, Wholey MH, Diethrich EB, Hopkins LN, Hobson RW, Leon MB, Myla SV, Shawl F, Ramee SR, Yadav JS, Rosenfield K, Liu MW, Gomez CR, Al Mubarak N, Gray WA, Tan WA, Goldstin JE, Stack RS. Safety, efficacy, and durability of carotid artery stenting for restenosis following carotid endarterectomy: A multicenter study. J Endovasc Ther 2000; 7(5):345–352.

68. Mukherjee D, Yadav JS. Percutaneous treatment for carotid stenosis. Cardiol Clin 2002; 20(4):589–597.

69. Wholey MH, Wholey MH, Eles G, Toursakissian B, Bailey S, Jarmolowski C, Tan WA. Evaluation of Glycoprotein IIb/IIIa inhibitors in carotid angioplasty and stenting. J Endovasc Ther 2003; 10(1):33–41.

70. Naylor AR, Bolia A, Abbott RJ, Pye IF, Smith J, Lennard N, Lloyd AJ, London NJ, Bell PR. Randomized study of carotid angioplasty and stenting versus carotid endarterectomy: A stopped trial. J Vasc Surg 1998; 28(2):326–334.

71. Alberts MJ. Results of a Multicenter Prospective Randomized Trial of Carotid Artery Stenting vs. Carotid Endarterectomy. Abstr. Int. Stroke Conf. 2001; 32(1):325.

72. Endovascular versus surgical treatment in patients with carotid stenosis in the Carotid and Vertebral Artery Transluminal Angioplasty Study (CAVATAS): A randomised trial [comment]. Lancet 2001; 357(9270):1729–1737.

73. Endovascular versus surgical treatment in patients with carotid stenosis in the Carotid and Vertebral Artery Transluminal Angioplasty Study (CAVATAS): A randomised trial. Lancet 2001; 357(9270):1729–1737.

74. Ouriel K, Yadav J, Wholey M, Katzen B, Fayad P. The SAPPHIRE randomized trial of carotid stenting versus endarterectomy: a subgroup analysis. Vascular annual meeting 2003, Chicago, IL, Jun 9 2003.

75. Ferguson GG, Eliasziw M, Barr HW, Clagett GP, Barnes RW, Wallace MC, Taylor DW, Haynes RB, Finan JW, Hachinski VC, Barnett HJ. The North American Symptomatic Carotid Endarterectomy Trial: Surgical results in 1415 patients. Stroke 1999; 30(9):1751–1758.

76. Randomised trial of endarterectomy for recently symptomatic carotid stenosis: final results of the MRC European Carotid Surgery Trial (ECST). Lancet 1998; 351(9113):1379–1387.

17

Balloon Angioplasty and Stent Placement in the Innominate and Common Carotid Arteries: Technique and Results

PETER A. SCHNEIDER

Hawaii Permanente Medical Group, Honolulu, Hawaii, U.S.A.

The purpose of this chapter is to update the technique and results of endovascular management of innominate and common carotid artery occlusive lesions. Prior chapters covered carotid bifurcation balloon angioplasty and stenting technique and results. Because the clinical syndromes, lesion considerations, and other factors are different with subclavian artery lesions, they are separately presented in Chap. 18. Although common carotid and innominate artery lesions are much less common than carotid bifurcation lesions, endovascular management is more widely accepted for the following reasons: Arch branch lesions are less accessible surgically; these lesions are less likely to present with embolization; and data has accumulated over a period of time about the results of this approach. In this chapter, the approach, supplies, technique, and results of endovascular treatment of common carotid and innominate artery lesions are discussed.

Approach to Lesions of the Common Carotid and Innominate Arteries

Arch branch lesions, such as those occurring in the innominate artery or the common carotid arteries, may be approached antegrade (with the direction of flow) from a

Table 1 Innominate and Common Carotid Artery Lesions: Best Indications for Antegrade and Retrograde Approaches

Retrograde (against flow) via distal common carotid artery
At the arch
Embolizing/friable lesion of proximal common carotid artery (can control outflow)
Combined with carotid endarterectomy
Unfavorable arch anatomy for access
Antegrade (with flow) via femoral approach
Close to bifurcation
Tandem distal CCA/ICA lesion (combine with stent of carotid bifurcation)
Favorable arch anatomy
Either retrograde or antegrade approach is acceptable
Innominate artery distal to origin
Origin of right common carotid artery to mid-right common carotid artery
Proximal left common carotid artery (distal to origin) to mid-left common carotid artery

femoral access site, or retrograde (against the direction of flow) from a distal carotid or axillary access site (in the case of the innominate artery). These two approaches substantially differ in terms of technical considerations. Although many lesions can be treated using either approach, there are some lesions that are well suited to one approach or the other (Table 1). Lesions of the innominate and common carotid arteries are represented in Fig. 1.

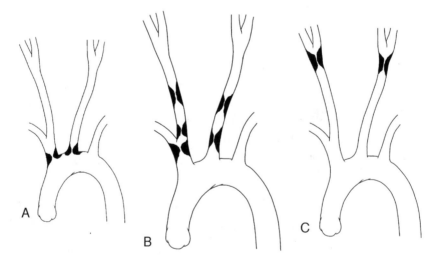

Fig. 1 Antegrade or retrograde approach to arch lesions? (A) Lesions of the origins of the innominate and left common carotid arteries are simplest and safest to treat using a retrograde approach. (B) Some occlusive lesions of the arch branches may be managed using either an antegrade approach or a retrograde approach. These include lesions that occur distal to the origins of the innominate and left common carotid arteries but proximal to the carotid bifurcations. (C) An antegrade approach works best for lesions of the distal common carotid arteries.

The retrograde approach can be used for lesions that occur at the origin of the arch branch. This approach permits secure access to the common carotid artery, and, when performed through open arterial access, provides the opportunity to control outflow if desired. This approach is particularly useful in patients with difficult arch anatomy. Patients who have a carotid bifurcation stenosis that requires endarterectomy can be treated with a combined procedure. This combined open and endovascular procedure is discussed in more detail later in this chapter. The major disadvantages of a retrograde approach through the common carotid artery are as follows. (1) It commits the patient to an incision for arterial access, albeit a small one. (2) Working room between the access site and the lesion is usually limited. (3) If there is any bifurcation disease, it must not be disrupted (unless it is severe enough to require treatment at the same time).

The antegrade approach is best for patients with favorable arch anatomy because the tip of the sheath, which has been placed transfemorally, must be securely anchored in the proximal common carotid artery. The antegrade approach is very functional for lesions that are distal to the vessel's origin at the arch. Perfect placement of a stent at the origin of the innominate or common carotid artery from the femoral artery is difficult because the sheath cannot be well anchored and an arch branch origin lesion treated at the same time. These arch lesions are best treated using a retrograde approach as mentioned above. When lesions of the distal common carotid artery occur with a bifurcation lesion, both can be treated with a carotid stent using the antegrade approach. The disadvantages of the transfemoral, antegrade approach are as follows: (1) The treatment of arteries that originate in segments IIb or III is very challenging. Maintaining a secure access in this situation requires passing the sheath at least a few centimeters into the artery to stabilize the tip of the sheath. This makes lesions of the innominate artery, which is more likely to originate in segments IIb or III, more difficult to treat. (2) The lesion must be crossed several times with catheters and guidewires to achieve sheath access from the groin.

Supplies

The equipment used for an antegrade approach to balloon angioplasty and stent placement in the innominate and common carotid arteries is similar to that used for carotid bifurcation angioplasty and stenting with a few additions (Table 2). Monorail balloons are available up to a diameter of 7 mm. Larger balloons are coaxial, and up to 8-mm diameter should be available for common carotid artery lesions and up to 12 mm for innominate artery lesions and can be obtained on a 0.035-in. platform. If a smaller platform guidewire is required, with the use of a distal protection device for example, the larger platform angioplasty catheters will usually track over it. Through an antegrade approach, either a balloon-expandable or a self-expanding stent may be placed. Each type of stent has technical considerations that are discussed in the next section. Lesions of the origin of the common carotid or innominate arteries are usually spillover plaque from the arch with a circumferential atherosclerotic ring. Much like for ostial subclavian or renal artery stenoses, balloon-expandable stents are most effective.

Table 2 Supplies for an Antegrade Approach to Common Carotid and Innominate Artery Lesions

Guidewires
    Angled tip, 0.035-in. steerable Glidewire, 260 cm
    Super-stiff Amplatz, 0.035, variable length floppy tip (1 or 6 cm), 260 cm
Catheters
    Angled tip, simple curve, 5-Fr selective catheter, 100 cm
    Complex curve, 5-Fr selective catheter, 100 cm
Sheaths
    Straight 90-cm shuttle sheath (Cook, Inc.), radiopaque tip, dilator, Tuohy Borst or hemostatic valve, Fr size of the sheath depends on the stent (usually 6 or 7 Fr)
Balloon catheters
    Up to 7 mm, rapid exchange, 0.014 or 0.018 in. (common carotid artery)
    Up to 12 mm, coaxial, 0.035 in., 120-cm length (common or innominate artery)
Stent
Common carotid artery
    Premounted, balloon-expandable 6, 7, 8 mm, 120-cm-length balloon catheter
    Self-expanding Nitinol, 8-, 10-, 12-mm-diameter, 120-cm-length delivery catheter
Innominate artery
    Premounted balloon-expandable 8, 10 mm, 120-cm-length balloon catheter
    Self-expanding 8-, 10-, 12-, 14-mm-diameter, 120-cm-length delivery catheter

Supplies for a retrograde approach are listed in Table 3. This approach is usually performed through a cutdown and may be combined with a carotid endarterectomy. The access is simple and the shortest sheath should be used to permit the most possible working room. The shortest guidewires and catheters are used to simplify the procedure. A super-stiff exchange guidewire is not required. A hockey stick or hook-shaped catheter is used to steer the guidewire into the descending thoracic aorta. Because no distal protection device or very small caliber angioplasty balloons are used, the 0.014-in.

Table 3 Supplies for a Retrograde Approach to Common Carotid and Innominate Artery Lesions

Guidewires
    Angled tip, 0.035-in. steerable Glidewire, 150 cm
    Wholey, steerable, 0.035 in., 145 cm
Catheters
    Angled tip, simple curve 5-Fr selective catheter, 40 or 65 cm
Sheath
    Straight 8- or 12-cm-length hemostatic access, 6 or 7 Fr, radiopaque tip
Balloon catheters
    6–8 mm, 0.035 in., coaxial, 40- or 75-cm length (common carotid artery)
    8–12 mm, 0.035 in., coaxial, 40- or 75-cm length (innominate artery)
Stent
    Premounted, balloon-expandable 6, 7, 8 mm (common carotid artery)
    Premounted balloon-expandable 8, 10 mm (innominate artery)
    Self-expanding 8-, 10-, 12-, 14-mm-diameter, 80-cm length

Table 4 Sheath Size Depends on the Stent Selected for Placement

Stent type	Diameter (mm)	Artery	Platform	Sheath size (Fr)
Balloon-expandable	6–8	CCA	0.018	6
	6	CCA	0.035	6
	7–8	CCA	0.035	7
	10	IA, CCA	0.035	7
	12	IA	0.035	8
Self-expanding	6–10	CCA	0.018	6
	6–10	CCA	0.035	6
	12–14	IA	0.035	7

CCA = common carotid artery; IA = innominate artery.

platform is not necessary, and because of the short distance, a 0.035-in. system is convenient. Sheath-sizing considerations are dependent on the type of stent used, either balloon-expandable or self-expanding (Table 4).

Technique

Arch aortography is performed, and the arch is assessed as described in Chap. 2. The approach to the lesion is considered as described in the previous sections. The approach selected will affect the room setup, method of anesthesia, and supplies required. Therefore a clear plan is required before initiating the procedure.

ANTEGRADE APPROACH

After arch aortography, heparin is administered. Placing an access sheath in this case is similar to the procedure used for carotid bifurcation angioplasty (see Fig. 3 of Chap. 6). The desired branch of the arch is catheterized. A disadvantage of the antegrade approach to the innominate and common carotid arteries is that the lesion intended for treatment must be crossed several times during the procedure. First, the selective guidewire, second the selective catheter, then the super-stiff guidewire must cross the lesion. The tip of the shuttle sheath must also cross if the stenosis is along the proximal part of the artery. Care must be taken while instrumenting the lesions to avoid embolization. The steerable Glidewire is placed into the external carotid artery. The selective catheter is advanced into the external carotid artery. The Amplatz super-stiff guidewire, or another stiff exchange guidewire, is placed through the selective cerebral catheter. The selective cerebral catheter is removed and the shuttle sheath is placed over the exchange guidewire. Another option is to place the selective cerebral catheter and advance the sheath over it (Fig. 2). Avoid crossing the lesion with the dilator or the shaft of the sheath, if possible, because this results in mechanical dilatation of the stenosis.

If a distal protection device is to be used, the appropriate small platform guidewire is passed. Whether using a distal occlusion balloon or a filter, they are all sized for the

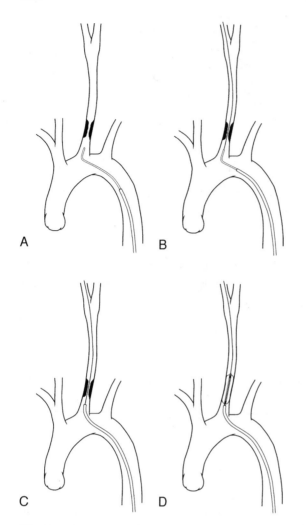

Fig. 2 Balloon angioplasty of the common carotid artery. (A) A sheath or guiding catheter has been placed in the proximal descending thoracic aorta and a selective catheter has been advanced through it. (B) The steerable guidewire is advanced across the lesion and placed in the external carotid artery. (C) The selective catheter is advanced, an exchange guidewire is placed, and the guiding sheath or guiding catheter is advanced into the origin of the common carotid artery. An arteriogram is performed that outlines the lesion. (D) Balloon angioplasty is performed. (From Schneider PA. Endovascular Skills. New York: Marcel Dekker, 2003.)

internal carotid artery. The guidewire is passed into the distal internal carotid artery and the distal protection device is deployed. Extreme caution must be used after this is performed because the distal protection device, no matter what kind, should not be moved while it is deployed. If the sheath must be moved or a larger caliber balloon catheter must be passed over the guidewire, these maneuvers will tend to move the distal protection device. If no distal protection device is used, the guidewire may be left in the external carotid artery.

The stenosis should be predilated, usually to 4 mm in diameter. Either balloon-expandable or self-expanding stents may be used. Figure 3 demonstrates antegrade placement of a balloon-expandable stent. As noted above, balloon-expandable stents are better for ostial lesions. These can be obtained premounted up to 10 mm in diameter. Balloon-expandable stents offer more precise placement than self-expanding stents. However, they are shorter (cover less distance) and more rigid (a disadvantage in a tortuous artery). Sizing for a balloon-expandable stent must be within 2 mm of the desired diameter. It must be large enough in diameter on initial deployment so that it

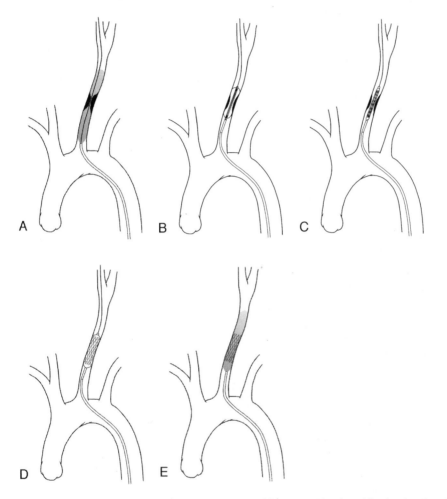

Fig. 3 Stent placement in the common carotid artery. (A) A guidewire is placed in the external carotid artery and a guiding sheath is advanced into the origin of the common carotid artery. (B) Balloon angioplasty is performed of the lesion in the proximal common carotid artery. (C) A premounted, balloon-expandable stent is advanced over the guidewire and across the lesion. The exact location of the tip of the sheath in relation to the lesion must be carefully confirmed before stent deployment. (D) The balloon-expandable stent is deployed by inflating the balloon. (E) A completion arteriogram is performed through the sheath.

does not migrate before another balloon can be placed to expand it further. On the other hand, if the initial diameter choice is a gross oversizing, the artery can be ruptured and there is no way to retract the stent. Self-expanding stents are easier to size but more difficult to deploy with accuracy. As long as the self-expanding stent is oversized to the artery, the diameter will be adequate. Because self-expanding stents deploy in the "tip to hub" direction, the first end of the stent can be very accurately deployed. This is the distal end of the stent when using a transfemoral, antegrade approach. However, it is not possible to predict exactly where the second end of the stent, the more proximal end, will be deployed. The concern is that if there is a short distance to the arch, the stent may hang out into the arch if deployed too low. If the stent is deployed too high, it may miss the lesion when the lesion is near the origin of the innominate or common carotid arteries. Because Nitinol stents foreshorten only a small amount when deployed, these are recommended when using a self-expanding stent in this position. A 120-cm-length coaxial delivery catheter is used. After the stent delivery catheter is in place, the proximal and distal markers on the constrained stent are matched up with the lesion. Double check the lower marker to make sure it does not pass into the arch. When deploying a self-expanding Nitinol stent, the leading end of the stent tends to jump forward a few millimeters, making it necessary to pull the whole catheter back a bit to readjust. Also, consider permitting the first few rings of the stent to flower out of the deployment catheter and waiting 20 or 30 sec for the Nitinol to warm up and stabilize. This will usually allow for a steadier deployment without the stent jumping forward. When withdrawing the stent delivery catheter, knowledge of the location of the artery origin is essential so the stent is not pulled back too far. Because many innominate arteries are relatively short and most of the lesions are near the artery origin, self-expanding stents are rarely used in this location. After the stent is deployed, poststent balloon angioplasty is performed. Completion arteriography is performed through the sheath.

RETROGRADE APPROACH

The common carotid artery is exposed through a short supraclavicular incision, either transverse or longitudinal (Fig. 4). Heparin is administered. The operator stands above the head of the bed. A long, sterile table is used as a working surface for guidewires and catheters and is placed contiguous with the head of the bed. A standard puncture needle is used to enter the artery. The puncture site should be at least a few centimeters from the bifurcation to avoid manipulating this area. The image intensifier is rotated into the LAO position as previously described. The guidewire is passed and fluoroscopy is immediately initiated because the distance to the lesion is very short. The distal common carotid artery may be clamped to control outflow. After the guidewire is across the lesion, advance it into the arch. Place a short access sheath. If a short access sheath is not available, the tip of a standard access sheath can be cut off. This should be performed over the dilator so that the tip of the sheath is not damaged. The sheath should be secured with a stitch because it is short and there is no subcutaneous tissue to hold it in place. The tip of the guidewire will tend to go into the ascending aorta and into the heart or bounce off the aortic valve. A hockey stick or hook-shaped catheter can be used to direct it into the descending thoracic aorta.

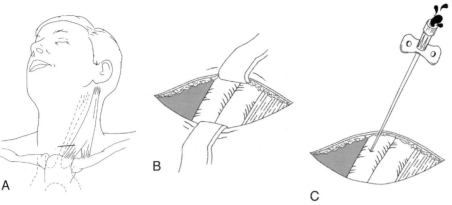

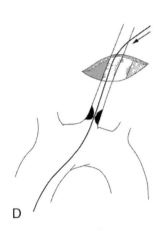

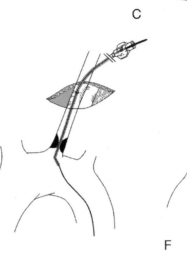

Fig. 4 Technique of retrograde approach to arch lesions. (A) A short, transverse incision is performed superior to the clavicle. (B) The common carotid artery is exposed. (C) A standard puncture needle is used to perform retrograde puncture of the common carotid artery. (D) Fluoroscopy is initiated during guidewire insertion. The guidewire tends to progress into the ascending aorta. (E) An angled-tip or hook-shaped catheter is used to direct the guidewire into the descending aorta. (F) The directional catheter is removed and a short standard access sheath is placed retrograde into the common carotid artery. (G) A balloon-expandable stent is placed in the proximal common carotid artery. (H) After the guidewire and sheath are removed, the arteriotomy is closed with a stitch.

A retrograde carotid arteriogram is performed through the sidearm of the sheath. If the lesion is preocclusive, sometimes the arch end of the lesion is difficult to delineate because only a wisp of contrast may go through and be immediately diluted by large volume blood flow in the arch. There are two options to manage this. (1) Predilate the lesion with a 4–6-mm diameter balloon and repeat the arteriogram. This usually provides an adequate lumen for retrograde flow of contrast. A high frame rate should be used because of the high flow in the arch. In addition, the impression of a waist along the partially inflated balloon can serve as a road map to the location of the lesion. (2) Place a pigtail catheter in the arch through a separate femoral puncture. If an arch aortogram has not already been performed to assess the case, it should be performed first anyway. If a pigtail is in place and a retrograde approach is selected, leave the catheter in place and use it during the case for interval arteriography.

After balloon angioplasty, the stent is placed. The principles of stent placement are the same as those for an antegrade approach, except that the working room is shorter. Ostial lesions are treated with premounted balloon-expandable stents. If self-expanding stents are used, assess the length of the stent before placement to be certain there is enough room to deploy it without having the upper end of the stent expand in the access sheath. The shortest available catheters and stent delivery devices are used. After stent placement, poststent balloon angioplasty is performed. Completion arteriography is performed through the retrograde sheath or through the transfemorally placed flush catheter. The carotid artery may be backbled and flushed through the arteriotomy after sheath removal. The arteriotomy is closed with a suture.

Results of Balloon Angioplasty and Stent Placement for Common Carotid and Innominate Artery Stenoses

Balloon angioplasty and stent placement has been used with success for innominate and common carotid artery lesions and reported in several single institution series. Although the studies tend to be small and to mix lesions of different arch branches, immediate and follow-up results are acceptable. The immediate technical success rate ranged from 92% to 100% (1–5). In most cases, a stent was placed. The patency ranged from 100% at 10 mo to 85% at 27 mo (4,5). This approach has been particularly successful for patients in whom open surgical options are limited, such as those with radiation injury and other types of arteritis (6,7).

Simultaneous Combined Carotid Endarterectomy and Retrograde Balloon Angioplasty and Stent of Proximal Stenosis of the Innominate or Common Carotid Artery

Among patients requiring carotid endarterectomy, a small percentage (approximately 1–2%) will have inflow disease at the arch that the operator may elect to treat at the same time as the bifurcation lesion (8). Over the past several years, the vast majority of patients requiring carotid endarterectomy have been treated on the basis of preoperative duplex evaluation. Because arch disease may be fairly severe and remain silent, it is quite likely that some arch lesions have been missed in patients requiring carotid endarterectomy. Arch disease should be evaluated with arteriography. Extrapolating from our experience in the lower extremities, it is an acceptable choice to leave a moderate isolated inflow lesion at the arch without intervention if the patient is not symptomatic. If this same lesion involves the inflow artery to an arterial reconstruction, it should be treated to

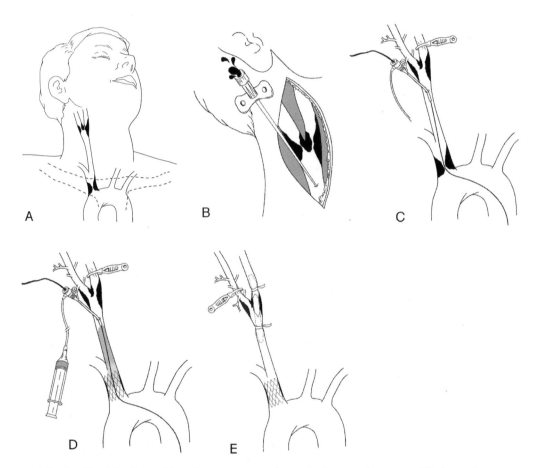

Fig. 5 Combined carotid endarterectomy and proximal stent placement. (A) An arch aortogram demonstrates an innominate artery stenosis and a carotid bifurcation stenosis. (B) The usual open exposure of the carotid bifurcation is performed. Heparin is administered. The entry needle is placed retrograde in the common carotid artery at the location where the lower end of the arteriotomy would usually be placed. (C) The guidewire is placed and directed into the descending aorta and a retrograde sheath is placed. The internal carotid artery is clamped to prevent emboli. (D) A balloon-expandable stent is placed in the origin of the innominate artery. A retrograde completion arteriogram is performed through the sheath. (E) The guidewire and sheath are removed. The arteriotomy is extended superiorly across the bifurcation. In this example, a shunt has been inserted across the bifurcation.

avoid compromising the more distally located open surgical reconstruction. This is the case for arch lesions proximal to a carotid endarterectomy.

The technique for the combined approach is described herein (Fig. 5). When positioning the patient for surgery, remove tubes, leads, and lines from behind the patient's head, neck, and upper chest. Ensure that this part of the patient is accessible to the image intensifier. Prepare the carotid artery for endarterectomy in the usual way. Perform the dissection and administer heparin. Because the artery will be clamped during angioplasty and stent placement, minimize the cross clamp time by getting everything out and ready. Clamp the internal carotid artery distal to the bifurcation lesion. The operator stands at the end of the head of the OR table. A long sterile table is placed contiguous with the head of the OR table to function as a workbench and to support the guidewires and catheters. Use the shortest available catheters and guidewires. Puncture the common carotid artery retrograde with an entry needle near the bifurcation where the lower end of the arteriotomy will be. Place the image intensifier in the left anterior oblique position. Pass the guidewire using fluoroscopy. Advance the guidewire into the descending thoracic aorta using a hook-shaped catheter. Place a short 7-Fr access sheath. Perform a retrograde carotid arteriogram. Advance the balloon angioplasty catheter and dilate the lesion. Use the waist on the balloon to road map the lesion and the origin of the artery. Advance a premounted, balloon-expandable stent over the guidewire. Puff contrast retrograde through the sheath to confirm the stent location before placement. Use the same deployment balloon to dilate the proximal and distal ends of the stent. Perform a completion arteriogram through the sidearm of the sheath. If the stent appears undersized, use a larger balloon to repeat the angioplasty. After a satisfactory completion study, remove the guidewire and sheath, bleed the artery, and crossclamp the common carotid artery proximal to the arteriotomy. Lengthen the arteriotomy across the bifurcation starting from the small hole in the artery made for the sheath. Place a shunt, if desired, in the usual way. If a very long shunt is used, it may catch on the upper end of the stent so do not force it if there is resistance. The remainder of the carotid endarterectomy procedure is performed as it usually would be. This procedure works best in patients who have proximal common carotid artery lesions. Although the working room from the endarterectomy site to stent site is short, the inflow lesion is not in the immediate surgical field.

Open Surgery vs. Endovascular Approach to Stenoses of the Innominate and Common Carotid Arteries

Although in-line, antegrade arch branch reconstructions are possible in most patients; this has largely fallen out of favor because of the magnitude of the operation. Morbidity and mortality rates have been reported in contemporary series that are substantially higher than those for either extra-anatomic bypass or endovascular repair. Most vascular surgeons are using extra-anatomic reconstructions when open repair is required. The most common of these extra-anatomic bypasses is the carotid–subclavian bypass, because subclavian lesions are more common than other arch branch lesions. The treatment of subclavian artery occlusive disease is discussed in the next chapter. Subclavian to carotid bypass, carotid to carotid bypass, and carotid to subclavian transposition are all used to treat common carotid and innominate artery lesions. It is difficult to assess the results of these procedures in comparison to balloon angioplasty and stent placement. In most series, the different types of operations are mixed. In general, the surgical series have a higher mortality rate, twice the complications, a longer length of stay, and only a slight improvement in long-term patency. There has not been a prospective comparison of these approaches.

What About Distal Protection Devices?

A distal protection device per se cannot be technically used with a retrograde approach but none is needed because outflow can be manually controlled. An antegrade approach may be accompanied by an adjunctive distal protection device. However, none of the existing devices are designed for deployment in the common carotid artery, with its larger diameter. Deployment of a protection device in the internal carotid artery during treatment of a proximal common carotid artery stenosis is possible, but may not be best because these devices have their own complication rates and it is not clear if this is necessary. Usage of cerebral protection devices in this setting has not been studied and the procedure has been performed for years without protection devices with authors reporting reasonable results. Case numbers are small and it is not certain that this will ever be studied. The disadvantages of a distal protection device in this situation are that it requires guidewire and device placement in the internal carotid artery that otherwise could be left alone; and it dictates the guidewire platform to be used (0.014 in.). The issue of guidewire platform does not make much difference for bifurcation stenting, but in the innominate and common carotid arteries, larger balloons and stents are required and a larger-caliber, 0.035-in. guidewire may be more suitable. The advantage of the distal protection device is that everything has been carried out, at least from a theoretical standpoint, to protect the patient form a neurological event. The author recommends that a distal protection device be used if the carotid bifurcation is free of disease and the catheters pass smoothly over the small caliber guidewire. Persisting with the use of a distal protection device is probably not warranted if it makes the procedure unnecessarily complicated.

References

1. Sullivan TM, Gray BH, Bacharach JM, Perl J, Childs MB, Modzelewski L, Beven EG. Angioplasty and primary stenting of the subclavian, innominate, and common carotid arteries in 83 patients. J Vasc Surg 1998; 28:1059–1065.
2. Ruebben A, Tettoni S, Muratore P, Rossato P, Savio D, Conforti M, Nessi F, Rabbia C. Feasibility of intraoperative balloon angioplasty and additional stent placement of isolated stenosis of the brachiocephalic trunk. J Thorac Cardiovasc Surg 1998; 115:1316–1320.

3. Criado FJ, Tweena M. Techniques for endovascular recanalization of supra-aortic trunks. J Endovasc Surg 1996; 3:405–413.
4. Lyon RD, Shonnard KM, McCarter DL, Hammond SL, Ferguson D, Rholl KS. Supra-aortic arterial stenoses: management with Palmaz balloon-expandable intraluminal stents. J Vasc Interv Radiol 1996; 7:825–835.
5. Queral LA, Criado FJ. The treatment of focal aortic arch branch lesions with Palmaz stents. J Vasc Surg 1996; 23:368–375.
6. Nomura M, Kida S, Yamashima T, Yamashita J, Yoshikawa J, Matsui O. Percutaneous transluminal angioplasty and stent placement for subclavian and brachiocephalic artery stenosis in aortitis syndrome. Cardiovasc Interv Radiol 1999; 22:427–432.
7. Al-Mubarak N, Roubin GS, Iyer SS, Gomez CR, Liu MW, Vitek JJ. Carotid stenting for severe radiation-induced extracranial carotid artery occlusive disease. J Endovasc Ther 2000; 7:36–40.
8. Arko FR, Buckley CJ, Lee SD, Manning LG, Patterson DE. Combined carotid endarterectomy with transluminal angioplasty and primary stenting of the supra-aortic vessels. J Cardiovasc Surg 2000; 41:737–742.

18

Balloon Angioplasty and Stent Placement in the Subclavian Arteries: Technique and Results

NICOLAS NELKEN

Hawaii Permanente Medical Group, Honolulu, HI, U.S.A.

Subclavian artery stenoses or occlusions can cause symptoms in both the cerebral and brachial territories. As in the carotid circulation, lesions in this territory are far more common than symptoms. The natural history of most symptomatic lesions is also usually more benign than in the carotid circulation. Intracerebral emboli are prevented by reversed flow in the vertebral arteries for the most part, so neurological symptoms are flow-related, generally reversible, and less likely to cause stroke. The prevalence of lesions, however, is quite high in certain populations, and with the increased use of internal mammary grafts for coronary artery bypass grafting, subclavian stenosis can have important consequences with respect to planning coronary revascularization. In patients with coronary ischemia who also demonstrated manifestations of peripheral vascular disease (PVD), 42% had some demonstrable subclavian stenosis, 35% had stenosis greater than 30%, and almost 20% had hemodynamically significant stenoses of >50% (1). In less highly selected populations (i.e., of all patients referred for coronary angiography), 3.5% demonstrate significant stenosis and, of those referred for coronary artery bypass grafting, 5.3%, or about 1 in 20, demonstrate hemodynamically significant stenosis (2), where a differential blood pressure of 20 mmHg defines a hemodynamically significant lesion at rest.

Hemodynamic significance on its own, however, does not usually require intervention. In fact, deliberate covering of the left subclavian artery orifice is sometimes performed in thoracic aortic stent grafting without either corrective surgery or subsequent disabling symptoms. Seventy-eight percent of these patients in one study suffered no symptoms whatsoever (3), some with brachio-brachial indices as low a 0.36. Therefore, mere identification of a hemodynamically significant stenosis is not an indication for intervention. Remember that for subclavian steal to produce vertebrobasilar symptoms, there needs to be a disease in the contralateral vertebral as well (Fig. 1).

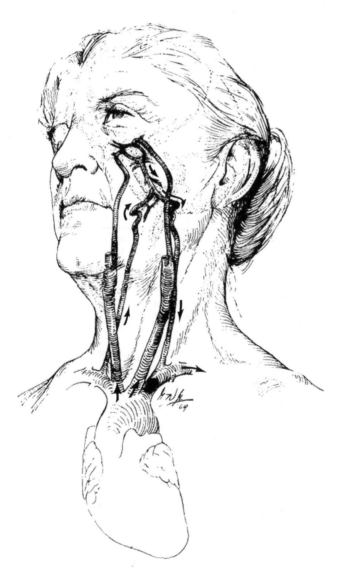

Fig. 1 Cartoon demonstrating the anatomy of subclavian steal phenomenon. For the syndrome to be clinically manifest, inflow stenosis on the contralateral side needs to be present as well.

Direct surgical approaches to the repair of subclavian origin stenosis requiring sternotomy or thoracotomy have been largely abandoned due to the magnitude of the operations necessary; however, extra-anatomical repairs are considerably less morbid and have excellent success rates. Carotid subclavian bypass and subclavian–carotid transposition are well tolerated, and it is against these historical successes that endoluminal management is to be compared.

Angioplasty of the subclavian artery was first described in 1980 (4). In reviewing the literature, numerous claims have been made for the relative safety of endoluminal management, with some authors going as far as to say that surgery is rarely indicated for this problem. The stroke rate in the literature, however, is not zero and hovers around 2% to 4% (see results below). In comparison to the preprotection device era in carotid stenting, this was an improvement, but now with distal protection devices used in the carotid circulation, there appears to be little difference in stroke rate between carotid and subclavian/inominate interventions.

The subclavian arteries are, in fact, generally good candidates for endoluminal intervention because they are large arteries with relatively high flow. Lesion length tends to be limited and the pathology atherosclerotic (except in Asian populations in which Takayasu may be present) (5). They are approachable, both antegrade and retrograde, and, in this location, endoluminal interventions require less hospitalization than bypass surgery.

From a surgeon's perspective, it is interesting to note excellent success rates in percutaneously dilating the subclavian artery, a structure universally recognized by vascular surgeons as particularly friable and susceptible to injury. Ruptures do occur, however (6).

Indications

Indications can be divided into therapeutic and preventative categories (Table 1). Indications for therapeutic interventions are really no different than for surgery. Indications for preventative interventions are somewhat more liberal. Note that all indications are functional or symptomatic, and none is based simply on degree of stenosis, hemodynamic significance, or appearance of the lesion.

Philosophy of Intervention

What follows is a discussion of our current approach at Kaiser Honolulu. The literature varies markedly in its recommendations, and other approaches are certainly possible and supportable.

We use an "endoluminal first" approach to subclavian stenosis and occlusion. Success rates of endoluminal interventions of the subclavian arteries are high, and *almost* all lesions can be approached with an endoluminal solution in mind. If the patient is likely to have a correctable lesion, we perform diagnostic angiography and endoluminal

Table 1 Indications for Subclavian Artery Interventions

Therapeutic
Subclavian steal syndrome
Posterior circulation transient ischemic attack
Upper extremity effort fatigue
Distal upper extremity embolization
Upper extremity resting critical ischemia, nonhealing ulcers, etc.
Coronary subclavian steal syndrome
Upper extremity steal syndrome in conjunction with ipsilateral dialysis access

Preventive
Preoperative coronary artery bypass grafting (CABG) if left internal mammary artery (LIMA)
   graft is planned (differential blood pressure 20 mmHg)
Saving of threatened dialysis access
Proximal to threatened axillo-femoral graft
Creation of upper extremity access for endoluminal interventions elsewhere
   (in very complex patients)

intervention at the same setting. The patient and family are counseled regarding risks, benefits, and potential outcomes. They are also told that an endoluminal solution may not be possible. This approach saves the patient a return to the endovascular suite and repeat hospitalization.

An alternative approach can be used if a combined endoluminal suite/operating room is used. Bring the patient into the room with the idea of performing an endoluminal procedure; if unsuccessful, then advance directly to bypass. The type of table, however, needs to be taken into account because radiolucent tables tend to have fewer features, which may be useful or necessary for open surgery. Choice of elevation of the head and positioning of self-retaining retractors are very personal. One should obviously never embark on a surgical approach without optimal equipment no matter what the cost-effectiveness of the plan. This also presupposes a clear preoperative diagnosis, as it is inefficient to fully prepare a patient for surgery before diagnosis is certain.

Given the difference in initial success rates between stenotic ($\sim 95\%$) and occluded ($\sim 50\%$) subclavian arteries, if an occluded lesion fails an initial guidewire traversal test, surgery is likely to be the best option, rather than performing difficult maneuvers to pass through a calcified plug. Complex lesions with high embologenic potential (i.e., thrombus as opposed to plaque) also suggest a surgical solution.

Preoperative Evaluation

Follow a suitable history with bilateral Doppler brachial blood pressures. If the history suggests effort fatigue and resting pressures are not what you expect, obtain post-exercise pressures as well. Perform duplex evaluation of the cerebrovascular arteries including bilateral carotids, vertebral arteries, and subclavian arteries, evaluating velocities, waveforms, and direction of flow. Reversal of flow in the vertebrals on rare occasions is noted only after exercise of the extremity in question.

Patients are routinely on aspirin. We add plavix for 30 days following the procedure.

Intraoperative Management

We favor local anesthesia with sedation, which is reserved for patients who demonstrate some need. In our hospital, we are blessed with anesthesiology coverage for these cases, although there have been issues related to reimbursement in some payer environments. Patients are complex with multiple medical problems. Having an anesthesiologist or certified registered nurse anesthetist (CRNA) present allows the surgeon to focus on the mechanics of the procedure.

Sedation can create difficulty in visualizing pathology because the patient is less able to breath-hold. As the lesions are within the chest, breath holding is often necessary for accurate positioning of stents and balloons, and is mandatory for digital subtraction. Instructing the patient to voluntarily alter chest expansion or head position can simplify access to a vessel compromised by tortuosity, and is impossible to do with a heavily sedated patient. Some patients have difficulty remaining still during attempts at breath holding. In these cases, delay injection of contrast for a second or two while acquiring multiple preinjection images. These can be used as alternative masks once the injection has been recorded, and can save valuable images that are unreadable using the first image mask.

Antegrade or Retrograde Access?

One of the advantages of treating subclavian artery pathology is that it can be approached from two different directions. Not only does this provide choice, but also offers a bailout in difficult cases. Much has been published on this and personal bias varies greatly (7–9). We do not believe that there is any intrinsic advantage to either technique in all cases. Table 2 includes the factors that we use to decide whether to approach a subclavian lesion antegradely or retrogradely, or to use both simultaneously.

Technique

As the subclavian artery orifices are proximal to the vertebral arteries, and antegrade access to the right subclavian artery requires crossing of all three supra-aortic trunks, control of potential air embolism is more important than in the periphery. Flushes must be performed with extreme care. Bubbles are obsessively eliminated from all lines, especially power injector circuits. Catheters are allowed to backbleed during all

Table 2 Approach to Subclavian Artery Lesions: Antegrade, Retrograde, or Both?

Antegrade (femoral puncture)

(1) Familiar setup, in patient with good lower extremity perfusion and good groin pulses
(2) Best for lesions with a cul de sac or lesions that are not flush with the arch wall; also easier for left-sided than right-sided lesions
(3) Depends on arch anatomy; some arches are considerably more difficult than others, especially with respect to the right side
(4) Generally better determination of arch anatomy, less favored for evaluation of anatomy distal to the lesion; does not require traversal of the lesion to obtain good arch anatomy
(5) Shaggy diseased arches increase the likelihood of embolization, especially when the lesion in question is on the right side where all three supra-aortic trunks are crossed in the approach; strokes do occur in other territories during access
(6) Best if brachial artery is very diseased, or if threatened dialysis access is present on the upper extremity in question (although dialysis grafts can also be great access routes in difficult cases, depending on their anatomy)

Retrograde (brachial artery puncture)

(1) Best for lesions flush with the aortic arch (harder to gain or maintain access via the antegrade approach)
(2) Better determination of the relationship of the distal portion of the lesion to the vertebral or internal mammary artery, using retrograde injection through the sheath
(3) Cutdown necessary if 8 F or larger system is used (rarely necessary)
(4) May be better for occlusions because instrumentation is forced in the direction of the occlusion by the distal artery, whereas the arch provides no stability for lesion traversal
(5) Even if your preference is to go from the femoral, if the procedure cannot be completed, this is an excellent backup strategy

Both simultaneously

(1) Allows best definition of anatomy upstream and downstream from the lesion; good for complex lesions that encroach both on the aortic arch and the vertebral artery orifice; eliminates the need to cross the lesion during diagnostic phase

exchanges. Touhy–Borst adaptors are carefully cleared, and may offer advantages over diaphragm-type check valves, which can allow air leakage to go undetected.

ANTEGRADE APPROACH

Obtain groin access with a single wall entry needle, and place a 5-F, 13-cm sheath. Introduce a floppy-tipped guidewire into the abdominal aorta after which the image intensifier is placed in the left anterior oblique projection (LAO) position (20–30°). Place a 5-F, 100-cm pigtail or tennis racquet catheter at the root of the aorta and rotate the image intensifier under active fluoroscopy to an obliquity that opens up the sweep of the aorta to its maximum width, using the catheter or guidewire as a visual guide. Obtain an arch aortogram to look for the shape and condition of the arch as well as a first view of the subclavian stenosis/occlusion. It is important to continue the exposure long enough to demonstrate possible late retrograde filling of the vertebral artery, as selective catheterization may not show the vertebral arteries at all if flow is reversed (Fig. 2). Tell the patient to breath-hold during the injection. Study the anatomical

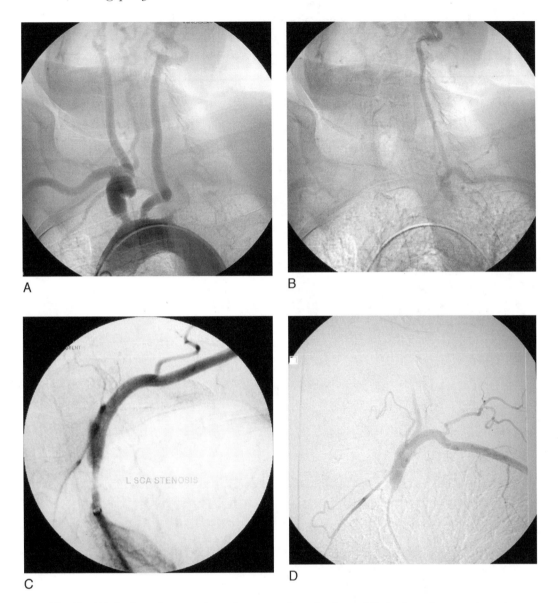

Fig. 2 (A) Arch angiogram via groin approach, early phase. (B) Arch angiogram via groin approach, late phase, showing retrograde flow in the left vertebral artery filling the subclavian and axillary arteries. (C) Antegrade injection through left subclavian stenosis in the same patient, demonstrating no filling of the vertebral artery because of retrograde flow. (D) Antegrade higher-pressure injection shows "puff" of contrast in vertebral artery in one frame despite primarily retrograde native flow, allowing definition of important anatomic landmarks.

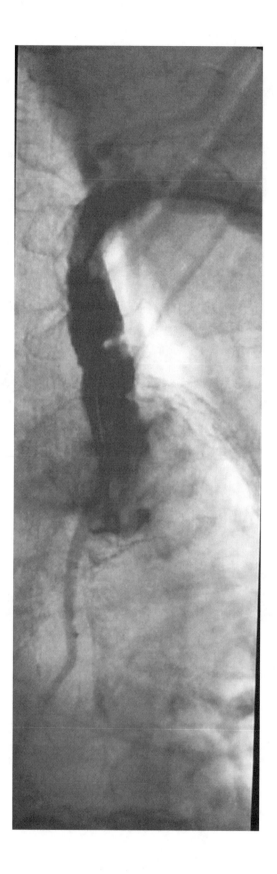

relationships and the association of the origin of the left subclavian or inominate artery with surrounding bony landmarks. Road mapping is not quite as useful in this position as selective catheterization is generally not done with the patient breath-holding. Therefore, the mask shifts as selective catheterization proceeds, obscuring the roadmap.

If it is decided to proceed, heparinize the patient at this point. The author uses 4000 U in this position, but some argue that all cerebrovascular procedures should undergo more complete anticoagulation.

Our choice of catheters for selective cannulation of the left subclavian is generally in the following order: 4-F (or 5-F tapered) angled glide catheter > 120-cm H1 "headhunter." Rarely does one need another catheter for this artery, although difficult arches require flexibility on the part of the surgeon. The 4-F glide catheter is soft enough that direct catheterization can be *carefully* performed without necessarily leading with a guidewire (a deviation from classical technique). We usually use an angled 0.035 hydrophilic guidewire as it is excellent for traversing tight stenoses, but can be difficult to maneuver. Another excellent guidewire for a difficult catheterization is the very steerable and deformable Wholey guidewire.

Inominate catheterization begins with the same catheters, but may require a Simmons 1 or 2. In rare cases, a Vitek catheter is needed. The rationale behind this progression of catheters is "direct" catheterization (angled glide, H1), followed by reverse "pullback" catheterization (Simmons) if direct catheterization fails, followed by antegrade "push forward" catheterization (Vitek). Simmons and Vitek catheters require reforming to use, thereby increasing their difficulty of use and the unlikely but real possibility of forming a knot, creating an arterial injury or embolizing with the catheter (see Chapter 4 for a more detailed discussion of the use of these different catheters).

Once you have entered the subclavian orifice, pass the guidewire far enough to advance the catheter within the artery beyond the stenosis. Remove the guidewire and further inject contrast if better definition of distal anatomy is necessary. An excellent demonstration of the relationship of the lesion to the arch as well as the vertebral and internal mammary arteries is mandatory before proceeding with intervention. Sometimes this requires the use of a straight, multiple-side hole catheter (5-F Beacon tip) to straddle the lesion and simultaneously opacify the arch origin and the distal extent of the stenosis (Fig. 3). Great care should be exercised in any potentially friable lesion; however, injection pressures should be low.

Place an Amplatz super stiff guidewire through the diagnostic catheter and park it deep within the brachial artery for support. The Amplatz is a reasonable guidewire for

Fig. 3 Retrograde injection straddling the lesion with a 5-F straight catheter with multiple side holes. This allows simultaneous opacification of areas upstream and downstream from the stenosis.

the subclavian territory because the tip is not parked in the cerebral circulation, and there is generally no need for a smaller platform unless the lesion is extremely tight. The 5-F short sheath is then removed and a 6-F or 7-F, 70- to 90-cm-long Shuttle or Raabe sheath (Cook, Inc., Bloomington, IN) is advanced to just proximal to the stenosis. Make sure that the dilator is in place before advancing the sheath, as it might otherwise shear plaque from the orifice. Another method is to advance the sheath over a front-loaded diagnostic catheter placed deep within the brachial artery over the Amplatz guidewire for extra support. This must be done cautiously because there is generally not a good caliber match between the catheter and the sheath tip, and shearing can occur. The advantage is more stability and fewer crossings of the lesion. The sheath tip should be close enough to the orifice to lend support for subsequent balloon or stent advancement, and also to inject enough contrast to adequately opacify the pathology, as this will be the final view before deployment.

The lesion can be predilated or directly stented, depending on the degree of stenosis. If balloon-expandable stents are to be used, the safest approach involves advancing the sheath through the lesion before the stent, and then pulling the sheath back, exposing the stent just before deployment. This decreases the risk of injury, lost stents, and embolization, although bareback stenting is currently practiced more frequently with newer devices. Inject contrast through the sheath immediately before deployment to ensure proper positioning of the balloon or stent.

RETROGRADE APPROACH

Prepare the appropriate upper extremity on a radiolucent arm board. After placing local anesthetic, use a Cook micropuncture set to cannulate the brachial artery near the antecubital fossa over the medial epicondyle of the humerus, which pushes the artery up closer to the skin and supports it during catheterization. This location also decreases the likelihood of nerve compression syndromes or postprocedure hematomas. Use ultrasound guidance, if necessary, as the pulse is often obliterated by the subclavian lesion. Knurled needles are available to assist in ultrasound localization (Cook MPIS-401-U). Some surgeons cut down on the brachial artery for more control (7), but we have not found this to be necessary. If the planned sheath is going to be larger than 7 F, however, cutdowns are necessary for hemostasis.

The micropuncture set consists of a 21-gauge needle, a short floppy-tipped 0.018-in. guidewire, and a coaxial catheter pair. The inner catheter and guidewire are removed, leaving a 4-F outer dilator through which an 0.035-in. guidewire can be placed. Catheterize the aorta by advancing the guidewire and 4-F angled glide catheter retrogradely through the lesion. Retrograde injection of contrast can help define the anatomy and set up roadmapping, if necessary. Place a flush catheter into the aortic root and perform arch angiogram in the LAO position (Fig. 4).

Place the guidewire in the descending aorta. It will almost always automatically go to the ascending aorta and will need to be guided selectively into the descending

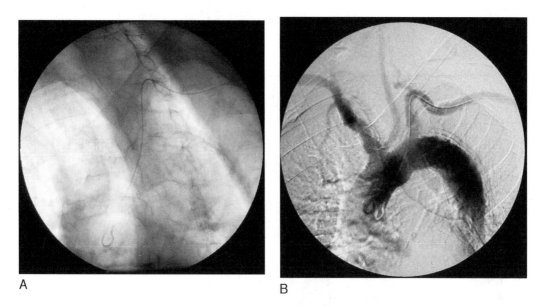

A   B

Fig. 4 (A) 4-F Omniflush catheter in the aortic root via retrograde brachial approach. (B) Arch angiogram via retrograde brachial approach.

aorta (so the tip of the guidewire does not irritate the heart during the procedure). Sometimes this will require an SOS Omni catheter or even a Sims catheter. Manipulate the lesion as little as possible. When the catheter is in the descending aorta, exchange the guidewire for an Amplatz super stiff guidewire to lend stability.

Place a 40-cm, 6-F straight sheath up to the lesion for retrograde injection of contrast (Fig. 5). Predilate if necessary, advance the sheath, place the stent, pull back the sheath, and deploy. If a balloon-expandable stent is being used, be absolutely certain that the location of the subclavian orifice at the arch as well as the vertebral and internal mammary arteries is known with certainty. Deployment of the stent with more than 2 mm of encroachment into the aorta can be problematical for subsequent cannulations. If it is not possible to precisely define the origin of the subclavian with retrograde injections of contrast because of the severity of the lesion, cannulate the arch via the groin and perform a simultaneous arch study from below and retrograde injection of the subclavian artery from above.

Axillary and high brachial puncture sites are considerably riskier with respect to possible hematoma and subsequent nerve compression syndromes. Radial approaches have been used in the coronary circulation, but probably are poor conduits for the larger stents required for subclavian intervention (10). The subclavian approach of Andros et al. (11) is an excellent choice for descending aortic access, but puts the tip of the sheath too close to most lesions to be useful in subclavian intervention.

After stent deployment, and especially if you decide to perform angioplasty alone, obtain cross-lesional pressures to make sure there is no gradient.

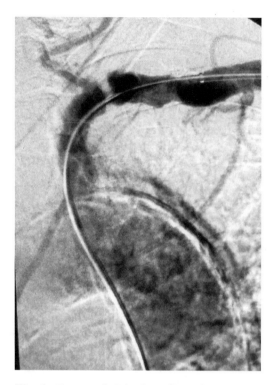

Fig. 5 Retrograde injection of contrast via 6-F sheath parked in the distal subclavian artery. More distal anatomy is seen more clearly than the aortic arch.

Balloon-Expandable Vs. Self-Expanding Stents

Subclavian lesions are short, frequently fairly calcifics and the tolerance for either proximal or distal misplacement is poor. The orifice of the vertebral artery is small and should not be "jailed." Therefore, we prefer balloon-expandable stents for subclavian intervention. They demonstrate greater radial strength and it is easier to predict both the leading and the trailing edges. Balloon-expandable stents are best for lesions of the subclavian artery origin. Newer deployment systems for self-expanding stents allow more exact final placement and can also be used in many cases. Self-expanding stents should be considered for use in tortuous subclavian arteries.

Results

The results of subclavian artery angioplasty and stenting should be evaluated in the context of the excellent results of surgery. AbuRahma et al.(12) demonstrated 6% morbidity without stroke or death in a 20-year series of para tetra fluoro ethylene (Teflon; PTFE) carotid subclavian bypasses. Primary patency of 1, 3, 5, and 10 years was an impressive 100%, 98%, 96%, and 92%, respectively; and secondary patency was 100%, 98%, 98%, and 95%, respectively. Late mean hospital stay was 2.1 days.

For subclavian transposition, Ballotta et al. (13) demonstrated 2.5% mortality and 2.5% morbidity (no strokes) with 100% immediate relief of symptoms in 39 patients followed for a mean 6.8 years. Their long-term follow-up data are the most impressive in the literature as "revascularization neither failed during the follow-up period, nor did patients have recurrent symptoms."

For angioplasty alone, Millaire et al. (14) demonstrated 6% acute thrombosis, 2% stroke, and 10% procedure failure. One complication was an aortic occlusion resulting in emergency aortobifemoral bypass. Late follow-up revealed 14% restenosis over 39 months. Burke et al. (15) reported a 4% stroke rate for a series of angioplasties published in 1987.

Relative safety of subclavian artery dilation has been ascribed to a phenomenon documented in a paper published in 1984 in which transcranial Doppler signals demonstrated delay in the reversal of vertebral artery flow following subclavian artery angioplasty between 20 sec up to 20 min (16). This report is interesting in that it has been used as a rationale for the safe deployment of devices in the subclavian artery, but makes little rational sense. We have personally seen cases in which flow reversal is noted almost immediately upon deployment of a stent, and worry that this initial report may relate to inadequate initial angioplasty, akin to "predilation" in current stented series, although the data are certainly very interesting (Fig. 6). Other transcranial Doppler series, however, show far fewer distal embolic "hits" in subclavian artery interventions vs. carotid territory interventions (17).

Series using selective angioplasty with or without stents include Motarjeme (8), who reported 100% procedural success with subclavian stenoses compared with only

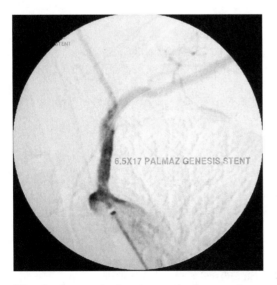

Fig. 6 Antegrade flow in vertebral artery demonstrated soon after deployment of stent in proximal subclavian artery.

47% with occlusions. The long-term outlook for total occlusions was even worse with 50% failure in successful cases in 1 year. Stenoses fared considerably better, however, with 7.5% restenosis in a 5-year follow-up period. Criado et al. (18) reported 80% patency at 2 years with more aggressive follow-up. Korner et al. (19) reported a 72% 100-month patency by life table analysis with an 84% initial success rate. Nine percent suffered thromboembolic events and 25% of patients had some residual symptoms.

Discussion

Although still imperfect, endoluminal intervention for subclavian artery lesions is reasonably safe, technically feasible, and effective. As patients' presentations and comorbidities vary so much, there is little place for dogma related to surgical vs. endoluminal approaches. Although considerably diminished in frequency, we still perform open surgical procedures in certain patients whom we feel are better suited, as history has shown these procedures to be durable, effective, and safe. Endoluminal techniques are evolving much more rapidly than open surgery, and the balance of this decision is likely to progressively point in the direction of endoluminal intervention. At this time in our institution, almost all stenoses are treated endoluminally, as are about half our occlusions. Being skilled in both approaches avoids at least one avenue of physician bias, and we think this ultimately benefits the patient.

References

1. Gutierrez GR, Mahrer P, Aharonian V, Mansukhani P, Bruss J. Prevalence of subclavian artery stenosis in patients with peripheral vascular disease. Angiology March 2001; 52(3):189–194.
2. English J, Donovan DJ, Guidera SA, Carell ES. Angiographic prevalence and clinical predictors of left subclavian stenosis in patients undergoing diagnostic cardiac catheterization. Abstracts for the 1999 Annual Scientific Session [abstr]. J Am Coll Cardiol 1999; 33(issue 2 supplement 1) Abstract 1193–72:292A.
3. Gorich J, Asquan Y, Seifarth H, Kramer S, Kapfer X, Orend KH, Sunder-Plassmann L, Pamler R. Initial experience with intentional stent–graft coverage of the subclavian artery during endovascular thoracic aortic repairs. J Endovasc Ther 2002; 9(suppl II):II39–II43.
4. Bachman DM, Kim RM. Transluminal dilatation for subclavian steal syndrome. AJR Am J Roentgenol 1980; 135:995–996.
5. Criado FJ, Twena M. Techniques for endovascular recanalization of supra-aortic trunks. J Endovasc Surg November 1996; 3(4):405–413. Review.
6. Lin PH, Bush RL, Weiss VJ, Dodson TF, Chaikof EL, Lumsden AB. Subclavian artery disruption resulting from endovascular intervention: treatment options. J Vasc Surg September 2000; 32(3):607–611.
7. Criado FJ. Endovascular intervention in the proximal brachiocephalic supra-aortic arteries. Chapter 15. In: Criado F, ed. Endovascular Intervention: Basic Concepts and Techniques. Armonk, NY: Futura Publishing Co., 1999:137–144.

8. Motarjeme A. Percutaneous transluminal angioplasty of supra-aortic vessels. J Endovasc Surg 1996; 3:171–181.

9. Henry M, Amor M, Henry I, Ethevenot G, Tzvetanov K, Chati Z. Percutaneous transluminal angioplasty of the subclavian arteries. J Endovasc Surg 1999; 6:33–41.

10. Kiemeneij F, Laarman GJ, de Melker E. Transradial artery coronary angioplasty. Am Heart J 1995; 129:1–7.

11. Andros G, Harris RW, Dulawa LB, Oblath RW, Schneider PA. Subclavian artery catheterization: a new approach for endovascular procedures. J Vasc Surg October 1994; 20(4):566–574, discussion 574–576.

12. AbuRahma AF, Robinson PA, Jennings TG. Carotid–subclavian bypass grafting with polytetrafluoroethylene grafts for symptomatic subclavian artery stenosis or occlusion: a 20-year experience. J Vasc Surg September 2000; 32(3):411–419.

13. Ballotta E, Da Giau G, Abbruzzese E, Mion E, Manara R, Baracchini C. Subclavian carotid transposition for symptomatic subclavian artery stenosis or occlusion. A comparison with the endovascular procedure. Int Angiol June 2002; 21(2):138–144.

14. Millaire A, Trinca M, Marache P, de Groote P, Jabinet JL, Ducloux G. Subclavian angioplasty: immediate and late results in 50 patients. Catheter Cardiovasc Diagn May 1993; 29(1):8–17.

15. Burke DR, Gordon RL, Mishkin JD, McLean GK, Meranze SG. Percutaneous transluminal angioplasty of subclavian arteries. Radiology September 1987; 164(3):699–704.

16. Ringelstein EF, Zeumer H. Delayed reversal of vertebral artery blood flow following percutaneous transluminal angioplasty for subclavian steal syndrome. Neuroradiology 1984; 26:189–198.

17. Jordan WD Jr, Voellinger DC, Doblar DD, Plyushcheva NP, Fisher WS, McDowell HA. Microemboli detected by transcranial Doppler monitoring in patients during carotid angioplasty versus carotid endarterectomy. Cardiovasc Surg January 1999; 7(1):33–38.

18. Criado FJ, Queral LA, Twena M. Is endovascular intervention justified for disease of the supra-aortic trunks? In: Greenhalgh RM, Fowkes FGR, eds. Trials and Tribulations of Vascular Surgery. London: WB Saunders, 1996:131–150.

19. Korner M, Baumgartner I, Do DD, Mahler F, Schroth G. PTA of the subclavian and innominate arteries: long-term results. Vasa May 1999; 28(2):117–122.

19

Management of the Complications of Carotid Interventions

PETER A. SCHNEIDER

Hawaii Permanente Medical Group, Honolulu, Hawaii, U.S.A.

The purpose of this chapter is to review the risks and complications of carotid angioplasty and stent placement (CAS). The concept of CAS is that it must have lower morbidity than carotid endarterectomy in a given patient to be an effective treatment. Therefore, avoiding or managing complications becomes crucial to the utility of CAS. Stroke and death rates in published studies have been reviewed in Chap. 16 on the results of CAS.

Complications can be divided into four general categories. These include systemic reactions and remote but major organ system problems, access site complications, complications at the carotid stent site, and neurologic/end organ complications (Table 1). Many of the complications associated with the first two categories, systemic and access site complications, are also associated with other endovascular procedures. Complications associated with the carotid stent site and its cerebral sequelae are almost uniformly unique to CAS. Systemic factors and medical comorbidities that increase the risk of carotid endarterectomy also generally increase the risk of CAS, although to lesser extent than that seen with open surgery. Anatomical and lesion factors may also increase the risk of CAS.

Systemic Complications

CAS has an associated cardiac risk, as demonstrated by the results of the SAPPHIRE Trial. The risk of perioperative myocardial infarction was 2.6% (1). Arrhythmias may be

Table 1   Complications Associated with Carotid Artery Balloon Angioplasty and Stent Placement

Systemic	Access site	Stent site	End organ/neuro
Bradycardia	Hematoma	Spasm	Stroke
Asystole	Hemorrhage	Occlude ECA	TIA
Hypotension	Retroperitoneal bleed	Carotid dissection	Hyperperfusion
Myocardial infarction	Pseudoaneurysm	Carotid perforation	Loss of consciousness
CHF	AV fistula	Stent thrombosis	Cerebral hemorrhage
Renal failure	Arterial infection	Filter thrombosis	Seizure
		Arch injuries	Multi-infarct dementia
		Kink above stent	

induced by guidewire placement in the arch, heart, or carotid bulb (2–4). Stretching of the carotid bifurcation with balloon angioplasty or stent placement has the potential to cause hypotension, bradycardia, and occasionally asystole, especially during the treatment of native bifurcation lesions. Arrhythmias are caused by stimulation of the carotid sinus by the balloon or stent. Hypotension is most often momentary but may last for several days. The management of these arrhythmias is described in Chap. 8. Congestive heart failure and myocardial infarction may result from these arrhythmias. The osmotic load associated with contrast administration may also contribute to the development of congestive heart failure. The usual amount of contrast administered is less than 100 ml for CAS. Renal failure or worsening renal insufficiency may also occur as a result of contrast administration.

Access Site Complications

Most CAS procedures are performed transfemorally. Total access site complications should be less than 10% and major access site complications have generally been less than 5% (5,6). This rate of complications would be consistent with a 6 to 8 Fr sheath in a fully anticoagulated patient on clopidogrel. As with most endovascular procedures, good results are enhanced by a clean and direct initial puncture into the anterior wall of a nondiseased common femoral artery followed by personal management of the puncture site. Closure devices have been used with increasing frequency following carotid stent placement. Although major complications of these devices appear to be infrequent (<1%), they can be limb threatening when they occur. When femoral access is managed diligently, it is rare for patients to require operative arterial repair and uncommon to require transfusion.

Complications Involving the Stent Site and the Surrounding Vasculature

The significance of these complications may range from inconsequential, as in the case of external carotid artery occlusion after carotid bifurcation stent placement, to devastating, as in the case of carotid perforation or distal carotid dissection. Table 2 briefly outlines the management of these complications and they are discussed in the paragraphs below.

Occlusion of the external carotid artery. This occurs in many patients who require a stent across the bifurcation. It is not associated with any reported disability except that if the carotid requires reintervention in the future, there is no external carotid branch in which to place the anchoring guidewire.

Spasm of the internal carotid artery. Spasm occurs frequently in a location distal to the site of the stent and, if severe, may stop antegrade flow altogether. It may result from guidewire placement alone but this is unusual. The most common scenario is spasm at or near the location of deployment of the distal protection device. Another vulnerable site is the flexible artery just distal to the stent. If there appears to be spasm along the stent itself, it is probably the wrong diagnosis. Nitroglycerine is administered directly into the internal carotid artery (500 µg is diluted in 10 mL and 2 mL or 100 µg are administered at a time). Additional doses may be administered every 3 to 5 min. The patient must be observed for the possibility of hypotension. If flow in the artery is decreased, consider administering additional heparin or initiating glycoprotein IIb/IIIa inhibitors. If the procedure is complete, remove the distal protection device. Differential diagnoses for spasm of the internal carotid artery include dissection, thrombosed filter, and stent thrombosis.

Carotid perforation. This is a rare complication. It results from overdilating the carotid artery. Considering the fact that many carotid bifurcation lesions are heavily calcified, bulky, and often shelflike, one might guess that perforation would occur more frequently in response to balloon dilatation. Most specialists do limit poststent angioplasty to a slightly smaller diameter than might be possible, both to avoid releasing debris from the stented lesion, and to avoid perforation. If carotid perforation does occur, the best thing to do is usually to proceed directly to open repair.

Carotid dissection. Dissection is most likely to occur in the same segments that are prone to spasm. Dissection may result from overdilating the internal carotid artery, elevation of plaque distal to the bifurcation that is not covered by the stent, and arterial

Table 2 Stent Site Complications and Their Management

Complication	Management
Occlude ECA	No treatment
ICA spasm	Nitroglycerine, additional anticoagulation
Carotid dissection	Medical (anticoagulation/antiplatelet/surveillance) vs. additional stent
Stent thrombosis	Heparin, IIb/IIIa inhibitors, aspiration, thrombolytic (chemical/mechanical)
Very slow flow	Troubleshoot (proximal or distal occlusion, filter thrombosis)
Thrombosed filter	Heparin, IIb/IIIa inhibitors, aspirate, remove
Kink after stent	Observation vs. another stent vs. surgery
Arch injury	Stent

injury, possibly from movement of the distal protection device while it is deployed. Carotid dissection may not require mechanical treatment if it is minimal, there is no significant stenosis, and there is no pooling of contrast in the arterial wall. If a dissection appears to be minor, consider waiting a few minutes and repeating the arteriogram to check for progression. If flow appears to be compromised, consider administering additional anticoagulation or IIb/IIIa inhibitors. A significant dissection should be treated with stent placement, usually a shorter and smaller diameter self-expanding stent than was placed at the bifurcation. Significant overlapping of stents in a small-caliber distal internal carotid artery is ill-advised. When the carotid stent is deployed across the bifurcation and the stent is not well opposed to the wall, completion arteriography occasionally produces flow streaming that mimics the appearance of a dissection.

Stent thrombosis. A stent may thrombose if it is not fully deployed. After a stent is placed, postplacement balloon angioplasty is usually performed immediately to ensure that the stent has achieved an acceptable minimum diameter. However, stent thrombosis is most often due to either mechanical problems proximally or distally, or a primary thrombotic problem. If thrombosis occurs, recheck the activated clotting time, administer heparin as appropriate, and administer IIb/IIIa inhibitors. If the stent thrombosis occurs while the distal protection device is deployed, the distal protection device itself may be the cause. Leave the distal protection device in place. Pass a 100 or 125-cm, 5 Fr straight or angled-tip catheter and perform aggressive aspiration of the stented segment and the artery proximal to the distal protection device. Leave the 0.014-in. guidewire across the stent and place the aspirating catheter along side. If thrombus remains after thorough aspiration, lace the clot with 1 to 2 mg of TPA in 5 ml. One might also consider a mechanical thrombectomy device, such as the Possis.

Very slow flow. This problem is almost always due to a mechanical problem, either proximal or distal to the stent site. Be certain to maintain access while trouble shooting. Slow flow can be caused by proximal or distal dissection, spasm, or occlusion, partial thrombosis of the stent, or massive cerebral embolization.

Thrombosed filter. Antegrade flow is stopped with a distal occlusion balloon, but if flow stops with a filter in place or is very sluggish, there is a likelihood of filter thrombosis. Leave the filter deployed and place an aspiration catheter, as described above. Aspirate the filter until no further debris can be removed. After thorough aspiration, remove the filter. If addition stenting or angioplasty is required, a new filter may be placed. If the aspirated material is primarily thrombus, rather than atherosclerotic debris, it may indicate that there is inadequate inhibition of coagulation and platelets.

Kink distal to the stent. This problem is usually due to an underestimation of the degree of tortuosity present in the carotid system prior to stent placement. The underlying curvature of the artery is displaced distally with stent placement, and a kink results in the segment distal to the stent. The worst ones are those that occur immediately adjacent to the stent. Minor kinks can be left behind. Moderate and non-hemodynamically significant kinks may be followed with duplex and considered for open repair later if worsening occurs or the stenosis is borderline. However, kinks that produce hemodynamically significant stenoses or cause sluggish flow require treatment. Adding stents in this situation is a potential trap, as the kink could be even worse when displaced more distally by another stent and also be out of reach for open surgery. The choice is either open surgery or additional stent placement. Sometimes a kink can mimic very focal spasm in its angiographic appearance.

Arch injury. The best way to manage arch injuries is to prevent them. When they do occur, they are usually caused on the way in due to difficulty with access. Check the anatomy before proceeding further into the case if there is concern about the possibility of an arch injury. Injury can also occur as a result of local damage at the location of a lesion, especially if the lesion is not apparent on the preoperative studies. If injury, such as local dissection, occurs to the arch itself, and is recognized prior to engaging the bifurcation lesion, consider abandoning the procedure and reversing the anti-coagulation. The treatment options for lesions in this location are limited and usually involve major, emergent surgery. Injury more commonly may occur to the proximal common carotid artery at the location of an underlying stenosis, kink, tortuous segment, or calcified plaque. This is usually best managed with stent placement at the site of arterial injury. A balloon expandable stent is used if the lesion is at the origin of the artery or is highly calcified. There is no general rule about whether to place the stent at the time of access sheath placement, which is usually when the injury occurs, or later, after the bifurcation lesion has been treated and it is time to remove the sheath.

Neurological and End Organ Complications

Concern about the potential for neurological complications has profoundly influenced the development of endovascular management of carotid bifurcation occlusive disease. Although the value of distal protection devices has not been proven in a direct comparison, the concept of stroke prevention during stenting by avoiding embolization is a driving factor in making CAS clinically relevant. Table 1 includes a list of some of the neurological complications that may occur with carotid stenting.

Neurological complications are best avoided by judicious patient selection, both from a standpoint of neurological status and carotid anatomy; achieving the appropriate level of anticoagulation and antiplatelet effect; careful control of blood pressure; rapid response to vital sign changes; and avoiding cerebral embolization.

In addition to the clinical circumstances of a neurological deficit, the time frame for a new occurrence is important for determining treatment (5,7). About half the perioperative events that occur present within the first 6 hr, and about one third occur after 24 hr. During the carotid stenting procedure, the development of a new local deficit, seizure, or change in the level of consciousness should prompt an immediate evaluation of the stent site, the cerebral runoff, and the anticoagulation status. There is no reliable way of detecting cerebral hemorrhage during the procedure; sometimes an extravascular contrast blush or a mass effect is present, but this is usually an advanced stage. If complications occur during balloon inflation, it may be a result of lack of cerebral collateral flow. New deficits that occur after the procedure are more likely to be due to cerebral hemorrhage or hyperperfusion syndrome and an emergent head CT should be performed. Delayed embolization may also occur from the stented bifurcation.

Transient ischemic attack/stroke. The development of a new focal deficit, loss of consciousness, or seizure may all be due to cerebral ischemia and may be the presenting symptoms for stroke (8). Evaluate the stent site and the distal runoff to check for a mechanical problem that could be responsible for an interruption of flow. If it is a focal deficit on exam, it is usually the result of an identifiable arterial lesion. If the patient cannot cooperate or protect the airway, general anesthesia is required. Once this step is taken, neurological evaluation is no longer possible. Thrombolysis and neurorescue for acute stroke are discussed in Chap. 14. If no evidence of focal embolization is present, consider the possibility of a diffuse embolic shower. This is manifested by slow flow in the cerebral vessels and smaller arterial branches. This is best managed with more aggressive use of anticoagulants and antiplatelet agents and maintaining a higher blood pressure. Administration of chemical thrombolysis should also be considered in this situation, although there are no data on the results of this approach.

Cerebral hemorrhage. A sudden loss of consciousness preceded by headache may be cerebral hemorrhage (9). This may be accompanied by a mass effect. If a cause for the new deficit cannot be located, finish the stent placement and obtain a brain CT scan. If cerebral hemorrhage has occurred, stop all anticoagulation, control blood pressure, and manage medically. Cerebral hemorrhage has been associated with the following factors; CAS of a preocclusive artery, excessive anticoagulation, excessive platelet inhibition, poorly controlled hypertension, and recent stroke (10). The use of intravenous glycoprotein IIb/IIIa inhibitors has also been associated with an increased incidence of cerebral hemorrhage when used routinely (11,12). Cerebral hemorrhage in this situation often has a poor outcome and may be fatal.

Hyperperfusion. Cerebral edema and hyperperfusion remains uncommon but may occur in the 2 weeks after CAS, and with a seemingly higher incidence than seen with carotid endarterectomy. The patient usually has focal headache and poorly controlled blood pressure. The worse the cerebral ischemia prior to the revascularization, the more likely that hyperperfusion will occur, since cerebral autoregulation does not improve for 2 to 3 weeks after arterial repair. If not recognized and treated early, decreased consciousness and brain swelling occurs and may result in permanent neurological damage.

What Is the Learning Curve for Carotid Stenting?

Every complex procedure has a learning curve, especially those that are relatively new and still under development. This describes carotid stent placement. The knowledge base for carotid stent placement comes from performing endovascular therapy in various vascular beds and from carotid arteriography. The more experience one has with balloon angioplasty, stents, and other endovascular surgical techniques prior to participation in CAS procedures, the shorter the learning curve will be. Carotid arteriography is also an essential part of the knowledge base to begin CAS training. Carotid arteriography provides an understanding of the following key factors for CAS; assessment of the aortic arch, remote access site cannulation of target arteries, selective catheterization of the carotid arteries, and arteriographic evaluation of the cerebral arteries. This experience, combined with the experience of endovascular therapy in other vascular beds, provides a foundation for CAS training.

The studies that have been performed have associated the learning curve with certain numbers of cases, and generally found decreasing morbidity with the greater number of cases (13). In the applications for the CREST Trial, operators who had performed 15 or more CAS procedures had a lower stroke rate (3.7%), than those who had done fewer procedures (7.1%) (14). The minimum number of cases required depends upon how much experience each surgeon has when these procedures are undertaken. Nevertheless, arbitrary minimum case numbers will likely be adopted by each of the societies and subsequently by the individual healthcare institutions.

Complications of Cerebral Protection Devices

Cerebral protection devices are reviewed in Chaps. 12 and 13. Distal protection devices are designed to prevent potentially embolic material from proceeding to the brain. Neurological events have been associated with the size and number of the embolic particles (15). Transcranial Doppler has been used to quantify the number of embolic particles that occur during carotid stent placement and to correlate them with the specific maneuver being performed during the procedure (16). Although CAS with distal protection has not been compared against CAS without distal protection in a randomized fashion, there is much evidence that embolization and neurological events are reduced but not completely eliminated (17,18). Most of these studies compare an earlier era with a more recent time frame, and other factors beside the development of distal protection devices are at play, such as more experience, better access devices, and improved stents. Therefore, it is not possible to know to what degree the distal protection devices improve neurological outcomes. In addition, it is very likely that there is some variation among devices with respect to the degree of protection (19).

Distal protection devices have their own unique complications. In one large series, the overall complication rate for CAS was excellent at 3.4%. However, about 30% of the major complications that occurred were attributed to the distal protection device. These included distal internal carotid artery occlusion, dissection, and arterial damage due to a trapped guidewire (20). In addition, approximately 15% of patients in whom distal occlusion balloons were used could not tolerate it and developed neurological deficits during the procedure. Although crossing profiles for distal protection devices have decreased significantly (several are < 3 Fr), critically stenotic lesions commonly have residual lumen diameters that are smaller. This requires predilatation or "forcing" the device across, both of which would likely produce emboli. The ideal filter pore sizes have not been worked out. Filters sometimes fill with debris and can overflow or thrombose. The capture efficiency of some devices is reduced due to poor wall apposition or pore sizes that are too large. As distal protection devices continue to be developed, they will likely improve.

Avoiding Complications in Carotid Artery Stenting

Technical experience and improved technical developments help to avoid complications in carotid artery stenting. However, on a case by case basis, clinical experience and patient selection seem to be the most important factors in avoiding complications. Patients at advanced age, with uncontrolled hypertension, frequent or severe neurological symptoms, renal insufficiency, or severe cardiac comorbidities, are at increased risk for CAS. Anatomic situations that increase risk are arch disease, long or preocclusive carotid stenosis, excessive tortuosity, and fresh thrombus at the lesion. These factors should be carefully considered in selecting patients for carotid stenting.

References

1. Yadav J. Stenting and angioplasty with protection in patients at high risk for endarterectomy (the SAPPHIRE trial). Presented, American Heart Association, Chicago, IL, November 19, 2002.
2. Mendelsohn FO, Weissman NJ, Lederman RJ, Crowley JJ, Gray JL, Phillips HR, Alberts MJ, McCann RL, Smith TP, Stack R. Acute hemodynamic changes during carotid artery stenting. Am J Cardiol 1998; 82:1077–1081.
3. Dangas G, Laird JR Jr, Satler LF, Mehran R, Mintz GS, Larrain G, Lansky AJ, Gruberg L, Parsons EM, Laureno R, Monsein LH, Leon MB. Postprocedural hypotension after carotid artery stent placement: predictors and short- and long-term clinical outcome. Radiology 2000; 215:677–683.
4. Qureshi AI, Luft AR, Sharma M, Janardhan V, Lopes DK, Khan V, Guterman LR, Hopkins LN. Frequency and determinants of postprocedural hemodynamic instability after carotid angioplasty and stenting. Stroke 1999; 30:2086–2093.
5. Tan KT, Cleveland TJ, Berczi V, McKevitt FM, Venables GS, Guines PA. Timing and frequency of complications after carotid artery stenting: what is the optimal period of observation? J Vasc Surg 2003; 38:236–243.
6. Roubin GS, New G, Iyer SS, Vitek JJ, Al-Mubarak N, Liu MW, Yadav J, Gomez C, Kunta RA. Immediate and late clinical outcomes of carotid artery stenting in patients with symptomatic and asymptomatic carotid artery stenosis: a five year prospective analysis. Circulation 2001; 103:532–537.
7. Wholey MH, Wholey MH, Tan WA, Toursarkissian B, Bailey S, Eles G, Jarmolowski C. Management of neurological complications of carotid artery stenting. J Endovasc Ther 2001; 8:341–353.
8. Wojak JC, Connors JJ. Management of stroke during carotid angioplasty and stenting. Techniques Vasc Interv Radiol 2000; 3:92–98.

9. McCabe DHJ, Brown MM, Clifton A. Fatal cerebral hemorrhage after carotid stenting. Stroke 1999; 30:2483–2486.

10. Al-Mubarak N, Roubin GS, Vitek JJ, Iyer SS, New G, Leon MB. Subarachnoid hemorrhage following carotid stenting with distal balloon protection. Catheter Cardiovasc Interv 2001; 54:521–523.

11. Wholey MH, Wholey MH, Eles G, Toursarkissian B, Baileys S, Jarmolowski C, Tan WA. Evaluation of glycoprotein IIb/IIIa inhibitors in carotid angioplasty and stenting. J Endovasc Ther 2003; 10:33–41.

12. Qureshi AI, Suri MF, Ali Z, Kim SH, Lanzino G, Fessler RD, Ringer AJ, Guterman LR, Hopkins LN. Carotid angioplasty and stent placement: a prospective analysis of perioperative complications and impact of intravenously administered abciximab. Neurosurgery 2002; 50:466–473.

13. Ahmadi R, Willfort A, Lang W, Schillinger M, Alt E, Gsehwandtner ME, Haumer M, Maca T, Ehringer H, Minar E. Carotid artery stenting: effect of learning curve and intermediate-term morphological outcome. J Endovasc Ther 2001; 8:539–546.

14. Al-Mubarak N, Roubin GS, Hobson RW. Credentialing of stent operators for the Carotid Revascularization Endarterectomy vs. Stenting Trial (CREST). Stroke 2000; 31:292.

15. Tubler T, Schluter M, Dirsch O, Sievert H, Bosenberg I, Grube E, Waigand J, Schofer J. Balloon protected carotid artery stenting: relationship of periprocedural neurological complications and the size of particulate debris. Circulation 2001; 4:2791–2796.

16. Al-Mubarak N, Roubin GS, Vitek JJ, Iyer SS, New G, Leon MB. Effect of the distal balloon protection system on microembolization during carotid artery stenting. Circulation 2001; 104:1999–2002.

17. Kastrup A, Groschel K, Krapf H, Brehm BR, Dichgans J, Schultz JB. Early outcome of carotid angioplasty and stenting with and without cerebral protection devices: a systematic review of the literature. Stroke 2003; 34:1941–1943.

18. McKevitt FM, Macdonald S, Venables GS, Cleveland TJ, Gaines PA. Complications following carotid angioplasty and stenting in patients with symptomatic carotid artery disease. Cerebrovasc Dis 2004; 17:28–34.

19. Ohki T. The dark side of cerebral protection devices. Endovasc Today 2003; 2: 54–64.

20. Cremonesi A, Manetti R, Setacci F, Setacci C, Castriota F. Protected carotid stenting: clinical advantages and complications of embolic protection devices in 442 consecutive patients. Stroke 2003;341936–1941.

20

How to Start a Carotid Stenting Program

PETER A. SCHNEIDER

Hawaii Permanente Medical Group, Honolulu, Hawaii, U.S.A.

MICHAEL B. SILVA, JR.

Texas Tech University, Lubbock, Texas, U.S.A.

Carotid stenting is likely to contribute significantly to the future management of carotid occlusive disease. The benefits of a carotid stent program are a shorter learning curve, patient safety, avoidance of adverse events, enhanced skill development, and education for staff. Vascular specialists possess varying degrees of preparedness for carotid artery stenting (CAS). Participation in the future care of carotid disease is dependent upon a strong commitment now to master the appropriate skills to be of value to the patient. Anyone intending to offer CAS to his or her patients should consider taking a programmatic approach. This chapter discusses training, hospital privileges, protocols, proctoring, quality assurance, and interdisciplinary issues.

What Is the Rationale for a Carotid Stent Program?

The reason to start a carotid stenting program is to ensure quality care for patients. The management of carotid bifurcation stenosis will likely change significantly over the next few years. Vascular surgeons have managed the medical and surgical aspects of carotid disease treatment in the past. Vascular surgeons have developed many skill sets that have permitted them to take clinical responsibility for patients with carotid artery occlusive disease. They have provided vascular patients with quality care up until the present era.

285

Carotid angioplasty and stent placement (CAS) may alter the management of carotid disease to an even greater extent than endovascular techniques have effected change in the management of many other arterial beds. Vascular specialists must adapt to this new era and advocate for high-quality vascular care.

The choice between carotid endarterectomy and carotid stenting is different from other open versus endovascular procedure debates. Carotid endarterectomy is well proven in preventing stroke. Carotid endarterectomy is an index vascular procedure, is the most commonly performed major vascular operation, and defines the field of vascular surgery. It is the most durable, successful, and best studied operation in open or endovascular practice. Vascular specialists have refined this procedure to minimize its cost, complications, and length of stay.

Many vascular surgeons do not believe that CAS can be performed safely. First-hand knowledge of embolizing carotid plaques and the clinical syndromes they cause has made vascular surgeons reluctant to acknowledge the potential value of CAS. This concern, combined with the success of carotid endarterectomy, has created an ethical dilemma for many vascular surgeons who are hesitant to consider CAS as a reasonable alternative.

Continued improvements are likely with respect to the miniaturization of access and platforms, the functional properties of stents, and the efficacy of distal protection devices. As clinical experience accumulates, the overall results and outcome of CAS procedures are likely to improve further, whereas the results of carotid endarterectomy, while excellent in many studies, are likely to remain static. Developing a programmatic approach is about embracing new technology while maintaining safe, appropriate, streamlined, and continuous care for patients with carotid occlusive disease.

Who Is Responsible for Patient Care?

Before describing a carotid stent program in detail, it is of value to consider who has clinical responsibility for the carotid patient. It is not logical for accomplished vascular clinicians who manage a disease process to send patients to technique-based physicians for treatment. This is a failed paradigm from a previous era, and it represents an inherent discontinuity of care. Providing seamless care for a complex process cannot be accomplished by arbitrarily dividing care among multiple disciplines. Nevertheless, many vascular specialists are faced with the potential of relinquishing the procedural aspects of carotid disease care to others that have never cared for carotid disease and are not clinically specialized in the care of vascular patients. Vascular surgeons have a responsibility to manage patients with carotid disease. Abdication of this responsibility to technicians and nonclinicians by failing to incorporate the necessary techniques is antithetical to the roles of surgeon and clinician. Vascular surgeons must adapt to remain the full-service vascular specialists.

The goal of care is a healthy patient, not the performance of any particular procedure. Focusing exclusively on a technique, as other disciplines have sometimes done, is rewarding in the short term but detrimental to care over the long run. New procedures should be introduced if they are safe and effective and they are only of value when they reach the right patients. This can only happen when the focus of clinical care is upon the patient and the vascular system. New procedures should be delivered in the context of a spectrum of various treatment options for a given patient. Vascular specialists should make the clinical and treatment decisions regarding vascular patient care. The physicians making the decisions should be the ones who know the disease process and the patients best.

The management of extracranial carotid occlusive disease has been performed up until now by the vascular surgeon, including consultation, evaluation, medical, and surgical treatment, preprocedure, intraprocedure, and postprocedure management, clinical and noninvasive follow-up, and surveillance. As endovascular carotid management develops, it should be included in the skill set of the vascular clinician. Vascular surgeons take personal responsibility for vascular patients and the long-term management of blood vessel problems.

What Might Be Included in a Carotid Stent Program?

Discussed in this section are some of the possible components of a carotid stent program. Which of the components that will require development is likely to vary from one institution to the next, depending upon the strength of the established vascular practice.

The first step is to honestly assess the available knowledge and skills. Training for carotid stent placement is discussed in the next section, but briefly, carotid stent placement is dependent upon experience with carotid arteriography and with endovascular therapy in other beds, such as the renal vasculature. Many practitioners will require specialized training in carotid arteriography to complement existing endovascular skills. Individuals must establish credentials for carotid arteriography and receive privileges to perform this procedure in their respective hospitals since this is the gateway to carotid stent placement. Most institutions do not have established credentials for carotid angioplasty and stent placement but eventually they will. Requirements should be established so that the necessary training is as clear as possible.

A specific inventory must be obtained to perform carotid arteriography and carotid stent placement and manage potential complications. Consider developing a protocol for patient selection, performance of the procedure, and patient management and follow-up. Seek dispassionate oversight of the carotid stent program until carotid stent systems are approved for routine use. Potential methods of participation in carotid stenting include an Institutional Review Board-approved study, participation in an FDA-approved IDE, or a carotid stent trial.

Create a system of proctoring the first cases. Establish a mechanism for quality assurance and ongoing education. Develop methods for introduction of new and developing technologies. Formalize an ongoing assessment of results.

Training

There are no formal training requirements as of yet. Training describes the skill development that prepares the operator to perform carotid angioplasty and stent placement. This experience comprises the basis upon which the operator qualifies for privileges at a specific institution. Carotid angioplasty and stenting has a learning curve associated with it, as discussed in Chap. 19. Many current fellowships are not able to provide substantial training in carotid angioplasty and stenting since it is not yet an approved procedure. This dearth of experience during fellowship is presently true for vascular surgery, cardiology, neuroradiology, neurointerventional radiology, and interventional radiology, unless the institution is enrolling patients in a clinical trial of carotid stenting. Few vascular specialists in current practice have extensive experience with carotid stenting, even among those who have recently trained. Therefore the necessary components for training in this area are an important issue. Training to perform CAS is dependent upon five knowledge areas.

1. Understanding the behavior of atherosclerotic lesions of the carotid arteries. Vascular surgeons have extensive experience with this.
2. Understanding the management options for carotid artery disease, including the long-term outcomes. This has traditionally been the role of the vascular surgeon.
3. Experience with arch anatomy and selective catheterization of arch branches that comes from carotid arteriography (1). This enables placement of an access sheath in the carotid artery. Many vascular surgeons do not have extensive experience with carotid arteriography. This experience could be gained by performing arteriography prior to carotid endarterectomy in patients in whom duplex alone is not adequate. Carotid arteriography may also be performed as a completion study after carotid endarterectomy.
4. Experience with angioplasty and stenting of other noncoronary arteries: transferring skills from other endovascular procedures shortens the learning curve, especially when using small platform devices.
5. Ability to evaluate cerebral runoff and use a cerebral protection device. Available data suggest that distal protection devices have resulted in a decrease in the incidence of perioperative stroke, and it is likely that they will be developed further in the next few years. The use of cerebral rescue techniques during CAS is not common and the results have been poor so far, but each program should include a protocol for use in the event of a perioperative cerebral embolus.

Specific knowledge areas that comprise training should be considered in planning a carotid stenting program. Operators who are performing carotid stent placement have used several different approaches to learning carotid angioplasty and stenting, including learning from colleagues, attending courses and meetings, and gaining practical experience (Table 1). It may help to write a plan for starting a program and analyze what is needed to accomplish this in the individual institution before embarking on the project.

Table 1 Methods of Obtaining Specialized Training in Carotid Stent Placement

---

Improve fund of knowledge
  Printed material
  Computer learning
  Self-study
Didactic courses, lab courses
Practice using simulators
Participation in live cases, either in home institution or as a visitor
Visiting fellowship
Perform cases in home institution with proctor

Finally, physician proctoring, careful record keeping and case follow-up, and a quality assurance plan are complementary to the training process.

At present, training for vascular specialists who already have essential knowledge of carotid disease and all other methods of management comes down to performing carotid arteriography, learning about and observing carotid stent cases, and performing them. In addition, any carotid stent and distal protection device approved by the FDA are likely to have formal training requirements mandated in association with its sale and use.

Hospital Privileges to Perform Carotid Interventions

Until the late 1980s, carotid arteriography was required for each carotid endarterectomy case to determine the degree of stenosis and to evaluate the surrounding anatomy. As less invasive tests for this task were developed, many vascular surgeons adopted the practice of performing treatment for most patients based upon noninvasive tests. Carotid arteriography was reserved for those with suspected intracranial or arch disease or other anatomic issues that could affect surgery. Most vascular surgeons who were performing carotid arteriography gave it up as its clinical importance diminished. In the era of carotid stent placement, carotid arteriography has made a resurgence, not to determine the degree of stenosis, but as a pathway to treatment. Carotid arteriography is the best method of determining whether a patient can be treated with a carotid stent. This presents a dilemma since many physicians have put in the effort to produce noninvasive studies that provide safe and excellent results. Nevertheless, the general reintroduction of carotid arteriography in the management of carotid occlusive disease appears to be inevitable.

Privileges to perform carotid arteriography are summarized in Chap. 4. Privileges to perform carotid angioplasty and stenting are granted to each practitioner through the credentialing mechanism of the hospital where their practice is located. Hospitals take into account multiple factors, including national standards, local practice patterns, standard of care, documentation of training and experience by the physician, and institutional politics among other things. The institution must ensure high standards, safe patient care, and appropriate qualification of physicians.

There are no generally accepted training requirements for carotid stent placement, but it is likely that future standards will require a specific number of cases to consider a practitioner qualified to perform CAS. Among vascular disease specialists who manage these patients and who perform a lot of endovascular procedures, the appropriate number of carotid stents is probably somewhere around 15 cases. Most institutions do not have established requirements for privileges to perform carotid angioplasty and stent placement as CAS remains investigational. Standards will be developed as CAS becomes accepted and as various disciplines vie for the privilege of caring for these patients. Credentials for carotid interventions should be based upon the following: (1) identification of a reasonable external standard (if possible); (2) demonstration of the ability to transfer existing skills; (3) documentation of additional training; and (4) a plan for patient safety.

After credentialing standards for noncoronary interventions became a contested issue among specialists of different disciplines in the late 1980s, national organizations representing vascular surgeons, interventional radiologists, and cardiologists published case requirements that serve as guidelines to acquire privileges to perform endovascular interventions. Credentialing standards for endovascular procedures are listed in Table 2. The recommended standards are similar, with the highest number of angiograms required by any criteria being 200 and the highest number of interventions required being 50 (2–5). These generally accepted guidelines treat all noncoronary vascular beds in the same manner. There is no specific differentiation between the aortoiliac, renal, carotid, tibial, and other vascular beds.

Among the many ongoing carotid stent trials in the United States, most of the trials had specific case requirements at 10–20 cases each. This case threshold is not a prerequisite to perform carotid stent placement, but is a threshold for demonstrating a high level of technical and clinical expertise consistent with the designation as a clinical trialist. The only NIH-sponsored trial, the Carotid Revascularization Endarterectomy versus Stent Trial (CREST Trial), initially require 20 carotid stent cases for an operator to demonstrate special expertise in this area and be admitted as a trial participant (6). The CREST Trial participant applicants included 103 physicians from 70 centers (7). The

Table 2 Credentialing Standards for Endovascular Procedures of the Noncoronary Arteries

Organization	Ref.	No. of angiograms	No. of interventions
Society of Interventional Radiology	2	200	25
American Heart Association	3	100(50)	50(25)
American College of Cardiology	4	100(50)	50(25)
Society for Vascular Surgery	5	100	50

Numbers in parentheses indicate the number required as primary operator.

mean number of carotid stent cases performed by each operator at the time of application was 13. The rate of perioperative stroke was lower after procedures performed by physicians who had performed 15 or more symptomatic carotid bifurcation cases (3.7%) than among those with fewer than 15 cases (7.1%).

A collaborative effort among radiologists American Society of Interventional and Therapeutic Neuroradiology (ASITN), American Society of Neuroradiology (ASNR), and Society of Interventional Radiology (SIR) recently resulted in the publication of recommendations for qualifications for carotid stenting without including the input of clinicians involved in the care of patients with cerebrovascular disease (8). These recommendations emphasize prerequisite numbers of carotid arteriograms: 200 for practitioners without catheter experience and 100 for physicians with catheter experience (defined as AHA criteria for noncoronary vascular interventions). In addition to carotid arteriography and other requirements, the following are also required: 25 noncarotid stents, plus 4 carotid stent cases, and 16 hr of CME, or 10 carotid stent cases as primary operator with acceptable results.

The introduction process for carotid stent placement should emphasize patient safety, careful patient selection, evidence-based implementation, and protocols for follow-up. It should be the goal of vascular specialists nationwide and in their specific institutions of practice to create the highest possible standards and provide the best possible care of patients based on those high standards. The likelihood is that each institution will develop case requirements for carotid stenting based upon national guidelines, local politics, and other factors. Carotid stent placement should be listed on the credentials and privileges for your vascular department and should be specifically approved as a privilege by the credentials committee.

Protocols

The protocol for carotid stent placement should describe the overall plan. Some factors to include are an outline of the training, a description of the procedure and perioperative management, a list of required inventory, requirements to consider in case selection, a clinical and duplex follow-up protocol, and possibly a mock procedure for staff preparation. The more of these factors that can be considered and decided upon ahead of time, the better. Some of this material may be required by the Institutional Review Board. Case selection for carotid stent placement is discussed in Chap. 7. The earliest cases should be those with straightforward access, minimal tortuosity, and a focal, easily traversed lesion. Get the staff involved in preparation for the procedure.

Proctoring

There is no national standard for proctoring prior to performing a new procedure independently. There is no requirement for what is included in proctoring a case. Check with the hospital to see if there are institutional requirements. Proctoring could include having the proctor assist in the case or observe the case and may include some pre-procedure or postprocedure evaluation of the patient, the chart, or both. However it is done, it should be established ahead of time. Proctoring adds an extra safety mechanism for the patients and the physician. A physician may be proctored at another center with expertise in carotid stenting where the proctored physician acquires privileges and performs the case. A physician may also be proctored at his or her own institution by an invited proctor. Make the process as deliberate and standardized as possible. If the home institution has a proctoring protocol or form, it should be used. If it does not, a simple, one-page form should summarize the case and its management. Consider adding proctoring to the requirements for acquiring privileges in this area.

Quality Assurance

Any new procedure must include a quality assurance mechanism. Most clinical departments already have some type of quality assurance program that includes re-cording and discussing complications and looking for opportunities to improve results. New procedures should receive special scrutiny within the department, especially when on the early phase of the learning curve. Consider discussing every case, whether complicated or not, for the first dozen.

Since carotid angioplasty and stent placement are investigational, Institutional Review Board approval should be obtained to offer this procedure. The Institutional Review Board provides additional patient protection and another level of quality assurance. Inquire with the IRB as to what the requirements are for initiating an application.

Dealing with Endovascular Realities

Before a carotid stent program can be initiated, there are multiple political issues that must be considered (Table 3). The solutions to these issues can only be achieved in each institution and usually depends upon local politics and physician leadership.

Table 3   Factors to Consider Before Initiating the Carotid Stent Program

- Patient selection is the key to early success.
- Obtain access to the best imaging equipment possible.
- Inventory must be studied and understood.
- Obtain as much training as possible prior to starting cases.
- Inform hospital administrators.
- Physician initiating carotid stent procedures is often the newest member of the group (with the least clout).
- Interdisciplinary issues can be contentious since many disciplines want to participate.
- Do you need "neuro rescue" capability?
- Payment issues must be considered in advance.
- Investigate the standards in your community and make sure they are met.
- Take every safety precaution on behalf of the patients.

Patient selection is the key to early success. Patients who are good stent candidates due to high medical comorbidities may not always have favorable anatomy for stent placement and they also have an elevated risk of periprocedural complications, even from a percutaneous procedure. Some candidates may have to be passed up for this procedure while early on the learning curve. The best early candidates for CAS are patients with focal recurrent stenosis. In many institutions, vascular surgeons do not have access to the best fluoroscopic imaging equipment. This does not prevent initiation of a carotid stent program. Portable digital C-arm fluoroscopy is adequate for imaging of the neck and skull. This process is facilitated by the concomitant use of a floating radiolucent table. Specific inventory for carotid arteriography, balloon angioplasty, and stent placement differs somewhat from that used in other vascular beds. The components of the carotid intervention inventory must be studied, understood, requested, and assembled before proceeding.

Hospital administrators need to know what is going on and it is best if they are supportive. Vascular specialists should focus on the following in presentations to administrators: providing new options in treating patients, offering treatment to patients who may not otherwise be candidates for intervention, and developing new areas of expertise. Payment issues must be considered in advance and require consulting with the local Medicare carrier and major private insurers. Often the leading physician role in initiating carotid stent procedures is the youngest/newest member of the group. Support from partners is essential.

Interdisciplinary issues associated with CAS have been as contentious as any in the past. Several specialties that have not treated carotid disease in the past are profoundly interested in carotid stenting. There is no universal solution for this conflict, and it will probably be solved in individual hospitals and communities by local physician leaders. It is hoped that opportunities to do a good job caring for patients will be the driving force.

In establishing this effort, existing standards in your community must be met or exceeded. For example, if stroke neurologists are involved in the care of patients re-

Table 4 Tips for Starting a Carotid Stent Program

- Be resourceful and inventive about training and participate in as many carotid angioplasty and stent cases as possible.
- Carotid arteriography.
- Establish specific endovascular credentialing requirements at your institution and gain as much experience as possible. Set the bar high and do what is required to exceed it.
- Include carotid arteriography and carotid angioplasty and stenting on the list of stated privileges in your department.
- Write a specific protocol for the procedure and the program.
- Arrange for proctoring.
- Institute quality assurance. This is a spotlight procedure.
- Dispassionate oversight/IRB approval until no longer investigational.
- Participate in a trial if possible.

quiring carotid endarterectomy, they should also participate when carotid stents are required. Focus most of all on patient safety in initiating a carotid stent program. Tips for initiating a carotid stenting program are summarized in Table 4.

References

1. Cooperative study between ASITN, ASNR, and SCVIR. Quality improvement guidelines for adult diagnostic neuroangiography. Am J Neuroradiol 2000; 21:146–150.
2. Spies JB, Bakal CW, Burke DR, et al. Standards for interventional radiology. Standards of Practice Committee of the Society of Cardiovascular and Interventional Radiology. J Vasc Interv Radiol 1991; 2:59–65.
3. Levin DC, Becker GJ, Dorros G, et al. Training standards for physicians performing peripheral angioplasty and other percutaneous peripheral vascular interventions. A statement for health professionals from the Special Writing Group of the Councils on Cardiovascular Radiology, Cardio-Thoracic and Vascular Surgery, and Clinical Cardiology, the American Heart Association. Circulation 1992; 86:1348–1350.
4. Spittell JA, Nanda NC, Creager MA, et al. Recommendations for peripheral transluminal angioplasty: Training and facilities. American College of Cardiology Peripheral Vascular Disease Committee. J Am Coll Cardiol 1993; 21:546–548.
5. White RA, Hodgson KJ, Ahn SS, et al. Endovascular interventions training and credentialing for vascular surgeons. J Vasc Surg 1999; 29:177–186.
6. Hobson RW. Update on the Carotid Revascularization Endarterectomy versus Stent Trial (CREST) protocol. J Am Coll Surg 2002; 194:S9–S14.
7. Al-Mubarak N, Roubin GS, Hobson RW, et al. Credentialing of stent operators for the Carotid Revascularization Endarterectomy vs. Stenting Trial (CREST). Stroke 2000; 31:292.
8. Barr JD, Connors JJ III, Sacks D, et al. Quality improvement guidelines for the performance of cervical carotid angioplasty and stent placement. J Vasc Interv Radiol 2003; 14:S321–S335.

21

Future Directions in the Management of Carotid Artery Occlusive Disease: The Era of Carotid Stenting

PETER A. SCHNEIDER and MICHAEL B. SILVA, JR.

The purpose of this chapter is to discuss how carotid artery occlusive disease might be managed in 5–10 years. Present-day techniques, the trajectory of current developments, and the importance of preventing stroke through carotid artery treatment are considered in developing a range of possibilities for future directions in this field.

How Did We Get Here?

Carotid occlusive disease was an untreated cause of stroke through history until the second half of the 20th century. Carotid endarterectomy was developed and performed in the early 1950s. (1) Carotid endarterectomy was a major conceptual advance in several ways: (1) the idea that the offending lesion could be removed from the flow-stream through mechanical intervention to benefit the patient would be the driving force behind the modern treatment of extracranial cerebrovascular disease; (2) the understanding that the plaque would separate from the carotid artery wall and that the new flow surface provided by the remaining artery would heal and maintain its integrity was new at the time; current concepts of remodeling the flow surface to achieve desired results are, at least in part, due to this advance; (3) carotid endarterectomy reinforced the fact that a preventive operation might be justified—even a major

295

one—when it prevented a potentially catastrophic event for the patient; and (4) the evolution of carotid endarterectomy has included refinement of technique, broad assessment of results, level 1 evidence from randomized controlled trials, and proof of cost-effectiveness (2–9). Carotid endarterectomy serves as a model for the modern development of efficacious clinical care and the dissemination of evidence-based medical treatment.

The number of carotid endarterectomies performed in the United States increased steadily from the 1950s to the mid-1980s. As with other prominent manifestations of atherosclerosis, such as coronary artery disease, the cost and complexity of care grew with an increasing incidence of carotid artery occlusive disease. Concern grew about the public health implications and efficacy of treatment of carotid disease, and the results of carotid endarterectomy were aggressively challenged (10–12). At that time, there was no level 1 evidence for carotid endarterectomy. The EC-IC bypass procedure had been routinely performed and was almost completely abandoned after being shown to be of no value in a prospective randomized controlled trial (13). In an effort to solve this problem, multiple randomized controlled trials of endarterectomy vs. medical management were established with the participation of vascular surgeons. These are reviewed in Chapter 16. Surgeons were generally convinced that carotid endarterectomy was efficacious, and were initially reluctant to consider randomizing patients to medical management. Other than neurologists, few other specialists were involved in the care of carotid disease; cardiologists did not play any significant role, and interventional and neurointerventional radiologists were not qualified or involved in the treatment of carotid bifurcation atherosclerosis.

The use of carotid endarterectomy decreased significantly during the trial period. It was not clear whether carotid endarterectomy had a future, and the distinct possibility had arisen that this procedure would become extinct, following the course of the EC-IC bypass. Carotid endarterectomy was subsequently validated as a beneficial treatment in appropriately selected patients in multiple randomized controlled trials of both symptomatic and asymptomatic patients (2–6).

Carotid endarterectomy is the most common major vascular procedure in the United States and the most common major operation performed by vascular surgeons (14). It is a procedure that has defined the field of vascular surgery for several decades and is an index procedure (15,16). Level 1 evidence supports its use. Since the early 1990s, the number of carotid endarterectomies has again risen steadily. Over the past dozen years, much understanding was gained, which has been put into action to benefit patients with carotid occlusive disease. These findings include the following facts: (1) the likelihood of embolization from a significant carotid lesion is associated with the degree of stenosis, even within smaller increments in the degree of stenosis as the narrowing progresses; (2) (2) the history of symptomatic, severe carotid stenosis is poor when treated medically (2); (3) carotid endarterectomy can be done safely and efficiently in most patients (17,18); (4) it is reasonable, safe, and cost-effective to perform carotid endarterectomy on the basis of duplex exam in most patients without preoperative carotid arteriography (19,20); (5) high-volume surgeons and institutions get better results (14,16,21,22); (6) practice guidelines were developed (15,23,24); (7) stroke-free and intervention-free survival after carotid endarterectomy is among the highest for any procedure in the vasculature (25–27); (8) excellent results may be obtained while maintaining a very short length of stay, thereby helping to minimize the cost of the surgery (9,28,29); (9) the composition of the lesion influences the likelihood of the lesion causing a stroke and could be used to select patients for intervention (30); and (10) despite practice guidelines and practice standards, there is a wide variation between hospitals and regions in the rate of carotid surgeries performed and the results obtained (31).

Carotid endarterectomy has been rigorously tested, both conceptually and technically, and is the best studied, most successful, most justified, and most common major vascular procedure.

So Why Is Carotid Stent Placement Here to Stay?

Carotid stent placement was first reported in 1994 (32). Early results demonstrated higher stroke rates than with carotid endarterectomy—but lower than many had anticipated. Carotid bifurcation lesions present with embolization; this is a major difference between carotid atherosclerosis and lesions requiring treatment in other vascular beds, which more often present with global end-organ ischemia. This feature of the disease has made surgeons reluctant to accept carotid stenting as an alternative to endartectomy because vascular surgeons usually manage the clinical sequelae of carotid bifurcation disease and routinely examine friable carotid plaque at the time of endarterectomy.

In the CAVATAS Trial, only a minority of patients received stents, whereas the majority had balloon angioplasty alone (33). The perioperative stroke risk with percutaneous carotid intervention was 10%. Case series have suggested that the addition of cerebral protection devices, and other advances, appears to have decreased the stroke risk by about half (34–39). Previous randomized controlled trials of carotid endarterectomy have indicated that acceptable stroke/death risk for mechanical intervention at the bifurcation is 6% or less for symptomatic patients and 3% or less for asymptomatic patients (15). The SAPPHIRE Trial of patients at high risk for carotid surgery (the majority were asymptomatic) demonstrated a 30-day stroke/death risk of 4.4% with carotid artery stenting (CAS) (40).

Multiple trials that will hopefully answer questions about which patients are best treated with carotid stent placement are in progress. These trials are summarized in Chapter 16. Carotid stent placement has also been shown to be of value in treating recurrent stenosis and patients with a hostile neck or an inaccessible lesion (41,42). Thousands of cases have been performed worldwide and many believe that it should be considered the treatment of choice for carotid occlusive disease on the basis of available data (43). Carotid stent placement is here to stay. The question is: How large an impact will it have?

Carotid stent placement represents the convergence of multiple factors. (1) Conceptually, carotid stent placement is a further refinement of the idea that the embolizing lesion must be taken out of the flow stream. It is an alternative method of mechanical intervention at the bifurcation. (2) Endovascular approaches to treatment are advancing with success in all other vascular beds and this progress provides encouragement in the cerebrovasculature. (3) Distal protection devices and other technical advances may be able to decrease stroke risk and make the neurological outcome of carotid stent placement competitive with carotid endarterectomy. In the case of carotid endarterectomy, it is not likely that any major technical advance, which is going to significantly improve stroke risk much further, will develop soon, whereas CAS is in a phase of rapid development and continued improvement. (4) Multiple specialists have claimed this vascular territory. Many among the traditional therapists of carotid occlusive disease—the vascular surgeons—are only able to offer endarterectomy and may lack the skills to perform carotid stent placement. Many physicians in the fields of cardiology and radiology have never managed carotid disease before and face significant challenges in learning and refining the clinical management of a complex medical problem. (5) Industry has a lot to gain from supporting this effort. It is likely that the huge carotid market will be even larger with the application of a less invasive procedure and that anything learned would be transferable to products designated for other vascular beds.

There is a likelihood that carotid stent placement will become the standard of care within the next 5 years, if not sooner. Carotid endarterectomy is likely to be the future treatment of choice in a small minority of patients with special circumstances

Table 1 Open Surgery Has Changed

Open operations that have almost disappeared	Open operations that are likely to decrease a lot	Open operations that are likely be around for awhile
Sympathectomy (1)	Aortic aneurysm (5)	Dialysis arteriovenous fistula
Peptic ulcer surgery (2)	Brain aneurysm (5)	Bypass to foot
Tuberculosis chest surgery (2)	Fem-pop bypass (5)	
Kidney stones (4,6)	Coronary bypass (5)	
Cholecystectomy (3)	Radical prostatectomy (3)	
Gastrointestinal polypectomy (4)	Bowel resection (3)	
Aortofemoral bypass (5)	Nephrectomy (3)	
Biliary drainage (4)	Brain tumor (6)	

Reasons why things have changed: (1) operation was of little value; (2) better medical treatment; (3) laparoscopic alternative; (4) endoscopic alternative; (5) endovascular alternative; (6) high-frequency ablation (e.g., lithotripsy).

that are yet to be determined. Table 1 shows a partial list of operations and their likely futures. Where on this table should carotid endarterectomy be listed?

Technical Aspects of the Carotid Stent Procedure: Developments in Progress

Many of the functional aspects of the devices used for carotid stenting are covered in detail in the descriptions of procedures in various chapters. What follows is the authors' wish list of near future developments.

ACCESS

Common contraindications to carotid stent placement at present are anatomical problems, many of which are related to access. When branch vessels originate in segment II or III, access can be challenging. The currently available sheaths are often too large and too stiff to work well across the fulcrum presented by the aortic arch. Once access is obtained, the procedures tend to be balloon angioplasty and stenting of a focal lesion. Access will likely be simplified in the future with stents and distal protection devices that are 5-F-compatible. A flexible 5-F guiding sheath would be much more trackable than presently available sheaths. A 5-F selective cerebral catheter can be placed in almost any carotid artery. A shaped 5-F guiding sheath could do the same. Shaped sheath tips will be required to help negotiate tortuous anatomy. The sheath will probably be placed over a directional guidewire with just enough stiffness to support a flexible 5-F guiding sheath. This will require less stiffness than an Amplatz guidewire and more than a standard Glidewire or starting guidewire. There is also a possibility that a sheath that was passed over a 5-F cerebral catheter, rather than in exchange for such a catheter, could be manufactured. Once access is achieved, the 0.014-in. guidewire would be the lowest-profile guidewire for initial crossing of the carotid lesion. Further development of guidewires that are compatible with the distal protection devices is required. Ideally, the guidewire used for the procedure would have an atraumatic steerable tip, would have a stiff shaft to facilitate exchanges, and be compatible with the distal protection device.

ANGIOPLASTY BALLOONS

Monorail or rapid exchange balloon catheters are used almost exclusively for coronary interventions, and these are the logical choice for carotid interventions. As the profile becomes lower, the guidewire smaller, the balloon catheter less bulky, and the distance greater, coaxial catheters lose pushability because they have the internal friction of the guidewire along the entire length of the catheter. The rapid exchange system is more pushable and trackable because the guidewire to catheter friction is limited to a short distance of 25 or 30 cm. This approach also permits use of a shorter guidewire (180 cm instead of 300 cm) and this helps to reduce the time it takes to exchange catheters (less time in the carotid bifurcation) and makes it easier to maintain the correct guidewire positioning during exchanges.

STENTS

A lot has already been learned about what is required in a carotid stent. It must be self-expanding, large enough to be able to bridge into the common carotid artery, and provide the opportunity for accurate deployment. Future stents are probably all going to be monorail and delivered on a 0.014-in. platform. They are likely to be very low-profile, so that primary stent placement at the carotid bifurcation without predilatation is possible in many cases. A 5-F delivery system is likely. Stents will be required in various lengths. Some will be tapered for arteries where stenting is required across the bifurcation, but the size mismatch between the common and internal carotid arteries is great. The intermediate term to long term is likely to foster the development of stents that elute drugs to prevent intimal hyperplasia/recurrent stenosis. It is not yet clear whether recurrent stenosis will be a significant problem with carotid stents. Stents may eventually be covered or biodegradable, but this will probably take a while because it would raise the profile considerably. The obvious attraction of a covered stent is the potential opportunity to prevent embolization of atherosclerotic debris from the interstices of the stent.

CEREBRAL PROTECTION DEVICES

Even in their current early form, distal protection devices appear to play an integral role in making carotid stent placement safer. Distal protection devices are discussed in detail in Chapters 12 and 13. A summary of developments that would significantly enhance the functionality of distal protection devices is presented in Table 2.

There are conceptual disadvantages to a distal occlusion balloon. Some patients (5–15%) cannot tolerate balloon occlusion of the carotid artery. There is no way to be certain that all released debris is aspirated after stent placement. Balloon inflation and/or movement of the inflated balloon in the distal internal carotid artery may cause either immediate or delayed arterial damage. During interrupted carotid flow, there is no way to perform interval evaluation of the internal carotid artery. Therefore, a balloon occlu-

Table 2 Developments That Will Make Protection Devices More Functional

Filter	Sump system
Lower profile/flexible	Control flow rate
Center itself for wall apposition	Less complicated
Optimal pore size	Atraumatic proximal occlusion
Large and secure catchment system	Smaller caliber sheath
Nonthrombogenic	Secure method of occluding inflow
Contingency for loose debris	

sion-based system is unlikely to be the mainstay for distal cerebral protection over the long run. Nevertheless, the occlusion balloon has the lowest profile of any distal protection devices. A temporary balloon occlusion system may be useful for protection during predilatation of the lesion to permit passage of a distal protection filter.

Filter devices are more attractive from a conceptual standpoint; cerebral blood flow is maintained, and debris is trapped as it is generated. Filter devices have other problems. These are mostly technical difficulties that will hopefully be worked out. Distal filters are currently too large and too stiff to pass routinely and safely across severely stenotic and friable carotid lesions. The balance between pore sizes that are too large (permit debris to pass) and pore sizes that are too small (impede blood flow) has not been clearly defined. In addition, the design must be such that the filter must be centered in the artery to be effective. There is no guarantee with any filter that all the debris will stay within the catchment mechanism. There is no very effective method for removing loose debris if the filter should become full. All vascular filters generate thrombus. Impeded distal flow could result in a tail of thrombus distal to the filter. The most functional filter must be simple, low-profile, compatible with a 0.014-in. platform, fit through a 5-F guiding sheath, have the optimal pore size, have a substantial catchment capacity, and be nonthrombogenic.

Sump systems or proximal protection systems have attractive attributes: there is no way for debris to get to the brain once flow in the ipsilateral internal carotid artery has been reversed, and the distal internal carotid artery does not require any instrumentation other than simple guidewire passage. The disadvantages of sump systems include the following: they are complicated; they raise the profile of the access sheath substantially; the rate of reversed flow from the internal carotid artery is not well controlled; many patients will not tolerate stoppage of forward cerebral blood flow, let alone a reversal of flow; and balloon occlusion of the inflow common carotid artery is likely to be unreliable and generate its own set of complications.

Table 3 Situations Where Different Distal Protection Devices May Be Indicated

---

Filter
    Contralateral carotid occlusion
    Contralateral critical stenosis
    Recent stroke
    Unfavorable arch anatomy (for sump)
Distal occlusion balloon
    Protection during predilatation
Sump system
    Preocclusive ipsilateral stenosis
    Small internal carotid artery distal to lesion
    Tortuous carotid artery
    Diseased distal internal carotid artery

Table 3 provides some examples of how filters and sump systems could be used in a complementary manner. For example, patients with a contralateral occlusion or critical lesion or recent stroke may be better candidates for filters that permit continued prograde carotid flow. Patients with preocclusive ipsilateral carotid stenosis may be better candidates for a sump system because only a 0.014-in. guidewire needs to be placed across the lesion. Patients with very tortuous or small distal internal carotid arteries that make filters impossible or less functional could be treated with a sump system during stent placement. As filters and sump systems are further developed, it is likely that some combination of these will be used to achieve nearly universal protection from carotid bifurcation emboli for all types of anatomy.

Improvements in Periprocedural Management

Optimal perioperative management, including preoperative testing, blood pressure control, antiplatelet agents, and postoperative monitoring, will require a few years to work out. It is likely that noninvasive preoperative assessment of the arch and carotid arteries with duplex and magnetic resonance angiography (MRA) or 3D computed tomography (CT) angiography will permit selection of patients for carotid stent placement without a separate preoperative carotid arteriogram at some point in the future. Better perioperative anticoagulants are likely to simplify care. Glycoprotein IIb/IIIa receptor inhibitors will not be used routinely. Better methods of extracting embolic debris are likely to be developed.

What Will Happen to the Trials?

The feasibility phase is over. The next focus will be on making carotid stent placement safer by defining operator qualifications, making the indications clear, and streamlining perioperative care and follow-up. Information from completed and ongoing trials will assist in this task. Indications for carotid stent placement will be determined by comparing it with carotid endarterectomy, rather than medical management. Although medical management has improved since Asymptomatic Carotid Atherosclerosis Study (ACAS) and North American Symptomatic Carotid Endarterectomy (NASCET), due to better oral antiplatelet agents, lipid-lowering agents, and antihypertensives, medical management alone as a comparison would probably not be ethical due to its poor performance in previous studies. The lower is the risk for the procedure (which is still technology-driven and operator-driven), the wider is the spectrum of patients that can be considered for treatment. The lower is the risk of treatment, the more sense it makes to perform screening for carotid occlusive disease.

The trials are expensive and may, in some cases, be redundant, and it is unlikely that all will finish. After some stents become approved for use in the carotid artery, the focus of clinical trials will shift away from comparisons with carotid endarterectomy and toward comparisons of various stent-protection device combinations for comparative efficacy and durability. Rather than look for groups that are uniquely well suited to stent placement, groups that do not fare well with stent placement will be identified so that these patients can consider medical management or carotid endarterectomy. These patients could include certain types of anatomy, or types of lesions that do not fare well with carotid stent placement.

Will Any Controversies Disappear? Will New Ones Develop?

The answer to combined coronary–carotid disease is likely to be stent placement prior to coronary intervention or surgery. The issue of how long one should wait to treat a carotid lesion after stroke might be possible to answer, in part, by analyzing data from the carotid stent trials. The patients referred for carotid endarterectomy are likely to be high-risk and in the spotlight, and a belt-and-suspenders approach will probably result in routine shunting and patching. The overall results of carotid endarterectomy are likely to worsen because the more favorable lesions are better for stents.

There will be lots of new controversies. Some issues are listed here. What are the various carotid stent training pathways in each of the disciplines? How will surgeons maintain skill with carotid endarterectomy if most lesions are eventually treated with stents? How will new surgeons be trained to proficiency to perform both methods of carotid repair? How and when should neurological deficits during or after the carotid stent procedure be treated? What are the qualifications for performing intracranial rescue? What is the protocol for rescue? How should carotid stent failure be treated? Will metal fatigue in this highly mobile location eventually result in stent fracture? When in the course of recurrent disease with a stent should the stented carotid artery be considered for replacement? What are the neuro-cognitive effects of the microemboli generated during most, if not all, carotid stent procedures? What is the long-term patency rate of CAS? Will the self-expanding carotid stents resist metal fatigue over a period of many years?

What Will the Management of Carotid Stenosis Look Like in 5–10 Years?

There will be more screening of patients for atherosclerosis, in general, and carotid occlusive disease, in particular. There will be better medications and more aggressive protocols for the management of atherosclerotic risk factors. Indications for treatment of carotid stenosis are likely to apply to a broad range of patients, even more so than is the current standard of care. Carotid stent placement will be the treatment of choice for mechanical intervention at the carotid bifurcation. Low-profile covered stents and drug-eluting stents will be available for special circumstances. Endarterectomy will most likely be used for some unusual cases, such as a failed stent, impossible access, too much distal internal carotid artery disease, tortuosity or kinks in the carotid artery, patient choice, or very young patients. Carotid surgery results will probably not be as good as they are now. Some practitioners will probably stop performing carotid endarterectomy due to inability to meet minimum-volume requirements. Aggressive evaluation of carotid and cerebral anatomy will lead to an increase in the identification and treatment of all kinds of intracranial lesions. Neurovascular anatomy, cerebral arteriography, and carotid interventions will be a standard part of clinical training in the treatment of vascular disease.

References

1. Eastcott HHG, Pickering GW, Rob C. Reconstruction of the internal carotid artery in a patient with intermittent attacks of hemiplegia. Lancet 1954; 2:994–996.
2. Beneficial effect of carotid endarterectomy in symptomatic patients with high-grade carotid stenosis. North American Symptomatic Carotid Endarterectomy Trial Collaborators. N Engl J Med 1991; 325(7):445–453.
3. Barnett HJ, Taylor DW, Eliasziw M, Fox AJ, Ferguson GG, Haynes RB, Rankin RN, Clagett GP, Hachinski VC, Sackett DL, Thorpe KE, Meldrum HE, Spence JD. Benefit of carotid endarterectomy in patients with symptomatic moderate or severe stenosis. North American Symptomatic Carotid Endarterectomy Trial Collaborators. N Engl J Med 1998; 339(20):1415–1425.
4. Endarterectomy for asymptomatic carotid artery stenosis. Executive Committee for the Asymptomatic Carotid Atherosclerosis Study. JAMA 1995; 273(18):1421–1428.
5. MRC European Carotid Surgery Trial: interim results for symptomatic patients with severe (70–99%) or with mild (0–29%) carotid stenosis. European Carotid Surgery Trialists' Collaborative Group. Lancet 1991; 337(8752):1235–1243.
6. Hobson RW, Weiss DG, Fields WS, Goldstone J, Moore WS, Towne JB, Wright CB. Efficacy of carotid endarterectomy for asymptomatic carotid stenosis. The Veterans Affairs Cooperative Study Group. N Engl J Med 1993; 328(4):221–227.
7. Mayberg MR, Wilson SE, Yatsu F, Weiss DG, Messina L, Hershey LA, Colling C, Eskridge J, Deykin O, Winn HR. Carotid endarterectomy and prevention of cerebral ischemia in symptomatic carotid stenosis. Veterans Affairs Cooperative Studies Program 309 Trialist Group. JAMA 1991; 266(23):3289–3294.
8. Young B, Moore WS, Robertson JT, et al. An analysis of perioperative surgical mortality and morbidity in the asymptomatic carotid atherosclerosis study. ACAS Investigators. Asymptomatic Carotid Artheriosclerosis Study. Stroke 1996; 27(12):2216–2224.
9. Kilaru S, Korn P, Kasirajan K, Lee TY, Beavers FP, Lyon RT, Bush HL, Kent KC. Is carotid angioplasty and stenting more cost effective than carotid endarterectomy? J Vasc Surg 2003; 37:331–339.
10. Chambers BR, Norris JW. The case against surgery for asymptomatic carotid stenosis. Stroke 1984; 15:964–967.
11. Beebe HG, Clagett GP, DeWeese JA, Moore WS, Robertson JT, Sandok B, Wolf PA. Assessing risk associated with carotid endarterectomy. Circulation 1989; 79:472–473.
12. Callow AD, Caplan LR, Correll JW, Fields WS, Mohr JP, Moore WS, Robertson JT, Toole JF. Carotid endarterectomy: what is its current status? Am J Med 1988; 85:835–838.
13. Failure of extracranial–intracranial arterial bypass to reduce the risk of ischemic stroke.

Results of an international randomized trial. The EC/IC Bypass Study Group. N Engl J Med 1985; 7:1191–1200.

14. Pearce WH, Parker MA, Feinglass J, Ujiki M, Manheim LM. The importance of surgeon volume and training in outcomes for vascular surgical procedures. J Vasc Surg 1999; 29(5):768–776.

15. Moore WS, Barnett HJ, Beebe HG, et al. Guidelines for carotid endarterectomy. A multidisciplinary consensus statement from the Ad Hoc Committee, American Heart Association. Circulation 1995; 91:566–579.

16. Hannan EL, Popp AJ, Feustel P, et al. Association of surgical specialty and processes of care with patient outcomes for carotid endarterectomy. Stroke 2001; 32:2890–2897.

17. Kresowik TF, Bratzler D, Karp HR, Hemann RA, Hendel ME, Grund SL, Brenton M, Ellerbeck EF, Nilasena DS. Multistate utilization, processes, and outcomes of carotid endarterectomy. J Vasc Surg 2001; 33(2):227–234.

18. Karp HR, Flanders WD, Shipp CC, et al. Carotid endarterectomy among Medicare beneficiaries: a statewide evaluation of appropriateness and outcome. Stroke 1998; 29: 46–52.

19. Dawson DL, Zierler RE, Strandness DE Jr, Clowes AW, Kohler TR. The role of duplex scanning and arteriography before carotid endarterectomy: a prospective study. J Vasc Surg 1993; 18(4):673–680.

20. Loftus IM, McCarthy MJ, Pau H, Hartshorne T, Bell PR, London NJ, Naylor AR. Carotid endarterectomy without angiography does not compromise operative outcome. Eur J Vasc Endovasc Surg 1998; 16(6):489–493.

21. Feasby TE, Quan H, Ghali WA. Hospital and surgeon determinants of carotid endarterectomy outcomes. Arch Neurol 2002; 58:1181–1877.

22. Cebul RD, Snow RJ, Pine R, Hertzer NR, Norris DG. Indications, outcomes, and provider volumes for carotid endarterectomy. JAMA 1998; 279(16):1282–1287.

23. Biller J, Feinberg WM, Castaldo JE, Whittemore AD, Harbaugh RE, Dempsey RJ, Caplan LR, Kresowik TF, Matchar DB, Toole JF, Easton JD, Adams HP Jr, Brass LM, Hobson RW II, Brott TG, Sternan L. Guidelines for carotid endarterectomy: a statement for healthcare professionals from the Special Writing Group of the Stroke Council, American Heart Association. Circulation 1998; 97:501–509.

24. Gorelick PB, Sacco RL, Smith DB, Alberts M, Mustone-Alexander L, Rader D, Ross JL, Raps E, Ozer MN, Brass LM, Malone ME, Golberg S, Boss J, Hanley DF, Toole JF, Greengold NL, Rhew DC. Prevention of first stroke: a review of guidelines and a multidisciplinary consensus statement from the National Stroke Association. JAMA 1999; 281:1112–1120.

25. Cunningham EJ, Bond R, Mehta Z, Mayberg MR, Warlow CP, Rothwell PM; European Carotid Surgery Trialists' Collaborative Group. Long-term durability of carotid endarterectomy for symptomatic stenosis and risk factors for late postoperative stroke. Stroke 2002; 33:2658–2663.

26. Rothwell PM, Eliasiw M, Gutnikov SA. Analysis of pooled data from the randomized controlled trials of endarterectomy for symptomatic carotid stenosis. Lancet 2003; 361:107–116.

27. Norman PE, Semmens JB, Laurvick CL, Lawrence-Brown M. Long-term relative survival in elderly patients after carotid endarterectomy: a population-based study. Stroke 2003; 34:95–98.

28. Kresowik TF, Hemann RA, Grund SL, Hendel ME, Brenton M, Wiblin RT, Adams HP, Ellerbeck EF. Improving the outcomes of carotid endarterectomy: results of a statewide quality improvement project. J Vasc Surg 2000; 31(5):918–926.

29. Hernandez N, Salles-Cunha SX, Daoud YA, Dosick SM, Whalen RC, Pigott JP, Seiwart AJ, Russell T, Beebe HG. Factors related to short length of stay after carotid endarterectomy. Vasc Endovasc Surg 2002; 36:425–437.

30. AbuRahma AF, Wulu JT, Crotty B. Carotid plaque ultrasonic heterogeneity and severity of stenosis. Stroke 2002; 33:1772–1775.

31. Huber TS, Seeger JM. Dartmouth Atlas of Vascular Health Care review: impact of hospital volume, surgeon volume, and training on outcome. J Vasc Surg 2001; 34:751–756.

32. Marks MP, Dake MD, Steinberg GK, Norbash AM, Lane B. Stent placement for arterial and venous cerebrovascular disease: preliminary experience. Radiology 1994; 191(2):441–446.

33. Endovascular versus surgical treatment in patients with carotid stenosis in the Carotid and Vertebral Artery Transluminal Angioplasty Study (CAVATAS): a randomised trial. Lancet 2001; 357(9270):1729–1737.

34. Kastrup A, Groschel K, Krapf H, Brehm BR, Dichgans J, Schulz JB. Early outcome of carotid angioplasty and stenting with and without cerebral protection devices: a systematic review of the literature. Stroke 2003; 34(3):813–819.

35. AlMubarak N, Colombo A, Gaines PA, Iyer SS, Corvaja N, Cleveland TJ, Macdonald S, Brennan C, Vitek JJ. Multicenter evaluation of carotid artery stenting with a filter protection system. J Am Coll Cardiol 2002; 39(5):841–846.

36. Guimaraens L, Sola MT, Matali A, Arbelaez A, Delgado M, Soler L, Balaguer E, Castellanos C, Ibanez J, Miquel L, Theron J. Carotid angioplasty with cerebral protection and stenting: report of 164 patients (194 carotid percutaneous transluminal angioplasties). Cerebrovasc Dis 2002; 13(2):114–119.

37. Henry M, Henry I, Klonaris C, Masson I, Hugel M, Tzvetanov K, Ethevenot G, Le BE, Kownator S, Luizi F, Folliguet B. Benefits of cerebral protection during carotid stenting with the PercuSurge GuardWire system: midterm results. J Endovasc Ther 2002; 9(1): 1–13.

38. Macdonald S, McKevitt F, Venables GS, Cleveland TJ, Gaines PA. Neurological outcomes after carotid stenting protected with the NeuroShield filter compared to unprotected stenting. J Endovasc Ther 2002; 9(6):777–785.

39. Whitlow PL, Lylyk P, Londero H, Mendiz OA, Mathias K, Jaeger H, Parodi J, Schonholz C, Milei J. Carotid artery stenting protected with an emboli containment system. Stroke 2002; 33(5):1308–1314.

40. Yadav J. Stenting and angioplasty with protection in patients at high risk for endarterectomy (the SAPPHIRE Trial). American Heart Association, Chicago, IL, November 19, 2002.

41. Hobson RW, Goldstein JE, Jamil Z, Lee BC, Padberg FT Jr, Hanna AK, Gwertzman GA, Pappas PJ, Silva MB Jr. Carotid restenosis: operative and endovascular management. J Vasc Surg 1999; 29(2):228–235.

42. Vitek JJ, Roubin GS, New G, Al Mubarek N, Iyer SS. Carotid angioplasty with stenting in post-carotid endarterectomy restenosis. J Invasive Cardiol 2001; 13(2):123–125.

43. Wholey MH, Jarmolowski CR, Wholey M, Eles GR. Carotid artery stent placement—ready for prime time. J Vasc Interv Radiol 2003; 14:1–10.

Appendixes

Appendix A. Inventory for Carotid Access and Interventions from Vascular Therapy at Kaiser Hawaii

Guidewires				
Starting	Bentson	180 cm	0.035 in.	Cook
Exchange	Amplatz	260 cm	0.035 in.	Cook, MediTech
	Nitinol	260 cm	0.035 in.	Microvena
	TAD (tapered)	260 cm	0.035–0.018	Mallinkrodt
	Supracore	260 cm	0.035 in.	Guidant
Selective	Glidewire	260 cm	0.015 in.	MediTech
Microguidewire	Spartacore	300 cm	0.014 in.	Guidant
	Ironman	190, 300 cm	0.014 in.	Guidant
	Transcend	190 cm	0.014 in.	MediTech
Catheters				
Flush	Pigtail	100 cm	4, 5 Fr	Cook
	OmniFlush	90 cm	4 Fr	Angiodynamics
Exchange	Straight Glide	120 cm	4 Fr	MediTech
	Straight Glide	100 cm	5 Fr	MediTech
	Beacon Tip	100 cm	5 Fr	Cook
Selective				
Simple curve	H1	100 cm	4, 5 Fr	Angiodynamics
	H1	100 cm	5, 6 Fr	Cook
	H1	125 cm	5 Fr	Cook
	Angled Glide	120 cm	4 Fr	MediTech
	Angled Glide	100 cm	5 Fr	MediTech
	MPB	100 cm	5 Fr	Cook
	JB1	100 cm	5 Fr	Angiodynamics
	Vertebral	125 cm	5 Fr	Cook

Complex curve	Simmons 1	100 cm	4, 5 Fr	MediTech, Cook
	Simmons 2	100 cm	5, 6 Fr	Cook
	H3	100 cm	5 Fr	Cook
	Vitek	100, 125 cm	5 Fr	Cook
	JB2	100 cm	5 Fr	Angiodynamics
Microcatheter	Renegade	150 cm	3 Fr	MediTech
Sheaths				
Access sheath	Pinnacle	4, 5, 6 Fr	15 cm	MediTech
Guiding sheath	Raabe	6, 7 Fr	70 cm	Cook
	Shuttle	6, 7 Fr	90 cm	Cook
	Destination	6, 7 Fr	90 cm	MediTech
Guiding catheter	Vista Brite Tip	8 Fr	90 cm	Cordis
	Veri-Path	7, 8 Fr	90 cm	Guidant
Balloons				
Monorail	Crossail	2.0–4.0	135 cm	Guidant
	Gazelle	2.0–6.0	135 cm	MediTech
Coaxial	Savvy	4.0–6.0	120 cm	Cordis
Stents				
Monorail	Wallstent	6 × 22	135 cm	MediTech
		8 × 21,		
		8 × 29,		
		8 × 36		
		10 × 24,		
		10 × 31,		
		10 × 37		
	Precise RX	7 × 20,	135 cm	Cordis
		7 × 40		
		8 × 20,		
		8 × 40		
		10 × 20,		
		10 × 40		
Coaxial	Precise	6 × 40	135 cm	Cordis
		7 × 40		
		8 × 40		
		10 × 40		
Distal protection devices				
PercuSurge	GuardWire		200, 300 cm	Medtronic
FilterWire	Filterwire EX	4 Fr	190, 300 cm	MediTech
	Bent tip retrieval sheath		150 cm	MediTech

Appendix B. Comparison of Monorail and Coaxial Systems

The most commonly used system for intervention in the noncoronary vasculature over the past several decades has been the coaxial, or over-the-wire, system. Coronary intervention has evolved in many institutions to the primary use of a monorail or rapid exchange system. The distinction between these different systems has implications in carotid intervention.

Coaxial systems have balloon catheters and stent delivery catheters with a guidewire lumen along the whole length of the catheter. The guidewire is inside the catheter for its entire length. Monorail systems have balloon catheters and stent delivery catheters with a short guidewire lumen, usually about 20 cm in length. The guidewire is inside the catheter for a short distance.

The coaxial system is precise and the balloon catheter or stent can be delivered without the proximity of a guiding sheath. This is an advantage when performing aortoiliac intervention. The access site is close to the site of intervention and larger caliber guidewires (0.035, 0.038 in.) are generally being used. As the access site becomes progressively more remote, the improved trackability of monorail systems over long distances (usually through a 90-cm sheath for carotid access) with lower profile catheters becomes an advantage. Because the length of catheter on the guidewire is less with monorail than with coaxial systems, the friction is decreased. Smaller-caliber guidewires (0.014, 0.018 in.) are typically used so the profile of the entire system is lower. This helps when treating an artery with a minimal residual lumen because the guidewire and catheter are likely to more easily traverse the lesion. When using a monorail system, the guiding sheath must be placed close to the target artery (i.e., coronary, carotid, renal guiding sheath) to deliver the catheter. Because the guidewire/catheter system is lower in profile, a 6-Fr sheath may be used for carotid, renal, or tibial intervention and still have adequate lumen in the sheath for interval arteriography at any juncture in the case. Monorail systems based on 0.014-in. guidewires usually offer balloon angioplasty catheters that are 2.8–3.0 Fr. Balloon-expandable and self-expanding stents may be delivered on 3.0–5.9-Fr shafts.

The difference in construction leads to some very practical differences in handling. The coaxial system has guidewire along its length. During catheter insertion, the guidewire must not be kinked because the entire length of catheter must be passed over the kinked segment of guidewire, both during insertion and removal of the catheter. The guidewire end that protrudes from the catheter must be pinned by an assistant during catheter insertion because it is usually not within the reach of the primary operator. Removing the catheter requires a two-handed technique, with one hand at all times preventing the guidewire from being inadvertently withdrawn and the other hand pulling back the catheter along the guidewire. The monorail system permits the primary operator to pin the guidewire during catheter insertion. During catheter removal, the primary operator may pin the guidewire with one hand and remove the catheter most of the distance (more than 90%) of the way out. Only the length of the catheter that carries

Table 1 Comparison of Coaxial and Monorail Systems

Coaxial	Monorail
Long guidewire lumen	Short guidewire lumen
Higher friction	Lower friction
Higher profile	Lower profile
Less trackable to remote location	More trackable to remote location
More precise catheter control	Less precise catheter control
Delivery with large caliber guidewire	Delivery with guiding sheath
Longer guidewire required	Shorter guidewire required

a guidewire lumen must be removed using the two-handed method described for the entire length of the coaxial system. Use of the monorail system also permits the use of short guidewires. In carotid stenting, this translates into the use of a 190-cm guidewire instead of a 300-cm guidewire. This is because the catheter when placed on the guidewire outside the patient before insertion takes up much less length when the guidewire lumen along the catheter is fairly short. For these reasons, the monorail system is described as "rapid exchange." When carotid stenting is performed in conjunction with distal balloon occlusion for cerebral protection (PercuSurge), the occlusion time may be shorter with rapid exchange systems. If the catheter becomes kinked while it is being inserted in a monorail system, it usually will still follow along the guidewire because it is housed parallel to the guidewire within the sheath.

Carotid stenting systems are likely to evolve toward monorail systems (Table 1).

Appendix C.   National Institute of Health Stroke Scale

The National Institutes of Health Stroke Scale (NIHSS) is a widely utilized method for assessing the severity of stroke. Instructions for its use are provided. An NIHSS score of 10 or higher represents a severe deficit. Patients with scores of 15 or higher have a very

Instruction	Scale definition
1a. Level of Consciousness: The investigator must choose a response, even if a full evaluation is prevented by such obstacles as an endotracheal tube, language barrier, orotracheal trauma/bondages. A 3 is scored only if the patient makes no movement (other than reflexive posturing) in response to noxious stimulation.	0 = Alert; keenly responsive. 1 = Not alert, but arousable by minor stimulation to obey, answer, or respond. 2 = Not alert, requires repeated stimulation to attend, or is obtunded and requires strong or painful stimulation to make movements (not stereotyped). 3 = Responds only with reflex or autonomic effects, or totally unresponsive, flaccid, areflexic.

Instruction	Scale definition

1b. LOC Questions:

The patient is asked the month and his/her age. The answer must be correct—there is no partial credit for being close. Aphasic and stuporous patients who do not comprehend the questions will score 2. Patients unable to speak because of endotracheal intubation, orotracheal trauma, severe dysarthria from any cause, language barrier, or any other problem not secondary to aphasia are given a 1. It is important that only the initial answer be graded and that the examiner not "help" the patient with verbal or nonverbal cues.

0 = Answers both questions correctly.
1 = Answers one question correctly.
2 = Answers neither question correctly.

1c. LOC Commands:

The patient is asked to be open and close the eyes and then to grip and release the nonparetic hand. Substitute another one-step command if the hands cannot be used. Credit is given if an unequivocal attempt is made but not completed because of weakness. If the patient does not respond to command, the task should be demonstrated to them (pantomime) and the result scored (i.e., follows none, one or two commands). Patients with trauma, amputation, or other physical impediments should be given suitable one-step commands. Only the first attempt is scored.

0 = Performs both tasks correctly.
1 = Performs one task correctly.
2 = Performs neither task correctly.

2. Best Gaze:

Only horizontal eye movements will be tested. Voluntary or reflexive (oculocephalic) eye movements will be scored but caloric testing is not performed. If the patient has a conjugate deviation of the eyes that can be overcome by voluntary or reflexive activity, the score will be 1. If a patient has an isolated peripheral nerve paresis (CN III, IV or VI), score a 1. Gaze is testable in all aphasic patients. Patients with ocular trauma, bandages, preexisting blindness, or other disorder of visual acuity or fields should be tested with reflexive movements and a choice made by the investigator. Establishing eye contact and then moving about the patient from side to side will occasionally clarify the presence of a gaze palsy.

0 = Normal.
1 = Partial gaze palsy. This score is given when gaze is abnormal in one or both eyes, but where forced deviation or total gaze paresis is not present.
2 = Forced deviation, or total gaze paresis not overcome by the oculocephalic maneuver.

3. Visual:

Visual fields (upper and lower quadrants) are tested by confrontation, using finger counting or visual threat as appropriate. Patient must be encouraged, but if they look at the side of the moving fingers appropriately, this can be scored as normal. If there is unilateral blindness or enucleation,

0 = No visual loss.
1 = Partial hemianopia.
2 = Complete hemianopia.
3 = Bilateral hemianopia (blind including cortical blindness).

Instruction	Scale definition

visual fields in the remaining eye are scored.
Score 1 only if a clear-cut asymmetry, including
quadrantanopia, is found. If patient is blind from
any cause score 3. Double simultaneous stimulation is performed at this point. If there is extinction patient receives a 1 and the results are used to
answer question 11.

4. Facial Palsy:
Ask or use pantomime to encourage the patient to
show teeth or smile and close eyes. Score sym-
metry of grimace in response to noxious stimuli in
the poorly responsive or noncomprehending patient. If facial trauma/bandages, orotracheal tube,
tape, or other physical barrier obscures the face,
these should be removed to the extent possible.

0 = Normal symmetrical movement.
1 = Minor paralysis (flattened nasolabial
fold, asymmetry on smiling).
2 = Partial paralysis (total or near total
paralysis of lower face).
3 = Complete paralysis (absence of facial
movement in the upper and lower face).

5 and 6. Motor Arm and Leg:
The limb is placed in the appropriate position:
extend the arms 90° (if sitting) or 45° (if supine)
and the leg 30° (always tested supine). Drift is
scored if the arm falls before 10 sec or the leg
before 5 sec. The aphasic patient is encouraged
using urgency in the voice and pantomime but not
noxious stimulation. Each limb is tested in turn,
beginning with the nonparetic arm. Only in the
case of amputation or joint fusion at the shoulder
or hip may the score be "9" and the examiner
must clearly write the explanation for scoring as
a "9."

0 = No drift, arm holds 90° (or 45°) for 10 sec.
1 = Drift, arm holds 90° (45°), but drifts
down before full 10 sec; does not hit bed
or other support.
2 = Some effort against gravity, arm cannot get
to or maintain (if cued) 90° (or 45°),
drifts down to bed, but has some effort
against gravity.
3 = No effort against gravity, arm falls.
4 = No movement.
9 = Amputation, joint fusion.
    Explain:
    5a = Left arm
    5b = Right arm

0 = No drift, leg holds 30° position for a full
    5 sec.
1 = Drift, leg falls by the end of the 5 sec
    period but does not hit bed.
2 = Some effort against gravity, leg falls to bed
    by 5 sec, but has some effort against gravity.
3 = No effort against gravity, leg falls to bed
    immediately.
4 = No movement.
9 = Amputation, joint fusion.
    Explain:
    6a = Left leg
    6b = Right leg

7. Limb Ataxia:
This item is aimed at finding evidence of a unilateral cerebellar lesion. Tests with eyes open. In

0 = Absent.
1 = Present in one limb.
2 = Present in two limbs.

Instruction	Scale definition

case of visual defect, ensure testing is carried out in intact visual field. The finger–nose–finger and heel-shin tests are performed on both sides, and ataxia is scored only if present out of proportion to weakness. Ataxia is absent in the patient who cannot understand or is hemiplegic. Only in the case of amputation or joint fusion may the item be scored "9," and the examiner must clearly write the explanation for not scoring. In case of blindness, test by touching nose from extended arm position.

If present, is ataxia in
  Right arm 1 = Yes, 2 = No
    9 = amputation or joint fusion.
    Explain:
  Left arm 1 = Yes, 2 = No
    9 = amputation or joint fusion.
    Explain:
  Right leg 1 = Yes, 2 = No
    9 = amputation or joint fusion.
    Explain:
  Left leg 1 = Yes, 2 = No
    9 = amputation or joint fusion.
    Explain:

8. Sensory:
Sensation or grimace to pinprick when tested, or withdrawal from noxious stimulus in the obtunded or aphasic patient. Only sensory loss attributed to stroke is scored as abnormal and the examiner should test as many body areas [arms (not hands), legs, trunk, face] as needed to accurately check for hemisensory loss. A score of 2, "severe or total," should only be given when a severe or total loss of sensation can be clearly demonstrated. Stuporous and aphasic patients will therefore probably score 1 or 0. The patient with brainstem stroke who has bilateral loss of sensation is scored 2. If the patient does not respond and is quadriplegic, score 2. Patients in coma (item 1a = 3) are arbitrarily given a 2 on this item.

0 = Normal; no sensory loss.
1 = Mild to moderate sensory loss; patient feels pinprick is less sharp or is dull on the affected side; or there is a loss of superficial pain with pinprick but patient is aware he/she is being touched.
2 = Severe to total sensory loss; patient is not aware of being touched.

9. Best Language:
A great deal of information about comprehension will be obtained during the proceeding sections of the examination. The patient is asked to describe what is happening in the attached picture, to name the items on the attached list of sentences. Comprehension is judged from responses here as well as to all of the commands in the preceding general neurological exam. If visual loss interferes with the tests, ask the patient to identify objects placed in the hand, repeat, and produce speech. The intubated patient should be asked to write. The patient in coma (question 1a = 3) will arbitrarily score 3 on this item. The examiner must choose a score in the patient with stupor or limited cooperation but a score of 3 should be used only if the patient is mute and follows no one-step commands.

0 = No aphasia; normal.
1 = Mild to moderate aphasia; some obvious loss of fluency or facility of comprehension, without significant limitation on ideas expressed or form of expression. Reduction of speech and/or comprehension, however, makes conversation about provided material difficult or impossible. For example, in conversation about provided materials, examiner can identify picture or naming card from patient's response.
2 = Severe aphasia; all communication is through fragmentary expression; great need for inference, questioning, and guessing by the listener. Range of information that can be exchanged is limited; listener carries burden of communication. Examiner

Instruction	Scale definition

cannot identify materials provided from patient response.

3 = Mute, global aphasia; no usable speech or auditory comprehension.

10. Dysarthria:

If the patient is thought to be normal, an adequate sample of speech must be obtained by asking patient to read or repeat words from the attached list. If the patient has severe aphasia, the clarity of articulation of spontaneous speech can be rated. Only if the patient is intubated or has other physical barrier to producing speech may the item be scored "9" and the examiner must clearly write an explanation for not scoring. Do not tell the patient why he/she is being tested.

0 = Normal.

1 = Mild to moderate: Patient slurs at least some words and, at worst, can be understood with some difficulty.

2 = Severe: patient's speech is so slurred as to be unintelligible in the absence of or out of proportion to any dysphasia, or is mute/anarthric.

9 = Intubated or other physical barrier. Explain:

11. Extinction and Inattention (formerly Neglect):

Sufficient information to identify neglect may be obtained during the prior testing. If the patient has severe visual loss preventing visual double simultaneous stimulation, and the cutaneous stimuli are normal, the score is normal. If the patient has aphasia but does appear to attend to both sides, the score is normal. The presence of visual spatial neglect or anosognosia may also be taken as evidence of neglect. Because neglect is scored only if present, the item is never untestable.

0 = No abnormality.

1 = Visual, tactile, auditory, spatial or personal inattention or extinction to bilateral simultaneous stimulation in one of the sensory modalities.

2 = Profound hemi-inattention or hemi-inattention to more than one modality. Does not recognize own hand or orients to only one side of space.

12. Distal Motor Function:

The patient's hand is held up at the forearm by the examiner and the patient is asked to extend his/her fingers as much as possible. If the patient cannot or does not extend the fingers, the examiner places the fingers in full extension and observes for any flexion movement for 5 sec. Only the patient's first attempts are scored. Repetition of the instructions, or of the testing, is prohibited.

0 = Normal (no flexion after 5 sec).

1 = At least some extension after 5 sec, but not fully extended. Any movement of the fingers that is not to command is not scored.

2 = No voluntary extension after 5 sec. Movements of the fingers at another time are not scored.

a. Left arm.

b. Right arm.

poor prognosis. In general, to demonstrate improvement, a decease in the score of 4 or more is required. Other important measures include the Modified Rankin Scale (Interobserver agreement for the assessment of handicap in stroke patients. Stroke 1987;19:604–697.) and the Glasgow Coma Scale (Assessment of outcome after severe brain damage: a practical scale. Lancet 1975;1:480–484.).

Appendix D. Conversion Table for French Sizes

French	Millimeters (OD)	Inches (OD)
1	0.33	0.013
2	0.67	0.026
3	1.0	0.039
4	1.33	0.053
5	1.67	0.066
6	2.0	0.079
7	2.33	0.092
8	2.67	0.105
9	3.0	0.118
10	3.33	0.131
12	4.0	0.158
14	4.67	0.184
15	5.0	0.197
16	5.33	0.210
18	6.0	0.236

3 Fr = 1 mm–0.0394 in.
OD = outer diameter.

Index